Clinical Management of Pregnancies following ART

Kanna Jayaprakasan • Lucy Kean
Editors

Clinical Management of Pregnancies following ART

Springer

Editors
Kanna Jayaprakasan, MD, MRCOG, PhD
Department of Maternity and Gynaecology
Royal Derby Hospital, University of Nottingham
Derby, United Kingdom

Lucy Kean, BM BCh, DM, FRCOG
Department of Obstetrics
Nottingham University Hospitals
Nottingham, United Kingdom

ISBN 978-3-319-42856-7 ISBN 978-3-319-42858-1 (eBook)
DOI 10.1007/978-3-319-42858-1

Library of Congress Control Number: 2016959591

Printed on acid-free paper

This Springer imprint is published by Springer Nature
The registered company is Springer International Publishing AG
The registered company address is Gewerbestrasse 11, 6330 Cham, Switzerland

To Rajisha, Jaidev and Jaishna

KJ

To my two lovely boys and husband and to all my patients who have been the inspiration for this book

LHK

Preface

Assisted reproduction treatment (ART) is increasingly used worldwide as it offers the greatest chances of success among all the fertility treatment options, regardless of the cause of infertility. Over the last two decades, there has been considerable advance in the field of ART, and its use has become more accessible worldwide. In vitro fertilization (IVF) is now almost synonymous with ARTs. It is estimated that more than five million babies have been born worldwide since the first IVF baby in 1978. In most countries, more than 1 % of the babies born are conceived by IVF, though in some IVF contributes to as many as 5 % of the national births.

While most pregnancies following ART will have a normal course, some ART pregnancies are at an increased risk of maternal and fetal complications with prolonged infertility itself being associated with poorer outcomes. There are many reasons why ART pregnancies may be at higher risk, with the risks potentially related to female and male age factor, increased rates of multiple pregnancies, underlying cause of subfertility, and potential increase in birth defects. Furthermore, IVF makes it possible to treat couples with severe comorbidity or a longer duration of infertility and complicated reproductive issues, all of which may pose risks to pregnancy.

As health professionals involved in the care of women undergoing ART, we need to understand the potential risks and problems, the psychological impact on prospective parents, when a pregnancy does not have increased risk, and the potentials for choice for parents.

We have aimed to provide a practical overview of clinical management ranging from pre-pregnancy care through pregnancy to birth and beyond. Special areas upon which we have focused include peri-conceptual psychological issues, pre-conceptual screening, surrogate pregnancy, strategies for risk reduction in women with medical problems, and ongoing developments in ART and associated pregnancy outcome.

We are extremely grateful to the authors who, having recognized as we have the need for an up-to-date and concise guide to pregnancy after ART, have contributed chapters for this book. We appreciate the valuable time and effort they have given to providing such excellent contributions despite the pressures of clinical work.

Derby, UK
Nottingham, UK

Kanna Jayaprakasan
Lucy H. Kean

Contents

Contributors

Catherine E.M. Aiken, PhD, MRCP, MRCOG Department of Fetal and Maternal Medicine, Addenbrooke's Hospital, Cambridge, UK

Janet R. Ashworth, BM, BS, BMedSci(hons), DM, FRCOG Department of Obstetrics and Gynaecology, Royal Derby Hospital, Derby, UK

Sonia Asif, MBChB, MRCOG Division of Obstetrics, Gynaecology, and Child Health, Queens Medical Centre, Nottingham, UK

Miriam N. Baumgarten, MD Department of Obstetrics and Gynaecology, Addenbrooke's Hospital, Cambridge, UK

Amarnath Bhide, MD, FRCOG Department of Obstetrics and Fetal Medicine, St George's University Hospital Foundation Trust, London, UK

Priya Bhide, MD, MRCOG Homerton University Hospital, London, UK

Queen Mary University of London, London, UK

Homerton Fertility Centre, London, UK

Jeremy Brockelsby, MBBS, PhD, MRCOG Department of Obstetrics and Gynaecology, Cambridge University Hospitals NHS Trust, Cambridge, UK

Lisa A. Joels, MB, ChB, MD, FRCOG, FHEA Royal Devon and Exeter NHS Foundation Trust, Centre for Women's Health, Wonford Hospital, Exeter, UK

Valarmathy Kandavel, MBBS, MRCOG, DGO Department of Obstetrics and Gynaecology, University Hospitals of Coventry and Warwickshire NHS Trust, Coventry, UK

Tülay Karasu, MRCOG, PhD Jessop Fertility, Sheffield Teaching Hospital, Sheffield, UK

Lisa J. Knight, BSc, BMBS, MRCOG, DipClinEd Department of Obstetrics and Gynaecology, Royal Devon and Exeter Hospital, Exeter, UK

Colleen Lynch, BSc, MSc Department of Embryology, Genesis Genetics Europe, CARE Fertility, Nottingham, UK

School of Biosciences, University of Kent, Canterbury, UK

Abha Maheshwari, MBBS, MD, MRCOG Aberdeen Royal Infirmary, Department of Gynaecology, Aberdeen Fertility Centre, Aberdeen, UK

Deivanayagam Maruthini, MBBS, DGO, MS(OG), MRCOG, MD Care Fertility, Nottingham, UK

Alec McEwan, BA, BM, BCh, MRCOG Department of Obstetrics and Gynaecology (Queens Medical Centre Campus), Nottingham University Hospitals NHS Trust, Nottingham, UK

Mostafa Metwally, MD, FRCOG Department of Obstetrics and Gynaecology, The Jessop Wing and Royal Hallamshire Hospital, Sheffield, UK

Scott M. Nelson, BSc, PhD, MRCOG School of Medicine, Glasgow Royal Infirmary, University of Glasgow, Glasgow, UK

Shobhana Parameshwaran, MBBS, MS, MRCOG Department of Obstetrics and Gynaecology, Sheffield Teaching Hospitals, Sheffield, UK

Lukasz T. Polanski, MD, PhD Department of Obstetrics and Gynaecology, Addenbrooke's Hospital, Cambridge, UK

Siobhan Quenby, BSC, MD, FRCOG Department of Reproductive Health, University of Warwick, University Hospitals Coventry and Warwickshire NHS Trust, Coventry, UK

Maha Ragunath, MB BS, DGO, MSc, FRCOG Department of Medicine and Gynaecology, CARE Fertility, Nottingham, UK

Margaret Mary Ramsay, MA, MB, BChir, MD, MRCP, FRCOG Department of Fetomaternal Medicine and Obstetrics, Nottingham University Hospitals, Queen's Medical Centre Campus, Nottingham, UK

Alison Richardson, MBChB, MA, MRCOG Division of Child Health, Obstetrics, and Gynaecology, School of Medicine, University of Nottingham, Nottingham, UK

Neelam Sisodia, MBBS, MA, FRCPsych Perinatal Psychiatric Service, Nottinghamshire Healthcare NHS Foundation Trust, Nottingham University Hospitals QMC Campus, Nottingham, UK

Myles J.O. Taylor, BA(Oxon), MRCGP, MRCOG, PhD Royal Devon and Exeter NHS Foundation Trust, Centre for Women's Health, Exeter, UK

Joo P. Teoh, MBBCh, MRCOG, MRCPI, MSc, MD Concept Fertility Centre, Subiaco, Perth, Australia

Srini Vindla, MB, BS, BSc, FRCOG, DM Department of Obstetrics and Gynaecology, Sherwood Forest Hospitals NHS Foundation Trust, Sutton-In-Ashfield, UK

Chapter 1
Pre-conception Risk Assessment: Medical Problems

Priya Bhide and Amarnath Bhide

Introduction

Since the first IVF baby was born in 1978 in the UK, more than five million babies have been born worldwide as a result of assisted reproductive technology (ART) [1]. Rapid advances in technology and treatments in this field and greater access to treatment have resulted in an increase in the number of women having fertility treatment [2]. There has also been a change in the demographic profile of these women. The average age of women having treatment has increased [2] in large part due to social factors. Body mass index has increased globally [3]. Furthermore, advances in medicine have made it possible for women with previously life limiting medical conditions to reach childbearing age and have fertility treatment. As a consequence more women seen in fertility clinics are likely to have pre-existing medical conditions or are at a greater risk of developing them in pregnancy.

Pre-existing medical conditions or risk factors for developing them may increase maternal and fetal risks during pregnancy. Conversely, the pregnancy may exacerbate the underlying medical disorder. Although uncommon, the presence of a systemic medical disorder may alert the clinician to a cause of sub fertility. Lastly, pre-existing medical disorders may necessitate alteration in the fertility treatment protocols in order to ensure safety of the treatment and prevent iatrogenic complications.

P. Bhide, MD, MRCOG (✉)
Homerton University Hospital, London, UK

Queen Mary University of London, London, UK

Homerton Fertility Centre, London, UK
e-mail: Priyabhide2002@yahoo.co.in

A. Bhide, MD, FRCOG
Department of Obstetrics and Fetal Medicine, St George's University Hospital Foundation Trust, London, UK
e-mail: abhide@sgul.ac.uk

K. Jayaprakasan, L. Kean (eds.), *Clinical Management of Pregnancies following ART*, DOI 10.1007/978-3-319-42858-1_1

Pre conception risk assessment before fertility treatment aims to identify and quantify the risks posed by pre-existing medical conditions to the fertility procedure and ensuing pregnancy in terms of severity and likelihood. This allows women planning fertility treatment to make informed choices. In some conditions, it may be possible to eliminate or reduce risk by various strategies detailed in later chapters of this book (see particularly Chaps. 9 and 13 on Maternal Medical Complications in Pregnancy following Assisted Reproductive Technology, and Strategies for Risk Reduction and Improving Success in Women with Medical Comorbidities, respectively). Where risks are considered acceptable, and the benefits of treatment outweigh the risks, women can be counselled appropriately. Certain medical conditions are associated with very high maternal morbidity and mortality in pregnancy; risk assessment will allow identification of such women in whom pregnancy would not be advised and hence fertility treatment not offered. Risk assessment should be done as a part of the routine fertility work up prior to the start of fertility treatment. It should be done by a multidisciplinary team of health professionals comprising the fertility clinician, obstetrician, physician, general practitioner and other relevant specialists where required.

Women with known medical conditions should be identified before the start of any fertility treatment. Details of their diagnosis and management should be sought from themselves and their treating clinicians. Further investigations and review of medications may be required in consultation with relevant specialities.

General Advice

Women should start pregnancy and hence fertility treatment in the best state of health. A full blood count should be done to exclude anaemia. Normal, up to date cervical smears and immunity to rubella should be confirmed. All women starting fertility treatment should be advised to take pre conception folic acid. Cessation of smoking should be advised and help to quit provided. The Royal College of Obstetricians and Gynaecologists (RCOG) recommends that there is no specific amount of alcohol intake that is proven to be safe in pregnancy, and the safest policy is not to drink at all during pregnancy and breastfeeding, particularly in the first 3 months of pregnancy [4]. The importance of an active lifestyle and a balanced good diet are also stressed.

Women with Pre-existing Medical Disorders

While it is not possible to present an exhaustive list of medical disorders that may present to a fertility clinic, we have tried to cover common conditions but the underlying principles of pre conception risk assessment essentially remain the same for all conditions.

Diabetes and Impaired Glucose Tolerance

Pre-existing diabetes may present in one of two forms; type I, insulin dependent diabetes mellitus (IDDM) or type II, non-insulin dependent diabetes mellitus (NIDDM). Out of the 650,000 women giving birth in England and Wales each year, 2–5 % of pregnancies involve women with diabetes. Approximately 87.5 % of pregnancies complicated by diabetes are estimated to be due to gestational diabetes (which may or may not resolve after pregnancy), with 7.5 % being due to type I diabetes and the remaining 5 % being due to type II diabetes [5]. The most serious pregnancy adverse outcomes with diabetes remain fetal abnormality, macrosomia, miscarriage and stillbirth. All of these are highly dependent on blood glucose control. Women with gestational diabetes with fasting hyperglycaemia and poorly controlled pre existing diabetes had significantly higher incidence of malformations (4.8 % and 6.1 % respectively) as compared to non diabetic women and women with gestational diabetes with normal fasting glucose (1.2 % and 1.5 % respectively) [6]. Poor glycaemic control in early pregnancy is associated with an increased risk of congenital heart disease (CHD) in offspring [7]. Starikov et al. [7] described 535 women with diabetes in pregnancy, 30 (5.6 %) of whom delivered an infant with confirmed congenital heart disease. Among the patients with poor glycaemic control ($n=331$), 17 (8.3 %) delivered an infant with CHD, whereas 13 (3.9 %) of those with an HbA1c level lower than 8.5 % ($n=205$) delivered an infant with CHD ($p=0.03$).

Hence, the importance of good blood glucose control and lower HbA1c in the peri-conception period in reducing the risk of congenital abnormalities should be highlighted. Pre-conception folic acid should be increased to 5 mg/day until 12 weeks of pregnancy. These women are also more likely to develop pre-eclampsia (18–20 %) and have a greater risk of developing infections [8]. The risk of IDDM in the child in parents with IDDM is 2–5 % and should be discussed [5].

As pregnancy is a state of physiological glucose intolerance and insulin resistance, target organ involvement is at a greater risk of worsening. A baseline screening for the presence of target organ damage (retinopathy and nephropathy) should be performed before treatment is started. Women should be informed about the role of diet, body weight and exercise, the risks of hypoglycaemia and hypoglycaemia unawareness and how morning sickness can affect diabetic control. Women who have a body mass index above 27 kg/m^2 should be offered advice on how to lose weight [5].

Gestational diabetes is seen in 3–6 % of women [5]. The incidence is higher in certain ethnic groups (e.g.: South East Asians), older women, obesity and women with a family history of diabetes. Women with these risk factors should be made aware of their chances of developing the condition. Although there is no greater risk of congenital abnormalities (unless there is fasting hyperglycaemia); the risk of developing pre-eclampsia is increased. Women developing gestational diabetes are at a higher risk of developing NIDDM in later life [5].

Women with diabetes who are planning to become pregnant should be informed that establishing good glycaemic control before conception and continuing this throughout pregnancy will reduce the risk of miscarriage, congenital malformation, stillbirth and neonatal death. It is important to explain that risks can be reduced but not completely eliminated [5].

Fertility treatment should be deferred until consistently good glycaemic control is achieved. If it is safely achievable, women with diabetes who are planning to become pregnant should aim to maintain their HbA1c below 6.1 % [5]. This may be difficult to achieve in a small minority of women and treatment may be started when an acceptable control of blood glucose as agreed by the multidisciplinary team is achieved. Women with diabetes whose HbA1c is above 10 % should be strongly advised to avoid fertility treatment and hence pregnancy [5]. Women with diabetes who are planning fertility treatment should be offered monthly measurement of HbA1c, and a meter to self-monitor blood glucose. They should be told to increase the frequency of self monitoring. Women with type 1 diabetes who are planning fertility treatment should be offered ketone-testing strips and advised to test for ketonuria or ketonaemia if they become hyperglycaemic or unwell. The other important concern for diabetic women planning fertility treatment is the medications used. Metformin may be continued, but all other oral hypoglycaemic agents should be stopped and substituted by insulin. Angiotensin-converting enzyme inhibitors and angiotensin-II receptor antagonists and statins should be discontinued before conception or as soon as pregnancy is confirmed. Women with diabetes should be offered a structured education programme as soon as possible if they have not already attended one [5].

Women with well-controlled diabetes are at no greater risk for the ART procedures and standard protocols may be followed. An anaesthetic review may be done prior to surgical procedures such as oocyte retrieval.

Thyroid Disorders

Thyroid disorders are the most common endocrine disorders affecting women of reproductive age. They may cause anovulatory infertility by interaction with the hypothalamic-pituitary axis. Thyroid disorders are associated with adverse reproductive outcomes such as early pregnancy loss, miscarriage, pre-term delivery, pre-eclampsia, growth restriction, stillbirth and adverse neonatal outcomes [9]. Women with known thyroid disorders should have thyroid function tests prior to commencing fertility treatment. Specialist advice and adjustment of drug dosages should be sought if the levels are abnormal. Women with thyroid disorders should continue their medication and should be explained the importance of frequent monitoring of thyroid function and adjustment of the doses if necessary [9]. The drug of choice for women with hyperthyroidism is propylthiouracil in view of lower levels of teratogenicity [10]. Treating hyperthyroidism should aim to achieve euthyroidism with the lowest possible doses of medication. In women with hypothyroidism treatment should aim to keep levels of thyroid stimulating hormone at the lower end of normal, below 2.5 mU/l, as this may improve pregnancy rates and reduce early pregnancy loss [11].

Women with hyperthyroidism should wait at least 4 months after radioiodine treatment before starting fertility treatment. Reliable contraception should be discussed [10]. Women with well-controlled thyroid disorders are at no greater risk for the ART procedures and standard protocols may be followed.

Essential Hypertension

Hypertension may be primary (essential hypertension) or secondary to renal, cardiac or endocrine disorders. During pregnancy, these women are at a greater risk of developing superimposed pre-eclampsia, small for gestational age (SGA) babies and placental abruption. The risk of super-imposed pre-eclampsia is approximately 25 % [8].

The other concern remains the safety of the antihypertensives used. The drugs with most safety data are methyldopa, beta-blockers (labetalol, metoprolol, propranolol), and hydralazine. If these drugs are ineffective, a modified-release preparation of nifedipine may be considered as a second-line alternative. Women taking thiazide diuretics, angiotensin converting enzyme (ACE) inhibitors and angiotensin II receptor blockers (ARBs) are at an increased risk of congenital abnormalities if these drugs are taken during pregnancy [12]. Risk assessment should aim to assess the severity and control of hypertension, review the current anti-hypertensive medication and assess the presence and severity of target organ involvement. Prior to becoming pregnant, women with a history of hypertension should be reviewed by a cardiac specialist [10]. The diagnosis should be reviewed and lifestyle changes discussed. Antihypertensive medication should be discussed with the responsible clinician and altered if necessary. An appropriate dosage to maintain consistently optimal blood pressure control is ensured. As an alternative to change of antihypertensive treatment with ACE inhibitors or ARBs before commencing fertility treatment, these should be stopped immediately if the woman became pregnant and alternatives should be offered [10]. Women should be told that there is an increased risk of adverse fetal outcomes if these drugs are taken during the second and third trimesters of pregnancy, but there is there is no strong evidence that first trimester exposure is associated with increased risk to the fetus. Women with chronic hypertension should be encouraged to maintain a low sodium diet. Fertility treatment may be commenced after optimal blood pressure control with appropriate antihypertensives. Women with well-controlled hypertension are at no greater risk for the ART procedures and standard protocols may be followed.

Cardiac Disease

Cardiac disease in pregnancy is a leading cause of maternal mortality in the UK and other developed countries [13]. Pregnancy is a stress on the cardiovascular system and deterioration of cardiac function during pregnancy remains a concern for these women seeking fertility treatment. The extent of this depends on the diagnosis and severity of the condition.

Women for fertility treatment may present with either congenital or acquired heart disease. Improved survival and developments in corrective surgery for congenital heart disease has led to an increase in the number of women with congenital heart disease presenting to the fertility clinic. Simple acyanotic defects, uncomplicated left to right shunts and defects with minimal haemodynamic changes are well tolerated and do not usually cause problems in pregnancy. However, conditions such as primary pulmonary hypertension, Marfan's syndrome and cyanotic heart diseases like Fallot's tetralogy and Eisenmenger's syndrome may be associated with significant problems during pregnancy and greater maternal mortality [13]. Women with congenital heart defect have a five times higher risk (3–5 %) of having a baby with a congenital heart defect [13]. The risk depends on the type of defect and these women will need a specialist detailed fetal cardiac assessment in pregnancy.

With increasing immigration and ethnic diversity, rheumatic heart disease is seen more often than before. The risks involved with rheumatic heart disease depend on the type and severity of the defect, stenotic lesions tending to develop greater problems than regurgitant ones. Ischaemic heart disease (IHD) is more commonly seen as older women are increasingly seeking fertility treatment. Associated risk factors in these women include obesity, hypertension, hyperlipidaemia, smoking and diabetes. A majority of these women are asymptomatic. Pregnancy increases the risk of myocardial infarction in women with IHD, and these women account for up to one-third of maternal deaths resulting from cardiac disease in pregnancy [13].

Lawley et al described 136 women with heart valve prosthesis. Although no maternal mortality was reported, major cardiovascular event was 35 times more likely than the general population [14]. Pregnancy is a stress on the cardiovascular system, and the life of a bio-prosthetic heart valve might be shortened because of the pregnancy. Cleuziou et al described 56 pregnancies in 33 women who conceived after valve replacement, and compared them to 67 women who did not get pregnant. They reported that age, valve type, valve position or pregnancy were not a risk factor for a valve re-replacement [15]. Women with mechanical heart valves are particularly problematic. They are on lifelong anticoagulation. They should have appropriate counselling regarding the high risks involved in the pregnancy to both mother and baby before embarking on fertility treatment. Switching treatment to low molecular weight heparin in the first and last trimester has been utilised to reduce the risk of warfarin embryopathy. However, Basude et al reported that although the rate of fetal loss in the warfarin group (n=22) was high, all women in the LMWH (n=4) and half of those in the combination group (n=6) had serious adverse maternal events, including valve thrombosis, maternal death and postpartum haemorrhage [16]. Both these studies show that pregnancy is a risky condition in women with artificial heart valves. The decision to embark on a pregnancy should only be taken after careful consideration.

Preconception risk assessment in women with cardiac disease aims to confirm the diagnosis, assess cardiac functional status and discuss the potential maternal and fetal risks in pregnancy. These women should be managed jointly by a cardiac, obstetric and fertility team. Preconception functional cardiac capacity remains an important predictor of a woman's ability to tolerate pregnancy. Consideration of the severity of the condition and cardiac function should dictate the multidisciplinary decision to proceed to fertility treatment and pregnancy. Women with pulmonary hypertension, an aortic aneurysm, severe aortic stenosis, or symptomatic ventricular dysfunction should be advised against becoming pregnant [10].

Women proceeding to fertility treatment should have an anaesthetic review prior to surgical procedures such as oocyte retrieval. In women on oral anticoagulants, anticoagulation should be temporarily replaced by LMWH and stopped for an appropriate duration prior to the procedure in conjunction with a haematologist.

Epilepsy

Epilepsy is the commonest chronic neurological disorder seen in women in the reproductive age group affecting about 0.5 % of women in this age group. The greatest concern in these women remains the teratogenicity of the anticonvulsant medications. All the major anti-epileptic medications cross the placenta and are teratogenic. Although the risks are similar for the individual drugs, they increase with the number of drugs and may be dose dependent for some such as sodium valproate (VPA). Holmes et al [17] described a cohort of 6857 women taking anti-epileptic drugs (AEDs). The risk of congenital malformations was 1.9 % and 2.9 % respectively, with Lamotrigine and Carbamazepine as mono-therapy, 2.5 % for Carbamazepine + any other AED but 15.4 % for Carbamazepine + Valproate, as polytherapy. They reported that the risk of malformations among infants exposed to Lamotrigine and Carbamazepine as poly-therapy was significantly higher than the corresponding mono-therapies only when the poly-therapy includes valproate.

Preconception assessment allows review of current medications to minimise teratogenicity coupled with the best seizure control. Most women with epilepsy should continue their medication during pregnancy as uncontrolled seizures carry a maternal risk. In a selected population of women it may be possible to discontinue medications with close supervision.

All women on anti-convulsant medication should be advised to take 5 mg/day of folic acid. The risk of a child developing epilepsy is greater if either of the parents have epilepsy. A Cochrane review reported on neurodevelopmental outcome of the child following in-utero exposure to AEDs. The most important finding was the reduction in IQ in the VPA exposed group, which was sufficient to affect education and occupational outcomes in later life [18]. However, for some women VPA is the most effective drug at controlling seizures. Informed treatment decisions require detailed counselling about these risks at treatment initiation and at pre-conceptual counselling. There are insufficient data about newer AEDs, some of which are commonly prescribed, and further research is required. The most common major malformations associated with AEDs include neural tube defects, orofacial defects, congenital heart abnormalities, and hypospadias. Minor malformations include hypertelorism, epicanthic folds, and digital hypoplasia [10].

Asthma

In women with mild-to-moderate asthma, good control of asthma should be ensured. Referral to a chest physician is recommended for women with severe asthma and those in whom asthma is poorly controlled. Women should be advised to continue asthma medicines both before and during pregnancy [10].

Connective Tissue and Auto-immune Disorders

Most women with rheumatoid arthritis improve during pregnancy and the arthritis does not affect pregnancy outcome negatively. The main concerns relate to the medications used. Referral to a rheumatologist is recommended for a review of the woman's medications. While several medications used are safe, chlorambucil, cyclophosphamide and methotrexate are contra-indicated in pregnancy due to their teratogenicity. In some cases, pregnancy is not advisable for several months after stopping medication. Hence a preconception assessment is necessary to review and allow modification of drug treatment suitable for pregnancy [10].

Women with systemic lupus erythematosus (SLE) should have investigations and assessment for the presence of anti Ro antibodies and target organ involvement. This allows appropriate counselling about the risks during pregnancy (fetal or neonatal death, preterm birth due to placental insufficiency, hypertension or pre-eclampsia and small-for-gestational-age neonate), which are better predicted after a complete assessment. Active disease during conception, anti-phospholipid antibodies, hypertension and renal involvement are associated with adverse pregnancy outcomes and hence fertility treatment and conception should take place in remission.

Sjogren syndrome is particularly common in young women. It is associated with the presence of Anti-Ro/Anti-La antibodies in the blood. These antibodies can lead to congenital complete heart block (CHB) in the fetus. The risk of CHB in antibody positive women is small (<5 %), but the implications are serious, and fetal mortality can be as high as 16–19 % [19].

Mental Disorders

In women suffering from depression requiring medical treatment, the risks of stopping any current antidepressant medication in relation to the woman's current mental state, her previous history of depression, and duration of current antidepressant medication and their safety in pregnancy should be assessed. Specialist help should be sought in severe cases. Women should be advised not to stop medications without specialist advice. The main concern is the possible risk of congenital malformations due to the medications used.

Extensive epidemiological studies have failed to show an association between tricyclic anti-depressant use and birth defects. A small increase in the risk of cardiovascular defects has been reported with Paroxetine, Fluoxetine, Sertraline and Citalopram. Use of mono-amine oxidase (MAO) inhibitors is not recommended in pregnancy. Other antidepressants such as Duloxetine, Mianserin, Reboxetine, and Trazodone should be avoided if possible as there is limited information about their use and safety [10].

Women with more serious disorders such as bipolar affective disorder or schizophrenia should have a consultation with a psychiatrist prior to attempting pregnancy. The chance of an episode of psychosis in the postnatal period is 50% in women with bipolar affective disorder [10] and there have been reported significant recurrences related to the hormonal manipulations of ART (see Chap. 3 on Psychological Issues of Preconceptual Period).

Patients at Higher Risk of Developing Problems due to Increased Age and BMI

Older women should be informed about the increased risk of chromosomal abnormalities in the fetus and available tests for screening and diagnosis (Table 1.1). The risk is related to the age of the egg, and is related to the age of the donor in cases of donor eggs [10].

Obese women (BMI $\geq$ 30 kg/m^2) should be informed that pre-pregnancy obesity is associated with an increased risk of the infant developing neural tube defects, heart defects, cleft palate and/ or cleft lip, anorectal atresia, hydrocephaly and limb reduction abnormalities [10]. Increasing obesity also increases the risk of pre-eclampsia, impaired glucose tolerance, gestational diabetes, gestational

Table 1.1 Risk of Down's syndrome with increasing maternal age

Age of the mother	Risk for Down syndrome
20 years	1:1500
30 years	1:800
35 years	1:270
40 years	1:100
45 years or older	1:50 or greater

Used with permission. National Institute for Health and Clinical Excellence (2012) Clinical Knowledge Summaries: Pre-conception: advice and management. Available from http://cks.nice.org.uk/pre-conception-advice-and-management Reproduced with permission. NICE guidance is produced for the National Health Service in England and Wales hypertension, miscarriage, stillbirth and maternal mortality [10]. They should be offered a weight loss support programme that includes advice about diet and physical activity as well as high dose (5 mg/day) folic acid. They should be informed that losing 5–10 % of their weight (a realistic target) would have significant health benefits [10].

Thrombo-Embolic Disease

A 2008 case control study from Norway [20] found that the OR for VTE with pregnancy following ART was 4.3 (95 % CI: 2.0–9.4). This risk is further increased in women with ovarian hyper-stimulation syndrome (OHSS).

Women with a personal or family history of venous thrombo-embolism should be screened for inherited and acquired thrombophilia. Women with a history of previous venous thromboembolism or asymptomatic inherited or acquired thrombophilias are at a greater risk of venous thrombosis in pregnancy [21]. Those with previous venous thrombosis are also at a risk of pulmonary embolism in pregnancy which remains one of the leading causes of maternal mortality in the UK [22]. Those with a positive screen need specialist advice and may need thromboprophylaxis during early pregnancy [10]. Some women may be on long-term oral anticoagulation with warfarin. The risks are that of warfarin embryopathy if the fetus is exposed, particularly in the first trimester. Warfarin should be substituted by LMWH before commencing fertility treatment. If this is not possible, stopping anticoagulation before the sixth week after conception may minimize the risk to the fetus [22].

Women proceeding to fertility treatment on anticoagulation should have an anaesthetic review prior to surgical procedures such as oocyte retrieval. In women on oral anticoagulants, anticoagulation should be temporarily replaced by LMWH and stopped for an appropriate duration prior to the procedure in conjunction with a haematologist.

Ovarian Hyperstimulation Syndrome

Ovarian Hyperstimulation Syndrome (OHSS) is an iatrogenic complication of controlled ovarian stimulation for IVF and occurs in about 3–8 % of these women [23]. It is triggered by endogenous or exogenous HCG and its effects mediated by the vascular endothelial growth factor. It is a potentially lethal condition, characterised by a third space fluid shift with intravascular volume depletion leading to electrolyte imbalance, haemoconcentration and compromise of vital systems. OHSS may pose a greater risk in women with pre existing conditions such as cardiac, renal and thrombo-embolic disease. IVF treatment protocols should be suitably tailored to avoid this complication.

Impact of Pre-conceptional Care

Pre-conception advice is not the same as prenatal care. Although the benefits appear obvious and logical, formal evidence of its benefit is difficult to come by.

A recent systematic review and meta-analysis by Wahabi et al [24] showed the impact of preconception care. This usually involved glycaemic control (with Insulin if necessary), self-monitoring of blood glucose levels and dietary advice. They concluded that pre-conception care is effective in reducing congenital malformations, RR:0.25 (95 % CI 0.15–0.42), NNT = 17 (95 % CI 14–24), preterm delivery, RR: 0.70 (95 % CI 0.55–0.90), NNT = 8 (95 % CI 5–23) and perinatal mortality RR: 0.35 (95 % CI 0.15–0.82), NNT = 32 (95 % CI 19–109). Preconception care lowers HbA1c in the first trimester of pregnancy by an average of 2.43 % (95 % CI 2.27–2.58). Women who received preconception care booked earlier for antenatal care by an average of 1.32 weeks (95 % CI 1.23–1.40). Hypoglycemia was, however, more common with pre-conceptional care group (RR = 1.51, 95 % CI: 1.15–1.99).

A Cochrane review [25] concluded that Folic acid, alone or in combination with vitamins and minerals, prevents NTDs but does not have a clear effect on other birth defects. Another Cochrane review [26] explored the effectiveness of preconception counselling for women with epilepsy, measured by a reduction in adverse pregnancy outcome in both mother and child. This review found no studies suitable for inclusion. Currently, a revision of this Cochrane review is in progress.

Summary

In summary, pre-conception advice is about what can be done before pregnancy to achieve the best outcome for the mother and the baby. This can be achieved by making sure that the mother enters a pregnancy in the best state of physical and mental health, providing lifestyle advice, optimising the management of chronic health problems, and identifying specific risks to a particular woman so as to enable her to make informed choices in pregnancy.

References

1. ART Factsheet. European Society of Human Reproduction and Embryology (ESHRE). 2014. http://www.eshre.eu/Guidelines-and-Legal/ART-fact-sheet.aspx.
2. Long term trends in fertility treatment. Human Fertilisation and Embryology Authority (HFEA). 2011. http://www.hfea.gov.uk/2585.html.
3. Obesity facts and figures World Health Organisation Fact sheet N°311. European Association for the Study of Obesity (EASO). http://easo.org/obesity-facts-figures.
4. RCOG release: Alcohol in pregnancy: information for you. The Royal College of Obstetricians and Gynecologists; 2015.

5. Diabetes in pregnancy. NICE clinical guideline No. 63. Issued March 2008, modified December 2014. http://www.nice.org.uk/guidance/cg63.
6. Sheffield JS, Butler-Koster EL, Casey BM, McIntire DD, Leveno KJ. Maternal diabetes mellitus and infant malformations. Obstet Gynecol. 2002;100(5 Pt 1):925–30.
7. Starikov R, Bohrer J, Goh W, Kuwahara M, Chien EK, Lopes V, Coustan D. Hemoglobin A1c in pregestational diabetic gravidas and the risk of congenital heart disease in the fetus. Pediatr Cardiol. 2013;34(7):1716–22.
8. Caritis S, Sibai B, Hauth J, Lindheimer MD, Klebanoff M, Thom E, VanDorsten P, Landon M, Paul R, Miodovnik M, Meis P, Thurnau G. Low-dose aspirin to prevent preeclampsia in women at high risk. National Institute of Child Health and Human Development Network of Maternal-Fetal Medicine Units. N Engl J Med. 1998;338(11):701–5.
9. Cignini P, Cafà EV, Giorlandino C, Capriglione S, Spata A, Dugo N. Thyroid physiology and common diseases in pregnancy: review of literature. J Prenat Med. 2012;6:64–71.
10. Pre-conception: advice and management. In Clinical Knowledge summaries. National Institute for Health and Care Excellence. Last revised 2015. http://cks.nice.org.uk/pre-conception-advice-and-management.
11. Stagnaro-Green A, Abalovich M, Alexander E, Azizi F, Mestman J, Negro R, et al. Guidelines of the American Thyroid Association for the diagnosis and management of thyroid disease during pregnancy and postpartum. Thyroid. 2011;21:1081–125.
12. Hypertension in pregnancy: the management of hypertensive disorders during pregnancy. NICE clinical guideline CG 107. 2010.
13. Cardiac disease and pregnancy. Good practice No 13. Royal College of Obstetricians and Gynaecologists. June 2011.
14. Lawley CM, Algert CS, Ford JB, Nippita TA, Figtree GA, Roberts CL. Heart valve prostheses in pregnancy: outcomes for women and their infants. J Am Heart Assoc. 2014;3(3), e000953.
15. Cleuziou J, Hörer J, Kaemmerer H, Teodorowicz A, Kasnar-Samprec J, Schreiber C, Lange R. Pregnancy does not accelerate biological valve degeneration. Int J Cardiol. 2010;145(3):418–21.
16. Basude S, Hein C, Curtis SL, Clark A, Trinder J. Low-molecular-weight heparin or warfarin for anticoagulation in pregnant women with mechanical heart valves: what are the risks? A retrospective observational study. BJOG. 2012;119(8):1008–13.
17. Holmes LB, Mittendorf R, Shen A, Smith CR, Hernandez-Diaz S. Fetal effects of anticonvulsant polytherapies: different risks from different drug combinations. Arch Neurol. 2011;68(10):1275–81.
18. Bromley R, Weston J, Adab N, Greenhalgh J, Sanniti A, McKay AJ, Tudur Smith C, Marson AG. Treatment for epilepsy in pregnancy: neurodevelopmental outcomes in the child. Cochrane Database Syst Rev. 2014;10, CD010236.
19. Costedoat-Chalumeau N, Amoura Z, Villain E, Cohen L, Piette JC. Anti-SSA/Ro antibodies and the heart: more than complete congenital heart block? A review of electrocardiographic and myocardial abnormalities and of treatment options. Arthritis Res Ther. 2005;7(2):69–73.
20. Jacobsen AE, Skjeldestad FE, Sandset PM. Ante- and postnatal risk factors of venous thrombosis: a hospital based case control study. J Thromb Haemost. 2008;6:905–12.
21. Reducing the risk of thrombosis and embolism during pregnancy and puerperium. Green top guideline N. 37a. RCOG, Nov 2009.
22. Schaefer C, Peters P, Miller RK, editors. Drugs during pregnancy and lactation: treatment options and risk assessment. 2nd ed. Oxford: Academic; 2007.
23. The management of ovarian hyperstimulation syndrome Green top guideline No. 5. RCOG Sept 2006.
24. Wahabi HA, Alzeidan RA, Bawazeer GA, Alansari LA, Esmaeil SA. Preconception care for diabetic women for improving maternal and fetal outcomes: a systematic review and meta-analysis. BMC Pregnancy Childbirth. 2010;10:63.

25. De-Regil LM, Fernández-Gaxiola AC, Dowswell T, Peña-Rosas JP. Effects and safety of periconceptional folate supplementation for preventing birth defects. Cochrane Database Syst Rev. 2010;10, CD007950.
26. Winterbottom JB, Smyth RM, Jacoby A, Baker GA. Preconception counselling for women with epilepsy to reduce adverse pregnancy outcome. Cochrane Database Syst Rev. 2008;3, CD006645.

Chapter 2
Pre-conception Risk Assessment: Gynaecological Problems

Tülay Karasu and Mostafa Metwally

Introduction

Infertility has increased in Western societies; one in six couples will encounter problems with fertility. Infertility is defined as failure to achieve a clinical pregnancy after regular intercourse for 12 months. Women are delaying childbearing due to life style changes like completing higher education, following a career and seeking for financial independence. Increasingly, infertile couples are using assisted reproductive technology (ART) in order to achieve a pregnancy. This chapter aims to cover gynaecological pathologies like fibroids, polyps, uterine anomalies, endometriosis, adenomyosis and hydrosalpinx which can adversely influence reproductive outcome. Furthermore, the pathology, effect on fertility and pregnancy and evidence based management of those gynaecological conditions are described here.

Fibroids

Uterine fibroids (leimyoma) are benign tumours of uterine smooth muscles and have an estimated prevalence of 20–40 % of women during their reproductive years [1]. Fibroids are classified according to their location in the uterus (submucous, intramural and subserous) and can be single or multiple. A relationship between uterine fibroids and infertility has been recognised. Women wishing to conceive are

T. Karasu, MRCOG, PhD (✉)
Jessop Fertility, Sheffield Teaching Hospital, Sheffield, UK
e-mail: karasut@doctors.org.uk

M. Metwally, MD, FRCOG
Department of Obstetrics and Gynaecology, The Jessop Wing and Royal Hallamshire Hospital, Sheffield, UK
e-mail: mmetwally@nhs.net

K. Jayaprakasan, L. Kean (eds.), *Clinical Management of Pregnancies following ART*, DOI 10.1007/978-3-319-42858-1_2

more likely to present with uterine fibroids due to the delay in childbearing. The effect of fibroids on fertility depends on the location of the uterine fibroid. Submucosal fibroids interfere with fertility and removal is recommended. Subserosal fibroids do not have an effect on fertility while the effect of intramural fibroids is controversial.

Most fibroids are asymptomatic, but they can also cause symptoms such as abnormal uterine bleeding, pelvic pressure and pain, infertility and miscarriage.

The diagnosis is made by ultrasound or magnetic resonance imaging (MRI). It is important to assess the number, size, location and any disruption of the junctional zone.

Effect on Fertility and Pregnancy

Submucous Fibroids

Submucous fibroids may contribute to miscarriage and infertility possibly by an effect on embryo implantation. The most common classification of submucous fibroids developed by the European Society of Gynaecological Endoscopy describes them according to the location to the uterine cavity. Type 0 fibroids are entirely in the uterine cavity, type 1 fibroids are ≥50 % and type 2 fibroids are ≤50 % located in the uterine cavity.

Improvement of reproductive outcomes has been shown after removal of submucous fibroids. A retrospective study observed a significant reduction in pregnancy loss and increase in live births after hysteroscopic myomectomy in women with infertility and recurrent pregnancy loss [2]. A prospective, randomised controlled study of hysteroscopic myomectomy versus hysteroscopy and biopsy in patients with unexplained primary infertility showed a statistically significant increase in spontaneous pregnancies in women following myomectomy (type 0: 57.9 % vs. 33.3 %, $p<0.001$; type 1: 35.7 % vs. 17.2 %, $p<0.001$) [3]. Women with submucosal fibroids undergoing IVF treatment have reduced pregnancy rates [4, 5] whereas hysteroscopic myomectomy improves pregnancy rates in women undergoing IVF treatment [6].

However, there is still controversy about the effect of intramural fibroids on reproductive outcomes. The exact mechanisms through which fibroids interfere with reproduction are not clear, but could include anatomical distortion, disruption of the uterine junctional zone, alteration of uterine contractility or endometrial blood supply or receptivity [7–9].

Intramural Fibroids

Some studies have shown a negative effect of intramural fibroids on IVF outcomes [10, 11] whereas other studies did not find an effect [12–15]. The first systematic review on fibroids and infertility did not show an effect of intramural fibroids on infertility [16]. An updated systematic review demonstrated a possible negative effect of intramural fibroids on reproductive outcomes [17]. Nevertheless, removal of intramural fibroids did not seem to improve significantly reproductive outcome [16, 17]. Another systematic review looked into the effect of intramural fibroids without cavity distortion and found a negative impact on IVF outcomes in women with intramural fibroids when compared to women without fibroids [18]. The most recent systematic review and meta-analysis initially confirmed a negative impact of intramural fibroids on clinical pregnancy rates, but not on live birth or miscarriage rates [19]. However, there was no significant effect of intramural fibroids on reproductive outcomes when only high quality studies were included and removal of intramural fibroids did not significantly improve clinical pregnancy or miscarriage rates [19]. This highlights the need for more good quality studies regarding the effect of intramural fibroids on reproductive outcomes.

In the meantime, the management of women with intramural fibroids needs to be individualised and any involvement of the uterine cavity needs to be excluded. However, many clinicians consider removal of intramural fibroids larger than 4 cm.

Subserosal Fibroids

Subserosal fibroids seem to interfere less with fertility unless they distort reproductive organs such as fallopian tubes. A prospective controlled study could not find a significant difference in pregnancy rates in women with removal of subserous fibroids compared to controls [20]. Other studies have also not demonstrated a negative effect of subserous fibroids on pregnancy rates following IVF [4, 5, 12]. Therefore, surgery for subserous fibroids in asymptomatic, infertile women is not recommended.

Management

Hormonal Treatment

Fibroids are hormone-sensitive tumours with sex steroid receptors [21]. Estrogens and progestogens enhance tumour growth. Medical treatment in the form of gonadotropin-releasing hormone analogue (GnRHa) can be given prior to myomectomy in order to reduce the size of the fibroid [22]. However, prolonged use can cause estrogen deficiency and a decrease in bone mineral density. Another medical treatment is the use of selective progesterone receptor modulators (SPRM) with mixed agonist/antagonist activity. Studies have confirmed the efficacy and safety of the SPRM ulipristal acetate (Esmya®) for the treatment of fibroids preoperatively [23–26]. However, the effect on subsequent fertility is as yet unknown.

Interventional Radiology

Uterine artery embolisation (UAE) occludes the uterine blood flow to the fibroid leading to necrosis and shrinkage [27]. Evidence suggests a 50–60 % reduction in fibroid size and 85–95 % symptom relief after UAE [28]. Complications include haematoma, thrombosis, pain, infection and vaginal discharge. The post-embolisation syndrome consists of pain, nausea, flu like symptoms, mild pyrexia and raised inflammatory markers.

UAE in women wishing to conceive is controversial. UAE has been associated with ovarian failure [29, 30] and the risk of infertility following the procedure is unknown. Pregnancies following UAE are at an increased risk of pre-term delivery, miscarriage, abnormal placentation and postpartum haemorrhage [31–34]. A randomised controlled trial looking into reproductive outcomes following UAE and myomectomy reported higher pregnancy and live birth rates and lower miscarriage rates in women following myomectomy [35]. Another study identified several atypical hysteroscopy findings 3–9 months following UAE including tissue necrosis, intracavitary fibroid protrusion and intrauterine adhesions [36].

A recent Cochrane review found low level evidence suggesting that myomectomy may be associated with better fertility outcomes than UAE [37]. Furthermore, women after UAE have an increased likelihood for further surgical intervention [37].

Magnetic resonance guided focused ultrasound surgery (MRgFUS) is a new method of thermal ablation for the treatment of fibroids beneath the anterior abdominal wall. However, only few patients are eligible for this new technique. Nevertheless, reproductive outcomes following this procedure are promising. A miscarriage rate of 26 % and a live birth rate of 41 % have been reported in women following this procedure [38].

Surgical Treatment

Hysteroscopic resection of a submucous fibroid is performed using a monopolar or bipolar resectoscopes. Complications include fluid overload that may lead to cerebral and pulmonary oedema, coagulopathy or death. Other complications are cervical laceration, bleeding, infection, uterine perforation (<1 %) and intrauterine adhesions. These risks are less with the use of bipolar technology.

Surgical treatment for intramural fibroids in the form of myomectomy can be performed abdominally or laparoscopically dependent on the position of the fibroid and the skills of the surgeon. Risks of myomectomy are intra-operative bleeding and formation of postoperative adhesions. The advantages of the laparoscopic procedure over an abdominal approach are reduction in postoperative pain, hospital stay and recovery [39]. However, laparoscopic myomectomy is technically challenging and time consuming. According to a systematic review there is no significant difference between those two approaches and fertility outcome [40].

Endometrial Polyps

Endometrial polyps are benign growths of the endometrium. Polyps can be single or multiple, sessile or pedunculated. Up to 25 % of women with unexplained infertility [41, 42] and 46.7 % of subfertile women with endometriosis [43] have endometrial polyps on hysteroscopy.

The relationship between endometrial polyps and subfertility is not entirely clear. However, endometrial polyps may affect fertility in many ways. They can interfere mechanically with sperm and embryo transport and implantation. Furthermore, polyps cause chronic inflammation and thereby make the endometrium unfavourable for implantation and interfere with the blood flow to the endometrium. A study suggested that endometrial polyps alter endometrial receptivity as reduced HOXA10 and HOXA11 mRNA levels, markers of endometrial receptivity, were found on endometrium with endometrial polyps [44]. In addition, the number, size or location may have an influence on reproductive outcome.

Endometrial polyps can present with irregular bleeding. However, most of them are asymptomatic and are found coincidentally as part of routine investigations for subfertility. They can be diagnosed by ultrasound, hysterosonography, hysterosalpingogram and hysteroscopy. The gold standard for the diagnosis of endometrial polyps is hysteroscopy and treatment can be offered at the same time.

Effect on Fertility

Observational studies suggest a better reproductive outcome following removal of polyps by operative hysteroscopy [45, 46]. A randomised controlled trial looked at the effect of endometrial polyps on the pregnancy rate in women undergoing intrauterine insemination (IUI) procedure [47]. These patients had a hysteroscopy and polypectomy or hysteroscopy and biopsy of the polyp. The spontaneous pregnancy rate and the pregnancy rate following IUI treatment were significantly higher in the group of women with polypectomy when compared to the group of women with only polyp biopsy (68 % vs 23 %, $p<0.001$) [47]. Another study looked at the location of the polyp and the effect on pregnancy and found that the removal of tubocornual polyps lead to higher pregnancy rates compared to the removal of polyps at other locations in the uterus [48].

A systematic review on the management of endometrial polyps in subfertile women included only 3 studies and found conflicting results with some evidence of an adverse effect of polyps on fertility [49]. Therefore, the review recommended removal of the polyp if detected prior to IVF treatment or an individualised approach when the polyp was detected during the IVF treatment cycle. The Cochrane review looked into hysteroscopy for treating subfertility associated with suspected major uterine cavity abnormalities and concluded that polypectomy in women prior to IUI treatment might improve the pregnancy outcome and that more good quality randomized controlled studies are necessary to assess the effectiveness of hysteroscopic polypectomy [50].

The effect of endometrial polyps on IVF remains unclear. Some studies suggest that endometrial polyps <2 cm in size have no impact on IVF outcome [51, 52]. Other studies could not confirm the effect of polyp size on fertility [47, 53, 54]. Stamatellos et al. demonstrated an increase in pregnancy rate following polypectomy independent of size or number of polyps [53]. Further studies are necessary to investigate the effect of large polyps, polyp location and number of polyps on IVF outcome.

Management

Polypectomy can be done by dilatation and curettage or hysteroscopy directed using scissors, loop electrode or morcellator. However, dilatation and curettage can remove endometrial polyps incompletely and is not recommended. Complication rates following hysteroscopic polypectomy are low with a polyp recurrence rate of 4.9 % [53].

If an endometrial polyp is detected during an IVF cycle treatment options include cycle cancellation and polypectomy or continuation of the cycle with cryopreservation and embryo transfer following polypectomy.

Overall, it is reasonable to remove an endometrial polyp prior to infertility treatment. This will provide a histological sample and also may improve reproductive outcome. Further studies on the effect of polyps on infertility and pregnancy are necessary.

Congenital Uterine Anomalies

Congenital uterine anomalies are mainly the result of a defect of development or fusion of the paired Mullerian ducts during embryogenesis. The most recent classification for uterine anomalies is the ESHRE/ESGE classification [55] (Table 2.1). The prevalence of uterine anomalies in the general population is between 1 and 3.5 %. Infertile women have a significantly higher incidence of Mullerian anomalies compared to fertile women [56].

Effect on Fertility and Pregnancy

The incidence of Mullerian anomalies in women with recurrent first trimester loss is estimated to be between 5–10 % and 25 % in recurrent second trimester loss [57]. Uterine anomalies are associated with infertility, miscarriage, malpresentations,

Table 2.1 Scheme of female genital tract anomalies according to the ESHRE/ESGE classification system

Uterine anomaly			Cervical/vaginal anomaly	
	Main class	Sub-class	Co-existant class	
U0	Normal uterus		C0	Normal cervix
U1	Dysmorphic uterus	(a) T-Shaped (b) Infantilis (c) Others	C1	Septate cervix
U2	Septate uterus	(a) Partial (b) Complete	C2	Double "normal" cervix
U3	Bicorporeal uterus	(a) Partial (b) Complete (c) Bicorporeal septate	C3	Unilateral cervical aplasia
U4	Hemi-uterus	(a) With rudimentary cavity (communicating or not horn) (b) Without rudimentary cavity (horn without cavity/no horn)	C4	Cervical aplasia
U5	Aplastic	(a) With rudimentary cavity (bi- or unilateral horn) (b) Without rudimentary cavity (bi- or unilateral uterine remnants/aplasia)	V0	Normal vagina
U6	Unclassified malformations		V1	Longitudinal non-obstructing vaginal septum
			V2	Longitudinal obstructing vaginal septum
			V3	Transverse vaginal septum
			V4	Vaginal aplasia

Used with permission of Oxford University Press from Grimbizis et al. [55]

placental abruption, intrauterine growth restriction, preterm labour, retained placenta and fetal mortality [56, 58]. This may be due to diminished muscle mass, abnormal uterine blood flow and cervical insufficiency. One study looked at IVF outcomes in women with untreated uterine malformations and found significantly lower implantation and pregnancy rates when compared to the general population [59]. A correct diagnosis of the malformation is important for correct treatment. Mullerian anomalies are often associated with kidney and skeletal malformations.

Septate Uterus

The septate uterus is the most common structural uterine anomaly [56] and is caused by an incomplete resorption of the partition between the fused Mullerian ducts. The diagnosis can be made by HSG with accuracy between 20–60 % and together with an ultrasound examination the diagnostic accuracy improves to 90 % [60]. It is difficult to distinguish between bicornuate uterus and septate uterus by HSG alone as the uterine fundus is not visualised. Transvaginal ultrasound has a sensitivity of

100 % and specificity of 80 % in the diagnosis of the septate uterus [61]. Three-dimensional (3D) ultrasound (92 % sensitivity) [62] and magnetic resonance imaging (MRI) (100 % sensitivity) can also be used as a diagnostic tool [61]. However, the gold standard is hysteroscopy and laparoscopy.

Among the different types of uterine anomalies, the septate uterus is associated with the poorest reproductive outcome. The septate uterus maybe associated with pregnancy loss [63] and infertility [64].

Management

Hysteroscopic metroplasty is performed with scissors, electrosurgery or laser under ultrasonographic or laparoscopic control. This improves pregnancy outcome in women with recurrent miscarriage and 80 % term live birth rate has been reported following the procedure compared to 3 % before the procedure [63]. Most studies of metroplasty have looked into women with recurrent miscarriage. There is controversy whether metroplasty is helpful in infertile patients. However, a prospective controlled study looked into women with a septate uterus and unexplained infertility who underwent metroplasty versus women where metroplasty was not performed found a significantly higher live birth rate following metroplasty (34.1 % vs. 18.9 %) [65]. Another study reported a 29.5 % live birth rate after hysteroscopic metroplasty in women with otherwise unexplained infertility [64]. Furthermore, IVF is more successful in women following metroplasty [59].

Unicornuate Uterus

Unicornuate uterus results from a fusion defect of the Mullerian ducts with one cavity being normal with a fallopian tube and cervix, whereas disrupted development is seen in the other horn. The other horn can be completely absent or rudimentary with or without a cavity that may connect to the primary horn. 40 % of women with a unicornuate uterus have an associated urinary tract anomaly [66].

Unicornuate uteri are more common in women with infertility and miscarriage than the general population. Furthermore, they are associated with poor obstetric outcome with a live birth rate of only 29.2 %, prematurity rate of 44 %, miscarriage rate of 29 %, and ectopic pregnancy of 4 % [67]. Another review of 151 women with a unicornuate uterus had 260 pregnancies and a mean miscarriage rate of 37.1 %, mean preterm delivery rate of 16.4 % and the mean term delivery rate of 45.3 % [68]. However, different types of unicornuate uterus are associated with different reproductive outcomes depending on the vascular supply, muscular mass of the myometrium and degree of cervical competence.

The rudimentary horn can contain functional endometrium which can lead to endometriosis, haematometra, pelvic pain and pregnancy with a risk of uterine rupture. Therefore, removal of the uterine horn containing endometrium by laparoscopy or laparotomy is recommended. However, there is no evidence that removal of the rudimentary horn improves reproductive outcome.

Bicornuate Uterus

The bicornuate uterus results from an incomplete fusion of the two Mullerian ducts and is a common uterine anomaly (46.3 %) [57].

Bicornuate uteri are more common in women with infertility and miscarriage than the general population. Women with a bicornuate uterus are at increased risk of second trimester miscarriage and preterm birth. They usually do not need any surgical intervention. The mildest form of the bicornuate uterus is the arcuate uterus and does not necessitate surgery. A systematic review showed an increased rate of second trimester miscarriage and fetal malpresentations at delivery in women with an arcuate uterus [69].

Uterus Didelphys

Complete failure of fusion of the two Mullerian ducts results in the uterus didelphys with a duplication of uterus and cervix and sometimes bladder, urethra, vagina and anus [70]. The uterus didelphys is more common in infertile women and women with a miscarriage than the general population. There is an increased risk of preterm birth and fetal malpresentations [68].

Intrauterine Adhesions

The main reasons for the formation of intrauterine adhesions are previous intrauterine surgical procedures such as curettage and hysteroecopic resection of fibroids or a uterine septum. It may also follow uterine infections [71]. Taskin et al. reported the presence of intrauterine adhesions in 6.7 % (1/15) of women after resection of septa, 31.3 % (10/32) after hysteroscopic resection of a solitary fibroid and 45.5 % (9/20) after resection of multiple fibroids [72]. These intrauterine adhesions are also known as Asherman Syndrome.

The patients can be assessed with transvaginal ultrasonography, saline infusion sonohysterography, hysterosalpingography (HSG) or hysteroscopy. Intrauterine adhesions appear as filling defects on HSG. HSG has a sensitivity of 75 % and a positive predictive value of 50 % in the detection of intrauterine adhesions [73]. On ultrasound, adhesions appear as dense echoes within the cavity with irregular thickness of the endometrium. Sometimes, there are echo lucent areas interrupting the endometrium which represent collected blood. However, ultrasound has a low sensitivity (52 %) in the diagnosis of intrauterine adhesions [74].

There is no clear consensus regarding the optimum classification of intrauterine adhesions. The widely used American Fertility Society classification includes the extent and type of the adhesions found on hysterosalpingography or hysteroscopy and the menstrual pattern (Table 2.2) [75]. The European Society of Gynaecological Endoscopy (ESGE) formulated a classification of intrauterine adhesions depending on the extent of intrauterine adhesions from findings at hysteroscopy and hysterography (Table 2.3).

Table 2.2 American Fertility Society classification of intrauterine adhesions 1988

Classification	Condition		
Cavity involved	<1/3	1/3-2/3	>2/3
	1	2	3
Type of adhesions	Filmy	Filmy and dense	Dense
	1	2	3
Menstrual pattern	Normal	Hypomenorrhoea	Amenorrhoea
	0	2	4
Prognostic classification		HSG score	Hysteroscopy score
Stage I (mild)	1–4		
Stage II (moderate)	5–8		
Stage III (severe)	9–12		

Used with permission of Elsevier from The American Fertility Society [75]

Table 2.3 European Society of Gynecological Endoscopy (ESGE) classification of intrauterine adhesions (IUA) (1995)

Grade	Extent of intrauterine adhesions
I	Thin or filmsy Easily ruptured by hysteroscope sheath alone, corneal areas normal
II	Singular dense adhesion Connecting separate areas of the uterine cavity Visualization of both tubal ostia possible Cannot be ruptured by hysteroscope sheath alone
IIa	Occluding adhesions only in the region of the internal cervical os Upper uterine cavity normal
III	Multiple dense adhesions Connecting separate areas of the uterine cavity Unilateral obliteration of ostial areas of the tubes
IV	Extensive dense adhesions with (partial) occlusion of the uterine cavity Both tubal ostial areas (partially) occluded
Va	Extensive endometrial scarring and fibrosis in combination with grade I or grade II adhesions with amenorrhea or pronounced hypomenorrhea
Vb	Extensive endometrial scarring and fibrosis in combination with grade III or grade IV adhesions with amenorrhea

Used with permission of Elsevier from Wamsteker and De Block [143]

Effect on Fertility and Pregnancy

The volume of menstrual bleeding can indicate the reproductive prognosis as it tells how much healthy endometrial tissue is present. Women with this condition can present with amenorrhoea, hypomenorrhoea, dysmenorrhoea, recurrent pregnancy loss and infertility [76, 77]. Poor implantation following ART and abnormal placentation has been reported in women with intrauterine adhesions [76].

Management

Hysteroscopy is the gold standard for diagnosis and treatment of intrauterine adhesions. Hysteroscopic adhesiolysis with scissors, electrosurgery or laser can restore the size of the uterine cavity. Severe intrauterine adhesions may require multiple operations. The division of adhesions can be performed under ultrasound or laparoscopic guidance to prevent perforation of the uterus. Other complications of the procedure include haemorrhage and infection. The reformation of adhesions seems to be related to the severity of the adhesions. There are a number of surgical and hormonal approaches in order to prevent postoperative adhesion formation. Estrogen is used to help with endometrial proliferation following the procedure [78]. An intrauterine placement of a device helps with the mechanical separation of the endometrial walls. This can be in the form of an intrauterine copper coil or an intrauterine triangular balloon [78, 79]. Furthermore, adhesion barriers such as hyaluronic acid seem to be promising. A systematic review looked at the effect of anti adhesion barrier gels following operative hysteroscopy and could find a reduction in adhesions at second look hysteroscopy 3 months later [80]. The postoperative assessment of the uterine cavity after adhesiolysis is recommended 1–2 months following the initial surgery and can be in the form of a midcycle ultrasound to measure the endometrial thickness, HSG and hysteroscopy [81]. Early recognition of recurrence of adhesions is important to achieve the best outcome and reduce obstetric risks [78].

An overall pregnancy rate from 40 to 63 % has been reported following adhesiolysis [77, 82–84]. More recently, intrauterine adhesion treatment with resectoscope or versapoint with subsequent hormone therapy and intrauterine copper coil placement showed to have an overall live birth rate of 41 % [83].

The reproductive outcome is dependent on the menstrual pattern, the severity of the adhesions and recurrence following treatment [85]. Nevertheless, pregnancies following treatment of intrauterine adhesions are at high risk of spontaneous miscarriage, preterm delivery, intrauterine growth restriction, abnormal placentation or uterine rupture and require careful monitoring [76].

Endometriosis

Endometriosis is a condition whereby endometrial like cells are found outside the uterus. It is an estrogen dependent chronic inflammatory condition in women of reproductive age. Endometriosis can lead to dysmenorrhoea, deep dyspareunia, chronic pelvic pain, cyclical pain and infertility [86]. However, some women do not have any symptoms. The prevalence of endometriosis depends on diagnostic methods, but ranges between 25–40 % of infertile women and 0.5–5 % of fertile women [87]. The pathogenesis is still not clear and several explanations exist. One theory for the development of endometriosis is retrograde menstruation [88]. However, most women have retrograde menstruation and only a few develop endometriosis. Another explanation is implantation of endometrial cells and coelemic metaplasia [89]. There is some evidence that there is a genetic component to the condition together with some environmental factors [90, 91]. Endometriosis may be a heterogeneous disease.

Common sites of endometriosis are pelvic peritoneum, ovaries and rectovaginal septum [92, 93]. An endometrioma is formed following the invagination of endometriotic deposits on the ovarian cortex, eventually forming what is commonly described as 'chocolate' cysts [93]. Ovarian endometriomas are found in 17–44 % of women with endometriosis [94, 95]. The gold standard to diagnose endometriosis is by laparoscopy and histological examination of the lesions. The extent of the disease has been classified in 4 stages (I–IV or minimal – severe) using the American Fertility (rAFS) System based on the laparoscopy findings. There is no correlation between the classification system and symptoms.

Effect on Fertility

Endometriosis is a chronic inflammatory condition. Moderate to severe endometriosis can lead to anatomical changes and thereby impair fertility. However, it is less clear how minimal to mild endometriosis interferes with fertility.

It has been suggested that ovulation, oocyte pick up by the fallopian tubes, fertilisation, embryo transport and implantation maybe disrupted in women with endometriosis [96].

Management

Hormonal medical treatment with progestins, oral contraceptives and gonadotropin releasing hormone agonists suppresses ovulation and menstruation and is not suitable for women seeking fertility. A Cochrane review showed that hormonal treatment in women diagnosed with minimal-mild endometriosis does not improve spontaneous conception [97, 98]. However, surgical treatment of minimal-mild endometriosis increases spontaneous conception rates compared to diagnostic laparoscopy (OR 1.64, 95 % CI 1.05–2.57) [99, 100]. Surgical treatment of infertile women with moderate to severe endometriosis also increases spontaneous pregnancy rates when compared to expectant management [101]. Surgery for deep infiltrating endometriosis is mainly performed to alleviate pain, but carries risk of major complications like ureteral and rectal injuries [102]. Furthermore, it may not greatly improve reproductive outcome [103]. Surgical treatment of endometriosis aims to remove visible endometriosis and restore the anatomy.

Assisted reproductive technology (ART) can be offered to infertile women with endometriosis. Stimulated IUI treatment in women with minimal to mild endometriosis maybe considered as it increases live birth rates compared to expectant management [104]. However, the most recent NICE guideline on fertility does not recommend routine IUI treatment in women with mild endometriosis [105]. They recommend IVF treatment after a total of 2 years without conception. IVF treatment is offered to women with endometriosis as it overcomes anatomical distortion and the abnormal peritoneal environment. Nevertheless, the pregnancy rates are lower compared to women with tubal factor infertility and women with severe endometriosis have even lower pregnancy rates than women with mild endometriosis [106]. A systematic review looked at the effect of endometriosis on IVF outcome and reported reduced fertilisation rates in women with stage I/II endometriosis (RR = 0.93, 95%CI 0.87–0.99) [107]. Women with stage III/IV endometriosis had low implantation (RR = 0.79, 95%CI 0.67–0.93) and clinical pregnancy rates (RR 0.79, 95%CI 0.69–0.91) [108]. Nonetheless, prolonged down-regulation with GnRH agonist 3–6 months prior to IVF improves clinical pregnancy rates as confirmed by a meta-analysis of three randomized trials [108].

The management of endometriomas depends on factors like size and previous ovarian surgery. Conservative treatment of endometrioma maybe considered with a small size (<3 cm). Surgical excision of endometrioma may lead to damage of healthy ovarian tissue and can reduce the ovarian reserve [109, 110]. Therefore, surgery should be avoided in women with previous ovarian surgery. Surgical treatment may be considered in women with large endometriomas (>3 cm) to improve endometriosis-associated pain or accessibility during egg collection for IVF treatment [111]. Laparoscopic excision of endometrioma is the preferred treatment as it has a lower recurrence and higher spontaneous pregnancy rate compared to drainage or coagulation of the endometrioma [112]. Furthermore, cystectomy gives a histological diagnosis. When the endometrioma is very large a two step procedure (surgery followed by 3 months GnRH agonist treatment and repeat surgery) may be considered. Medical management in the form of GnRH analogue can reduce the size of the endometrioma. A study showed that the presence of endometrioma affected the number of oocytes collected for IVF treatment, but oocyte quality or clinical pregnancy rate was not affected when compared to women without endometrioma [113]. Studies have demonstrated that there is no cumulative recurrence risk of endometriosis following assisted reproductive technology (ART) [114–116].

Overall it is important to take into account the benefits and risks of surgery, medical treatment and ART when managing couples with endometriosis associated infertility.

Adenomyosis

Adenomyosis is a condition whereby ectopic endometrial islands are found in the myometrium and causes dysmenorrhoea, abnormal uterine bleeding and infertility. A recent meta-analysis confirmed a reduced clinical pregnancy rate and an increased miscarriage rate after IVF/ICSI treatment in women with adenomyosis [117]. There are several possible explanations for this detrimental effect, including a chronic inflammatory condition [118], increased local estrogen production [119], uterine dysperistalsis leading to impaired utero-tubal sperm transport [120] and lower uterine receptivity suggested by the presence of implantation marker defects [121] and abnormal levels of intrauterine free radicals [122]. Adenomyosis is most commonly localised in the posterior uterine wall and can be diffuse or with focal nodules, also called adenomyoma. Adenomyosis is frequently encountered with other pathologies like endometriosis, polyps or fibroids. The diagnosis can be made with 2D/3D transvaginal ultrasound and MRI. 2D ultrasound criteria are globular uterus, asymmetry of uterine walls, poorly defined junctional zone and myometrial cysts [123]. An MRI is recommended if the uterus is enlarged or associated with a fibroid.

Pathogenesis

Multiple factors could be contributing to the pathogenesis of adenomyosis. One theory is that the basal layer of the endometrium invaginates between smooth muscle cell bundles or along lymphatic vessels into the myometrium [124]. Another theory is that adenomyosis may develop de novo through metaplasia of Mullerian remnants [125]. The relationship between adenomyosis and fertility is not exactly clear. On one hand adenomyosis is found in multiparous women and on the other hand it is seen in women with infertility and miscarriages [126].

Management

Medical and surgical treatments are available. Medical treatment is in the form of NSAIDs, progestogens and GnRH agonists. Women undergoing IVF treatment benefit from long agonist stimulation protocols with GnRH agonists [127]. However, women with adenomyosis had a lower clinical pregnancy rate on the antagonist cycle compared to women without adenomyosis (OR 0.4, 95%CI 0.18–0.92) [128]. A systematic review about adenomyosis and IVF outcome showed a 28 % reduction in the likelihood of a clinical pregnancy following IVF/ICSI [117].

Hydrosalpinx

Hydrosalpinges are found in 10–30 % of couples with tubal factor infertility and can be diagnosed by ultrasound or hysterosalpingogram.

Hydrosalpinx is a fluid collection in the fallopian tube due to distal tubal occlusion. The most common cause is pelvic inflammatory disease from Chlamydia trachomatis or Neisseria gonorrhoeae. A hydrosalpinx can also be a result of tubal tuberculosis, endometriosis, appendicitis or following abdomino-pelvic surgery.

Effect on Fertility and Pregnancy

It has been shown that implantation, pregnancy, and live birth rates are reduced by 50 % in women with hydrosalpinx [129–131]. Furthermore, miscarriage rates are doubled [130]. The presence of hydrosalpinx fluid in the uterine cavity is embryotoxic and alters the embryo endometrium receptivity as well as the tubo-uterine flow dynamics [132, 133].

Management

The management of hydrosalpinges involves the disruption of the tubo-uterine communication. A randomised controlled trial found that women following laparoscopic salpingectomy for hydrosalpinx prior to IVF doubled their live birth rates compared to women without surgery [134]. This interrupts the communication between the fallopian tube and the uterine cavity. A systematic review confirmed a doubling of clinical pregnancy rates following surgical treatment of hydrosalpinges (OR 2.14, 95 % CI 1.23–3.73) [135]. However, salpingectomy can reduce the blood supply to the ovary and thereby reduce the ovarian reserve. Studies looking into the ovarian response during IVF treatment did not show a significant difference in women who had a previous salpingectomy [136, 137]. If the surgical skills are present the tubal mucosa could be assessed and if found to be healthy a salpingostomy could be attempted. These patients need to be informed about the risk of an ectopic pregnancy. Laparoscopic tubal occlusion is possible if there are severe pelvic adhesions present. A systematic review confirmed a significant increase of pregnancy rates following this approach [135]. Laparoscopic tubal occlusion is as effective as laparoscopic salpingectomy in improving clinical pregnancy rates (RR 1.1, 95%CI 0.85–1.6) [138].

Hysteroscopic occlusion of the tube with the help of Essure® (Bayer, Whippany, NJ, USA) can be considered in women when laparoscopy is contraindicated. Essure® is a 4 cm long microinsert with polyethylene terephthalate fibres that induce a tissue reaction resulting in tubal occlusion. It is used for hysteroscopic tubal sterilisation. Initially there were concerns about the possible effect of the coils from the Essure® device protruding into the uterine cavity on implantation and pregnancy [139]. However, a study assessed the pregnancy outcome of 50 pregnancies following Essure® insertion and concluded that the device is unlikely to interfere with implantation and pregnancy [140]. A systematic review looked into the efficacy of Essure in the management of hydrosalpinx before IVF and found a 27.9 % live birth rate per embryo transfer (95 % CI 21.7–36.6 %) [141]. It appears that Essure ® is an effective treatment option for women with hydrosalpinges before IVF when the laparoscopic approach is contraindicated.

If a hydrosalpinx is detected during the IVF cycle freezing of all embryos can be considered followed by treatment of the hydrosalpinx. Transvaginal aspiration of the fluid after egg collection and embryo transfer showed a trend in increasing the clinical pregnancy rate compared to no treatment, but this was statistically not significant (RR 1.7, 95 % CI 0.69–4.0) [142]. Further research is needed to assess the value of aspiration of hydrosalpinges.

In summary, laparoscopic surgical treatment should be considered for all women with hydrosalpinx before IVF. When laparoscopy is not recommended, hysteroscopic tubal occlusion seems the most effective option for the management of hydrosalpinx before IVF.

Conclusion

Gynaecological pathologies are frequently found in infertile women. The correct diagnosis is essential in order to counsel the couple on risks and benefits of treatment alternatives to allow informed choices. Medical and/or surgical and/or ART are available to increase the chances for a healthy pregnancy and live birth.

References

1. Cramer SF, Patel A. The frequency of uterine leiomyomas. Am J Clin Pathol. 1990;94(4):435–8.
2. Roy KK, Singla S, Baruah J, Sharma JB, Kumar S, Singh N. Reproductive outcome following hysteroscopic myomectomy in patients with infertility and recurrent abortions. Arch Gynecol Obstet. 2010;282(5):553–60.
3. Shokeir T, El-Shafei M, Yousef H, Allam AF, Sadek E. Submucous myomas and their implications in the pregnancy rates of patients with otherwise unexplained primary infertility undergoing hysteroscopic myomectomy: a randomized matched control study. Fertil Steril. 2010;94(2):724–9.
4. Farhi J, Ashkenazi J, Feldberg D, Dicker D, Orvieto R, Ben RZ. Effect of uterine leiomyomata on the results of in-vitro fertilization treatment. Hum Reprod. 1995;10(10):2576–8.
5. Eldar-Geva T, Meagher S, Healy DL, MacLachlan V, Breheny S, Wood C. Effect of intramural, subserosal, and submucosal uterine fibroids on the outcome of assisted reproductive technology treatment. Fertil Steril. 1998;70(4):687–91.
6. Surrey ES, Minjarez DA, Stevens JM, Schoolcraft WB. Effect of myomectomy on the outcome of assisted reproductive technologies. Fertil Steril. 2005;83(5):1473–9.
7. Buttram Jr VC, Reiter RC. Uterine leiomyomata: etiology, symptomatology, and management. Fertil Steril. 1981;36(4):433–45.
8. Donnez J, Jadoul P. What are the implications of myomas on fertility? A need for a debate? Hum Reprod. 2002;17(6):1424–30.
9. Brosens I, Derwig I, Brosens J, Fusi L, Benagiano G, Pijnenborg R. The enigmatic uterine junctional zone: the missing link between reproductive disorders and major obstetrical disorders? Hum Reprod. 2010;25(3):569–74.
10. Hart R, Khalaf Y, Yeong CT, Seed P, Taylor A, Braude P. A prospective controlled study of the effect of intramural uterine fibroids on the outcome of assisted conception. Hum Reprod. 2001;16(11):2411–7.
11. Khalaf Y, Ross C, El-Toukhy T, Hart R, Seed P, Braude P. The effect of small intramural uterine fibroids on the cumulative outcome of assisted conception. Hum Reprod. 2006;21(10):2640–4.

12. Oliveira FG, Abdelmassih VG, Diamond MP, Dozortsev D, Melo NR, Abdelmassih R. Impact of subserosal and intramural uterine fibroids that do not distort the endometrial cavity on the outcome of in vitro fertilization-intracytoplasmic sperm injection. Fertil Steril. 2004;81(3):582–7.
13. Ng EH, Ho PC. Doppler ultrasound examination of uterine arteries on the day of oocyte retrieval in patients with uterine fibroids undergoing IVF. Hum Reprod. 2002; 17(3):765–70.
14. Bozdag G, Esinler I, Boynukalin K, Aksu T, Gunalp S, Gurgan T. Single intramural leiomyoma with normal hysteroscopic findings does not affect ICSI-embryo transfer outcome. Reprod Biomed Online. 2009;19(2):276–80.
15. Surrey ES, Lietz AK, Schoolcraft WB. Impact of intramural leiomyomata in patients with a normal endometrial cavity on in vitro fertilization-embryo transfer cycle outcome. Fertil Steril. 2001;75(2):405–10.
16. Pritts EA. Fibroids and infertility: a systematic review of the evidence. Obstet Gynecol Surv. 2001;56(8):483–91.
17. Pritts EA, Parker WH, Olive DL. Fibroids and infertility: an updated systematic review of the evidence. Fertil Steril. 2009;91(4):1215–23.
18. Sunkara SK, Khairy M, El-Toukhy T, Khalaf Y, Coomarasamy A. The effect of intramural fibroids without uterine cavity involvement on the outcome of IVF treatment: a systematic review and meta-analysis. Hum Reprod. 2010;25(2):418–29.
19. Metwally M, Farquhar CM, Li TC. Is another meta-analysis on the effects of intramural fibroids on reproductive outcomes needed? Reprod Biomed Online. 2011;23(1):2–14.
20. Casini ML, Rossi F, Agostini R, Unfer V. Effects of the position of fibroids on fertility. Gynecol Endocrinol. 2006;22(2):106–9.
21. Tamaya T, Fujimoto J, Okada H. Comparison of cellular levels of steroid receptors in uterine leiomyoma and myometrium. Acta Obstet Gynecol Scand. 1985;64(4):307–9.
22. Lethaby A, Vollenhoven B, Sowter M. Pre-operative GnRH analogue therapy before hysterectomy or myomectomy for uterine fibroids. Cochrane Database Syst Rev. 2001;(2):CD000547.
23. Donnez J, Tatarchuk TF, Bouchard P, Puscasiu L, Zakharenko NF, Ivanova T, et al. Ulipristal acetate versus placebo for fibroid treatment before surgery. N Engl J Med. 2012;366(5):409–20.
24. Donnez J, Tomaszewski J, Vazquez F, Bouchard P, Lemieszczuk B, Baro F, et al. Ulipristal acetate versus leuprolide acetate for uterine fibroids. N Engl J Med. 2012;366(5):421–32.
25. Donnez J, Hudecek R, Donnez O, Matule D, Arhendt HJ, Zatik J, et al. Efficacy and safety of repeated use of ulipristal acetate in uterine fibroids. Fertil Steril. 2015;103(2):519–27.e3.
26. Donnez J, Vazquez F, Tomaszewski J, Nouri K, Bouchard P, Fauser BC, et al. Long-term treatment of uterine fibroids with ulipristal acetate. Fertil Steril. 2014;101(6):1565–73. e1–18.
27. Freed MM, Spies JB. Uterine artery embolization for fibroids: a review of current outcomes. Semin Reprod Med. 2010;28(3):235–41.
28. Hald K, Klow NE, Qvigstad E, Istre O. Laparoscopic occlusion compared with embolization of uterine vessels: a randomized controlled trial. Obstet Gynecol. 2007;109(1):20–7.
29. Tulandi T, Sammour A, Valenti D, Child TJ, Seti L, Tan SL. Ovarian reserve after uterine artery embolization for leiomyomata. Fertil Steril. 2002;78(1):197–8.
30. Amato P, Roberts AC. Transient ovarian failure: a complication of uterine artery embolization. Fertil Steril. 2001;75(2):438–9.
31. Homer H, Saridogan E. Uterine artery embolization for fibroids is associated with an increased risk of miscarriage. Fertil Steril. 2010;94(1):324–30.
32. Torre A, Paillusson B, Fain V, Labauge P, Pelage JP, Fauconnier A. Uterine artery embolization for severe symptomatic fibroids: effects on fertility and symptoms. Hum Reprod. 2014;29(3):490–501.
33. Mara M, Kubinova K. Embolization of uterine fibroids from the point of view of the gynecologist: pros and cons. Int J Womens Health. 2014;6:623–9.

34. Pron G, Mocarski E, Bennett J, Vilos G, Common A, Vanderburgh L, et al. Pregnancy after uterine artery embolization for leiomyomata: the Ontario multicenter trial. Obstet Gynecol. 2005;105(1):67–76.
35. Mara M, Maskova J, Fucikova Z, Kuzel D, Belsan T, Sosna O. Midterm clinical and first reproductive results of a randomized controlled trial comparing uterine fibroid embolization and myomectomy. Cardiovasc Intervent Radiol. 2008;31(1):73–85.
36. Mara M, Horak P, Kubinova K, Dundr P, Belsan T, Kuzel D. Hysteroscopy after uterine fibroid embolization: evaluation of intrauterine findings in 127 patients. J Obstet Gynaecol Res. 2012;38(5):823–31.
37. Gupta JK, Sinha A, Lumsden MA, Hickey M. Uterine artery embolization for symptomatic uterine fibroids. Cochrane Database Syst Rev. 2014;12, CD005073.
38. Rabinovici J, David M, Fukunishi H, Morita Y, Gostout BS, Stewart EA, et al. Pregnancy outcome after magnetic resonance-guided focused ultrasound surgery (MRgFUS) for conservative treatment of uterine fibroids. Fertil Steril. 2010;93(1):199–209.
39. Mais V, Ajossa S, Guerriero S, Mascia M, Solla E, Melis GB. Laparoscopic versus abdominal myomectomy: a prospective, randomized trial to evaluate benefits in early outcome. Am J Obstet Gynecol. 1996;174(2):654–8.
40. Metwally M, Cheong YC, Horne AW. Surgical treatment of fibroids for subfertility. Cochrane Database Syst Rev. 2012;11, CD003857.
41. Shokeir TA, Shalan HM, El-Shafei MM. Significance of endometrial polyps detected hysteroscopically in eumenorrheic infertile women. J Obstet Gynaecol Res. 2004; 30(2):84–9.
42. de Sa Rosa e de Silva AC, Rosa e Silva JC, Candido dos Reis FJ, Nogueira AA, Ferriani RA. Routine office hysteroscopy in the investigation of infertile couples before assisted reproduction. J Reprod Med. 2005;50(7):501–6.
43. Kim MR, Kim YA, Jo MY, Hwang KJ, Ryu HS. High frequency of endometrial polyps in endometriosis. J Am Assoc Gynecol Laparosc. 2003;10(1):46–8.
44. Rackow BW, Jorgensen E, Taylor HS. Endometrial polyps affect uterine receptivity. Fertil Steril. 2011;95(8):2690–2.
45. Spiewankiewicz B, Stelmachow J, Sawicki W, Cendrowski K, Wypych P, Swiderska K. The effectiveness of hysteroscopic polypectomy in cases of female infertility. Clin Exp Obstet Gynecol. 2003;30(1):23–5.
46. Varasteh NN, Neuwirth RS, Levin B, Keltz MD. Pregnancy rates after hysteroscopic polypectomy and myomectomy in infertile women. Obstet Gynecol. 1999;94(2):168–71.
47. Perez-Medina T, Bajo-Arenas J, Salazar F, Redondo T, Sanfrutos L, Alvarez P, et al. Endometrial polyps and their implication in the pregnancy rates of patients undergoing intrauterine insemination: a prospective, randomized study. Hum Reprod. 2005;20(6):1632–5.
48. Yanaihara A, Yorimitsu T, Motoyama H, Iwasaki S, Kawamura T. Location of endometrial polyp and pregnancy rate in infertility patients. Fertil Steril. 2008;90(1):180–2.
49. Afifi K, Anand S, Nallapeta S, Gelbaya TA. Management of endometrial polyps in subfertile women: a systematic review. Eur J Obstet Gynecol Reprod Biol. 2010;151(2):117–21.
50. Bosteels J, Kasius J, Weyers S, Broekmans FJ, Mol BW, D'Hooghe TM. Hysteroscopy for treating subfertility associated with suspected major uterine cavity abnormalities. Cochrane Database Syst Rev. 2013;1, CD009461.
51. Isikoglu M, Berkkanoglu M, Senturk Z, Coetzee K, Ozgur K. Endometrial polyps smaller than 1.5 cm do not affect ICSI outcome. Reprod Biomed Online. 2006;12(2):199–204.
52. Lass A, Williams G, Abusheikha N, Brinsden P. The effect of endometrial polyps on outcomes of in vitro fertilization (IVF) cycles. J Assist Reprod Genet. 1999;16(8):410–5.
53. Stamatellos I, Apostolides A, Stamatopoulos P, Bontis J. Pregnancy rates after hysteroscopic polypectomy depending on the size or number of the polyps. Arch Gynecol Obstet. 2008;277(5):395–9.
54. Preutthipan S, Herabutya Y. Hysteroscopic polypectomy in 240 premenopausal and postmenopausal women. Fertil Steril. 2005;83(3):705–9.

55. Grimbizis GF, Gordts S, Di Spiezio Sardo A, Brucker S, De Angelis C, Gergolet M, et al. The ESHRE/ESGE consensus on the classification of female genital tract congenital anomalies. Hum Reprod. 2013;28(8):2032–44.
56. Raga F, Bauset C, Remohi J, Bonilla-Musoles F, Simon C, Pellicer A. Reproductive impact of congenital Mullerian anomalies. Hum Reprod. 1997;12(10):2277–81.
57. Acien P. Incidence of Mullerian defects in fertile and infertile women. Hum Reprod. 1997;12(7):1372–6.
58. Green LK, Harris RE. Uterine anomalies. Frequency of diagnosis and associated obstetric complications. Obstet Gynecol. 1976;47(4):427–9.
59. Lavergne N, Aristizabal J, Zarka V, Erny R, Hedon B. Uterine anomalies and in vitro fertilization: what are the results? Eur J Obstet Gynecol Reprod Biol. 1996;68(1–2):29–34.
60. Reuter KL, Daly DC, Cohen SM. Septate versus bicornuate uteri: errors in imaging diagnosis. Radiology. 1989;172(3):749–52.
61. Pellerito JS, McCarthy SM, Doyle MB, Glickman MG, DeCherney AH. Diagnosis of uterine anomalies: relative accuracy of MR imaging, endovaginal sonography, and hysterosalpingography. Radiology. 1992;183(3):795–800.
62. Wu MH, Hsu CC, Huang KE. Detection of congenital mullerian duct anomalies using three-dimensional ultrasound. J Clin Ultrasound. 1997;25(9):487–92.
63. Homer HA, Li TC, Cooke ID. The septate uterus: a review of management and reproductive outcome. Fertil Steril. 2000;73(1):1–14.
64. Pabuccu R, Gomel V. Reproductive outcome after hysteroscopic metroplasty in women with septate uterus and otherwise unexplained infertility. Fertil Steril. 2004;81(6):1675–8.
65. Mollo A, De Franciscis P, Colacurci N, Cobellis L, Perino A, Venezia R, et al. Hysteroscopic resection of the septum improves the pregnancy rate of women with unexplained infertility: a prospective controlled trial. Fertil Steril. 2009;91(6):2628–31.
66. Fedele L, Bianchi S, Agnoli B, Tozzi L, Vignali M. Urinary tract anomalies associated with unicornuate uterus. J Urol. 1996;155(3):847–8.
67. Akar ME, Bayar D, Yildiz S, Ozel M, Yilmaz Z. Reproductive outcome of women with unicornuate uterus. Aust N Z J Obstet Gynaecol. 2005;45(2):148–50.
68. Grimbizis GF, Camus M, Tarlatzis BC, Bontis JN, Devroey P. Clinical implications of uterine malformations and hysteroscopic treatment results. Hum Reprod Update. 2001;7(2):161–74.
69. Chan YY, Jayaprakasan K, Tan A, Thornton JG, Coomarasamy A, Raine-Fenning NJ. Reproductive outcomes in women with congenital uterine anomalies: a systematic review. Ultrasound Obstet Gynecol. 2011;38(4):371–82.
70. Patton PE. Anatomic uterine defects. Clin Obstet Gynecol. 1994;37(3):705–21.
71. Schenker JG, Margalioth EJ. Intrauterine adhesions: an updated appraisal. Fertil Steril. 1982;37(5):593–610.
72. Taskin O, Sadik S, Onoglu A, Gokdeniz R, Erturan E, Burak F, et al. Role of endometrial suppression on the frequency of intrauterine adhesions after resectoscopic surgery. J Am Assoc Gynecol Laparosc. 2000;7(3):351–4.
73. Soares SR, Barbosa dos Reis MM, Camargos AF. Diagnostic accuracy of sonohysterography, transvaginal sonography, and hysterosalpingography in patients with uterine cavity diseases. Fertil Steril. 2000;73(2):406–11.
74. Salle B, Gaucherand P, de Saint Hilaire P, Rudigoz RC. Transvaginal sonohysterographic evaluation of intrauterine adhesions. J Clin Ultrasound. 1999;27(3):131–4.
75. The American Fertility Society classifications of adnexal adhesions, distal tubal occlusion, tubal occlusion secondary to tubal ligation, tubal pregnancies, mullerian anomalies and intrauterine adhesions. Fertil Steril. 1988;49(6):944–55.
76. Yu D, Wong YM, Cheong Y, Xia E, Li TC. Asherman syndrome – one century later. Fertil Steril. 2008;89(4):759–79.
77. Deans R, Abbott J. Review of intrauterine adhesions. J Minim Invasive Gynecol. 2010;17(5):555–69.

78. March CM. Management of Asherman's syndrome. Reprod Biomed Online. 2011;23(1):63–76.
79. Polishuk WZ, Weinstein D. The Soichet intrauterine device in the treatment of intrauterine adhesions. Acta Eur Fertil. 1976;7(3):215–8.
80. Bosteels J, Weyers S, Mol BW, D'Hooghe T. Anti-adhesion barrier gels following operative hysteroscopy for treating female infertility: a systematic review and meta-analysis. Gynecol Surg. 2014;11:113–27.
81. Kodaman PH, Arici A. Intra-uterine adhesions and fertility outcome: how to optimize success? Curr Opin Obstet Gynecol. 2007;19(3):207–14.
82. Capella-Allouc S, Morsad F, Rongieres-Bertrand C, Taylor S, Fernandez H. Hysteroscopic treatment of severe Asherman's syndrome and subsequent fertility. Hum Reprod. 1999;14(5):1230–3.
83. Zikopoulos KA, Kolibianakis EM, Platteau P, de Munck L, Tournaye H, Devroey P, et al. Live delivery rates in subfertile women with Asherman's syndrome after hysteroscopic adhesiolysis using the resectoscope or the Versapoint system. Reprod Biomed Online. 2004;8(6):720–5.
84. Roy KK, Baruah J, Sharma JB, Kumar S, Kachawa G, Singh N. Reproductive outcome following hysteroscopic adhesiolysis in patients with infertility due to Asherman's syndrome. Arch Gynecol Obstet. 2010;281(2):355–61.
85. Yu D, Li TC, Xia E, Huang X, Liu Y, Peng X. Factors affecting reproductive outcome of hysteroscopic adhesiolysis for Asherman's syndrome. Fertil Steril. 2008;89(3):715–22.
86. Giudice LC, Kao LC. Endometriosis. Lancet. 2004;364(9447):1789–99.
87. Buck Louis GM, Hediger ML, Peterson CM, Croughan M, Sundaram R, Stanford J, et al. Incidence of endometriosis by study population and diagnostic method: the ENDO study. Fertil Steril. 2011;96(2):360–5.
88. Sampson JA. Peritoneal endometriosis due to the menstrual dissemination of endometrial tissue into the peritoneal cavity. Am J Obstet Gynecol. 1927;14:422–69.
89. Burney RO, Giudice LC. Pathogenesis and pathophysiology of endometriosis. Fertil Steril. 2012;98(3):511–9.
90. Stefansson H, Geirsson RT, Steinthorsdottir V, Jonsson H, Manolescu A, Kong A, et al. Genetic factors contribute to the risk of developing endometriosis. Hum Reprod. 2002;17(3):555–9.
91. Nyholt DR, Low SK, Anderson CA, Painter JN, Uno S, Morris AP, et al. Genome-wide association meta-analysis identifies new endometriosis risk loci. Nat Genet. 2012;44(12):1355–9.
92. Koninckx PR, Martin DC. Deep endometriosis: a consequence of infiltration or retraction or possibly adenomyosis externa? Fertil Steril. 1992;58(5):924–8.
93. Nisolle M, Donnez J. Peritoneal endometriosis, ovarian endometriosis, and adenomyotic nodules of the rectovaginal septum are three different entities. Fertil Steril. 1997;68(4):585–96.
94. Redwine DB. Ovarian endometriosis: a marker for more extensive pelvic and intestinal disease. Fertil Steril. 1999;72(2):310–5.
95. Busacca M, Vignali M. Ovarian endometriosis: from pathogenesis to surgical treatment. Curr Opin Obstet Gynecol. 2003;15(4):321–6.
96. de Ziegler D, Borghese B, Chapron C. Endometriosis and infertility: pathophysiology and management. Lancet. 2010;376(9742):730–8.
97. Hughes E, Fedorkow D, Collins J, Vandekerckhove P. Ovulation suppression for endometriosis. Cochrane Database Syst Rev. 2003;(3):CD000155.
98. Hughes E, Brown J, Collins JJ, Farquhar C, Fedorkow DM, Vandekerckhove P. Ovulation suppression for endometriosis. Cochrane Database Syst Rev. 2007;(3):CD000155.
99. Jacobson TZ, Duffy JM, Barlow D, Farquhar C, Koninckx PR, Olive D. Laparoscopic surgery for subfertility associated with endometriosis. Cochrane Database Syst Rev. 2010;(1):CD001398.

100. Duffy JM, Arambage K, Correa FJ, Olive D, Farquhar C, Garry R, et al. Laparoscopic surgery for endometriosis. Cochrane Database Syst Rev. 2014;4, CD011031.
101. Vercellini P, Fedele L, Aimi G, De Giorgi O, Consonni D, Crosignani PG. Reproductive performance, pain recurrence and disease relapse after conservative surgical treatment for endometriosis: the predictive value of the current classification system. Hum Reprod. 2006;21(10):2679–85.
102. Vercellini P, Somigliana E, Vigano P, Abbiati A, Barbara G, Crosignani PG. Surgery for endometriosis-associated infertility: a pragmatic approach. Hum Reprod. 2009;24(2): 254–69.
103. Emmanuel KR, Davis C. Outcomes and treatment options in rectovaginal endometriosis. Curr Opin Obstet Gynecol. 2005;17(4):399–402.
104. Tummon IS, Asher LJ, Martin JS, Tulandi T. Randomized controlled trial of superovulation and insemination for infertility associated with minimal or mild endometriosis. Fertil Steril. 1997;68(1):8–12.
105. National Collaborating Centre for Women's and Children's Health (UK). Fertility: assessment and treatment for people with fertility problems. 2013.
106. Barnhart K, Dunsmoor-Su R, Coutifaris C. Effect of endometriosis on in vitro fertilization. Fertil Steril. 2002;77(6):1148–55.
107. Harb HM, Gallos ID, Chu J, Harb M, Coomarasamy A. The effect of endometriosis on in vitro fertilisation outcome: a systematic review and meta-analysis. BJOG. 2013;120(11):1308–20.
108. Sallam HN, Garcia-Velasco JA, Dias S, Arici A. Long-term pituitary down-regulation before in vitro fertilization (IVF) for women with endometriosis. Cochrane Database Syst Rev. 2006;(1):CD004635.
109. Benaglia L, Somigliana E, Vighi V, Ragni G, Vercellini P, Fedele L. Rate of severe ovarian damage following surgery for endometriomas. Hum Reprod. 2010;25(3):678–82.
110. Hwu YM, Wu FS, Li SH, Sun FJ, Lin MH, Lee RK. The impact of endometrioma and laparoscopic cystectomy on serum anti-Mullerian hormone levels. Reprod Biol Endocrinol. 2011;9:80. doi:10.1186/1477-7827-9-80.
111. Dunselman GA, Vermeulen N, Becker C, Calhaz-Jorge C, D'Hooghe T, De Bie B, et al. ESHRE guideline: management of women with endometriosis. Hum Reprod. 2014;29(3):400–12.
112. Hart RJ, Hickey M, Maouris P, Buckett W. Excisional surgery versus ablative surgery for ovarian endometriomata. Cochrane Database Syst Rev. 2008;(2):CD004992.
113. Benaglia L, Bermejo A, Somigliana E, Faulisi S, Ragni G, Fedele L, et al. In vitro fertilization outcome in women with unoperated bilateral endometriomas. Fertil Steril. 2013;99(6):1714–9.
114. Benaglia L, Somigliana E, Vercellini P, Benedetti F, Iemmello R, Vighi V, et al. The impact of IVF procedures on endometriosis recurrence. Eur J Obstet Gynecol Reprod Biol. 2010;148(1):49–52.
115. D'Hooghe TM, Denys B, Spiessens C, Meuleman C, Debrock S. Is the endometriosis recurrence rate increased after ovarian hyperstimulation? Fertil Steril. 2006;86(2):283–90.
116. Benaglia L, Somigliana E, Santi G, Scarduelli C, Ragni G, Fedele L. IVF and endometriosis-related symptom progression: insights from a prospective study. Hum Reprod. 2011;26(9):2368–72.
117. Vercellini P, Consonni D, Dridi D, Bracco B, Frattaruolo MP, Somigliana E. Uterine adenomyosis and in vitro fertilization outcome: a systematic review and meta-analysis. Hum Reprod. 2014;29(5):964–77.
118. Tremellen KP, Russell P. The distribution of immune cells and macrophages in the endometrium of women with recurrent reproductive failure. II: adenomyosis and macrophages. J Reprod Immunol. 2012;93(1):58–63.
119. Brosens J, Verhoeven H, Campo R, Gianaroli L, Gordts S, Hazekamp J, et al. High endometrial aromatase P450 mRNA expression is associated with poor IVF outcome. Hum Reprod. 2004;19(2):352–6.

120. Kissler S, Hamscho N, Zangos S, Wiegratz I, Schlichter S, Menzel C, et al. Uterotubal transport disorder in adenomyosis and endometriosis – a cause for infertility. BJOG. 2006;113(8):902–8.
121. Campo S, Campo V, Benagiano G. Adenomyosis and infertility. Reprod Biomed Online. 2012;24(1):35–46.
122. Benagiano G, Brosens I, Habiba M. Structural and molecular features of the endomyometrium in endometriosis and adenomyosis. Hum Reprod Update. 2014;20(3):386–402.
123. Bazot M, Cortez A, Darai E, Rouger J, Chopier J, Antoine JM, et al. Ultrasonography compared with magnetic resonance imaging for the diagnosis of adenomyosis: correlation with histopathology. Hum Reprod. 2001;16(11):2427–33.
124. Benagiano G, Habiba M, Brosens I. The pathophysiology of uterine adenomyosis: an update. Fertil Steril. 2012;98(3):572–9.
125. Bergeron C, Amant F, Ferenczy A. Pathology and physiopathology of adenomyosis. Best Pract Res Clin Obstet Gynaecol. 2006;20(4):511–21.
126. Parazzini F, Vercellini P, Panazza S, Chatenoud L, Oldani S, Crosignani PG. Risk factors for adenomyosis. Hum Reprod. 1997;12(6):1275–9.
127. Costello MF, Lindsay K, McNally G. The effect of adenomyosis on in vitro fertilisation and intra-cytoplasmic sperm injection treatment outcome. Eur J Obstet Gynecol Reprod Biol. 2011;158(2):229–34.
128. Thalluri V, Tremellen KP. Ultrasound diagnosed adenomyosis has a negative impact on successful implantation following GnRH antagonist IVF treatment. Hum Reprod. 2012;27(12):3487–92.
129. Vandromme J, Chasse E, Lejeune B, Van Rysselberge M, Delvigne A, Leroy F. Hydrosalpinges in in-vitro fertilization: an unfavourable prognostic feature. Hum Reprod. 1995;10(3):576–9.
130. Zeyneloglu HB, Arici A, Olive DL. Adverse effects of hydrosalpinx on pregnancy rates after in vitro fertilization-embryo transfer. Fertil Steril. 1998;70(3):492–9.
131. Camus E, Poncelet C, Goffinet F, Wainer B, Merlet F, Nisand I, et al. Pregnancy rates after in-vitro fertilization in cases of tubal infertility with and without hydrosalpinx: a meta-analysis of published comparative studies. Hum Reprod. 1999;14(5):1243–9.
132. Strandell A, Lindhard A. Why does hydrosalpinx reduce fertility? The importance of hydrosalpinx fluid. Hum Reprod. 2002;17(5):1141–5.
133. Strandell A. The influence of hydrosalpinx on IVF and embryo transfer: a review. Hum Reprod Update. 2000;6(4):387–95.
134. Strandell A, Lindhard A, Waldenstrom U, Thorburn J. Hydrosalpinx and IVF outcome: cumulative results after salpingectomy in a randomized controlled trial. Hum Reprod. 2001;16(11):2403–10.
135. Johnson N, van Voorst S, Sowter MC, Strandell A, Mol BW. Surgical treatment for tubal disease in women due to undergo in vitro fertilisation. Cochrane Database Syst Rev. 2010(1):CD002125.
136. Strandell A, Lindhard A, Waldenstrom U, Thorburn J. Prophylactic salpingectomy does not impair the ovarian response in IVF treatment. Hum Reprod. 2001;16(6):1135–9.
137. Bredkjaer HE, Ziebe S, Hamid B, Zhou Y, Loft A, Lindhard A, et al. Delivery rates after in-vitro fertilization following bilateral salpingectomy due to hydrosalpinges: a case control study. Hum Reprod. 1999;14(1):101–5.
138. Bosteels J, Weyers S, Mathieu C, Mol BW, D'Hooghe T. The effectiveness of reproductive surgery in the treatment of -female infertility: facts, views and vision. Facts Views Vis Obgyn. 2010;2(4):232–52.
139. Kerin JF, Cattanach S. Successful pregnancy outcome with the use of in vitro fertilization after Essure hysteroscopic sterilization. Fertil Steril. 2007;87(5):1212.e1–4.
140. Veersema S, Mijatovic V, Dreyer K, Schouten H, Schoot D, Emanuel MH, et al. Outcomes of pregnancies in women with hysteroscopically placed micro-inserts in situ. J Minim Invasive Gynecol. 2014;21(3):492–7.

141. Arora P, Arora RS, Cahill D. Essure((R)) for management of hydrosalpinx prior to in vitro fertilisation-a systematic review and pooled analysis. BJOG. 2014;121(5):527–36.
142. Hammadieh N, Coomarasamy A, Ola B, Papaioannou S, Afnan M, Sharif K. Ultrasound-guided hydrosalpinx aspiration during oocyte collection improves pregnancy outcome in IVF: a randomized controlled trial. Hum Reprod. 2008;23(5):1113–7.
143. Wamsteker K, De Block S. Diagnostic hysteroscopy: technique and documentation. In: Sutton C, Diamond M, editors. Endoscopic surgery for gynecologists. London: WB Saunders; 1998. p. 511–24.

Chapter 3
Psychological Difficulties and Mental Ill-Health Associated with ART

Neelam Sisodia

Introduction

Artificial reproductive techniques (ART) have advanced a great deal over the course of the last 30 years or so and treatment for infertility or sub-fertility has become more easily accessible to "ordinary" couples, both through the national health service (e.g., NHS in the UK) and private fertility clinics world-wide. Alongside the technical advances in assisted reproduction, there has been a burgeoning in literature about the psychological difficulties associated with the inability to conceive a child when a couple wishes to do so, as well as the psychological distress consequent on undergoing any treatment necessary, whether this is successful or not [1–5].

In addition to the impact of stress on the quality of life of any individuals undergoing treatment for reproductive difficulties, there is the very important issue of how to screen for and manage the mental health of patients who have a pre-existing significant mental illness (usually moderate to severe anxiety and mood disorders, but also more serious and enduring conditions such as mood related and schizophrenia-like psychoses) or those who develop such illnesses during the course of treatment with ART or after the delivery of a much wanted and long-awaited child (or children, in the case of twin or triplet pregnancies).

The biochemical changes that occur in the pituitary as a result of the "down-regulation" and "up-regulation" of the ovulation cycle in women and the subsequent use of large quantities of hormones for stimulating the production of ova in preparation for egg harvesting and IVF are likely to be significant in the aetiology of first onset severe mood disorders and mood related psychoses, as well as the trigger for recurrent episodes in those with pre-existing illnesses of this kind [6]. However, a

N. Sisodia, MBBS, MA, FRCPsych
Perinatal Psychiatric Service, Nottinghamshire Healthcare NHS Foundation Trust, Nottingham University Hospitals QMC Campus, Nottingham, UK
e-mail: neelam.sisodia@hotmail.com

K. Jayaprakasan, L. Kean (eds.), *Clinical Management of Pregnancies following ART*, DOI 10.1007/978-3-319-42858-1_3

review and discussion of this topic is beyond the scope of this chapter. Therefore I will briefly discuss the issue of screening for a personal or family history of moderate to severe mood disorders and psychoses, before going on to describe some anthropological and socio-cultural considerations that may help health professionals to understand a couple's or an individual patient's response to the stresses of infertility (or sub-fertility) and treatment for this with ART. I will end with a number of clinical scenarios, which demonstrate the way in which patients may present to the treating fertility specialist, whilst they are attempting to conceive, or to a family physician, obstetrician, midwife or psychiatrist, in pregnancy or postpartum.

Brief Discussion About Screening for a Mental Health Problem Which May Be Impacted Upon by Treatment with ART

Those working in the United Kingdom will be familiar with the kind of screening pro-forma used by midwives at booking for antenatal care, which prompt them to ask a pregnant woman about a personal or family history of mental health problems and more serious mental illness, as the NICE guidelines for antenatal and postnatal mental health, first published in 2007, and updated in 2015, recommend this [7, 8]. Over the last 10 years, and longer than this in areas at the forefront of developing Obstetric Liaison and Perinatal Psychiatric Services, such screening methods have been used to identify those women who are at increased risk of developing a significant mental illness during the course of their pregnancy or in the early weeks after delivery of a child, whether this be a relapse of a pre-existing serious mental disorder, most often mood related, or the first onset of such an illness. It is noteworthy that the latter group of women often have a strong family history of serious mood disorder or psychosis and their genetic vulnerability to these conditions seems to be impacted on by the physiological changes that occur in late pregnancy and early postpartum, leading to a greatly increased risk for first onset psychosis at this time in their lives [9–11].

Ideally a woman who has a pre-existing serious mental illness, who is taking maintenance treatment for this, should have access to pre-conceptual advice about the management of her psychiatric disorder and treatment, in case of an accidental or planned pregnancy. This is particularly relevant to fertility treatments with ART, where there is time for advanced planning. It is to be hoped that such individuals would contact their general practitioner before starting ART or at least on the discovery of a pregnancy rather than waiting for screening in antenatal clinic, allowing for an early psychiatric review or assessment (ideally from a psychiatrist with experience in the sub-speciality of Perinatal Psychiatry or from another mental health professional working in a specialised multi-disciplinary Perinatal Psychiatric Service) and to advise them about the use of psychotropic medication and treatment planning for the remainder of the pregnancy and the early weeks after delivery [12, 13]. For those women who are currently well and not taking medication, screening at around 12 weeks gestation allows for assessment by the beginning of the second trimester of pregnancy, so that the patient and her family know how any emerging symptoms, recurring or new in onset, can be managed robustly, in order to reduce the impact of serious mental illness on the woman and her baby, during pregnancy and afterwards.

The screening that has been developed for antenatal identification of women with a potential for becoming significantly mentally unwell in pregnancy and afterwards, is also useful when a woman or a couple attend a fertility clinic, so that plans can be made for any potential relapse of symptoms during the course of treatment with ART. There may be fertility clinics where such programmes exist and those accessing them feel comfortable enough to reveal their personal or family history of psychiatric disorder. However, I have come across a number of patients who were asked questions about their personal or family history of mental illness, but who chose not to reveal this, for the fear that they would not be able to access the fertility treatment they so desperately wished for; their mental state subsequently deteriorated in pregnancy or the weeks after giving birth, leading them to present acutely to Psychiatric Services. Having talked to a number of colleagues working as fertility specialists locally, my personal experience is that questions about a past history of mental health problems are not asked routinely. Given the potential for difficulties both during treatment with ART and any pregnancy conceived, consideration should be given to making this a formal part of the pre-treatment assessment, so that fertility specialists can work closely with colleagues in Obstetric Liaison or Perinatal Psychiatry in their area, to ensure that patients undergoing fertility treatment receive the same kind mental health care and support as those who present to antenatal clinic following natural conceptions [6, 14].

Anthropological and Socio-Cultural Considerations That May Help a Fertility Specialist Understand a Couple's or an Individual Patient's Response to the Stresses of Infertility (or Sub-fertility) and Its Treatment with ART[1]

Perhaps many people would say, or at least think, that anthropological and socio-cultural considerations are not relevant in the twenty-first century. The rapid developments in and spread of communication technologies (be they satellites which beam radio and television programmes into once remote towns and villages, or mobile phones, for which there are apparently an estimated seven billion subscriptions around the world) have led to a "globalisation" of scientific ideas and understandings once felt to belong exclusively to those raised in technologically advanced

[1] A significant portion of the material used in this particular section of the chapter was put together for an original but unpublished essay submitted for my Masters in Medical Anthropology (1997); it has been updated with new material and references where appropriate.

nations. However, it is my experience of living and working in a very multicultural city in the United Kingdom that even when individuals are educated to a level that would include some basic facts about human biology and physiology, their understanding of fertility and what will lead to conception, is influenced by things other than their formal education.

Religious teachings, which in certain communities of all the world's major religions, may be taken from texts many centuries old, may influence individuals in their beliefs about procreation. For others, there may be cultural traditions or folk-myths that underlie their understanding about such matters, and they continue to hold these ideas, passed on to them by parents, grandparents and members of the larger community, despite their education in an urban environment in their own or an adopted country. Then again, for some people, traditional beliefs and ideas may be replaced by "modern" or "scientific" explanations about their bodies and the world around them, only to re-surface at times of acute distress or active mental illness (and then these ideas may be described by those treating them, according to a strictly medical model, as "over-valued" ideas or "delusional" beliefs). I have therefore included some ethnographic material in this section, related to beliefs and practices that may now be considered outmoded and irrelevant, but which nevertheless may continue to influence the ideas of individuals with their origins in these communities and geographical locations.

As stated in the introduction above, the subject of infertility has generated a vast literature in biomedicine, and this has been fuelled by the rapid development of artificial reproductive technology (ART) since the 1970s, although artificial insemination by donor (AID) in humans was first performed successfully in 1799 and has been used consistently in Western biomedical practice since the 1920s [15]. There had been relatively little written about infertility and reproductive morbidity in general in the field of medical anthropology until the early 1990s [16]. This is in sharp contrast to the wide ranging exploration of human reproduction by anthropologists with regards to theories of conception across cultures, fertility and birthing practices and more recently, with a rising world population, the thorny issue of family planning.

In a world that is seen as overpopulated, the distress and suffering of those unable to conceive for whatever reason, is largely submerged. Inhorn argues that the gap in medical anthropological knowledge about infertility will become even more important in the light of the increasing incidence of reproductive failure worldwide [16]. One cited example of this trend is of selected populations in the AIDS endemic "infertility-belt" of Central Africa. In this region not only has there been a high mortality from AIDS, but other sexually transmitted infections (STIs) such as gonorrhoea and genital chlamydial infections cause secondary infertility thereby further threatening depopulation. In this region, one-third to one-half of couples are infertile [17, 18], compared to an average of one in six couples in the USA and Europe. Inhorn further argued that there are major gender issues surrounding reproductive morbidity: "Women worldwide appear to bear the major burden of reproductive setbacks of all kinds" [16]. This is in terms of blame for reproductive failure as well as shouldering the engendered personal grief and frustration, marital strain, social stigma and ostracism [1, 19]. This remains the case in the twenty-first century

[18]. Where ART is available, although it holds out the hope of a "cure," it can also be a great iatrogenic source of further distress, both physical and psychological.

Despite widely differing geographical and cultural milieus, women's experience of infertility is a shared one in which the normative pressures are to conceive. For those who cannot, there is fear, anxiety and isolation generated at times by a sense that the problem is so shameful that it should be kept a secret [1] from family and friends, the very people who would usually be a source of support. Women are described across cultures going to great lengths to overcome what is seen as "their" infertility. The endless search for treatment may take the form of elaborate locally practised de-polluting or fertility enhancing rituals or "high-tech," invasive ART. Globally, societies give pre-eminence to women's role as mother and it is women's bodies that are seen as the locus of the "disease" of infertility. Even when there is a male factor involved in a couple's inability to conceive, men in many cultures find this hard to acknowledge, such is the socio-cultural determination that infertility is always women's fault [18, 20]. Therefore it is women's bodies that are most often the site of surveillance and intervention. Women are most often stigmatized whether it is they who are infertile or not [16, 18, 21].

Studies across cultures show how intimately infertility is linked with other important areas of social life. Kinship, marriage, divorce, inheritance, household residence patterns, economic productivity, gender relations, notions of body, health and illness are examples of the domains involved. Exploring infertility leads to the discovery of many important fertility related beliefs. Theories about how conception occurs and how it may be prevented, intentionally or unintentionally, lead to an understanding of attitudes towards contraception and its perceived dangers. These theories may also shed light on what is believed to cause infertility and what measures are taken to rectify the situation. Infertility highlights the importance societies give to parenting and children and the perceptions of risk and risk-taking with regards to the body and its reproductive processes. In many cultures, infertility is not just a threat to the individual but also a threat to the extended family [18, 19], the community [22], and society itself.

Socio-Cultural Factors Which Interact with Biology to Modify an Individual's Natural Fertility

Natural fertility depends on a set of biological variables: monthly probability of conceiving, uterine receptivity, duration of breast-feeding in the post-partum period and the incidence of sterility. All of these factors are modified by cultural practices and social circumstances [23]. There is considerable variation between societies in the age at which women are allowed to marry or become sexually active. Societies may practice monogamy, polygyny, or polyandry. Extra-marital sex may or may not be permissible. Divorce and residence patterns and the economic climate (when and where it may be necessary for large numbers of men to live away from home for long periods, as migrant workers) will also affect a group's natural fertility.

In societies that practice polyandry the procreative ability of the husbands is limited by the fertility of their one wife. Although this is a less common arrangement than polygyny, it has the advantage of masking any male infertility factors that may exist as long as the wife herself is fertile. In polygynous arrangements, for the wives, there is the reduced probability that coitus will take place during days of the cycle when conception may occur. This may be accentuated when, as often happens with groups of women living together, their menstrual cycles become synchronous. Access to the husband can be a source of friction between co-wives, particularly if one is thought to be favoured above others. When infertility exists in these circumstances a wife may accuse a co-wife of "stealing" her chances of conceiving [24, 25]. Male infertility will be more obvious too in polygynous marriages, if successive wives fail to conceive.

Extra-marital sex may also be a factor influencing a group's natural fertility. Male infertility could be masked if a wife chose to look outside the marriage to help her conceive. The structure of some societies seems to allow for this. For instance, amongst the Nuer, a husband and his lineage received the fertility of a woman's womb in return for paying the bride-wealth. Any child which is issue of that womb is of the lineage regardless of who the genitor is. Adultery is considered illegal but not immoral. Fines of cattle imposed on the discovery of adultery are returned if a healthy child is born as a result of it. Otherwise, payment of cattle could be seen as a legitimatization fee and give the genitor a claim on the child [25]. In most societies, however, there are harsh penalties for extra-marital sex. The importance of the husband in having sole sexual access to the wife to ensure paternity is seen as paramount. The notions of honour and shame in studies of Mediterranean culture exemplify this. Women are fields to be fenced off and only ploughed by the owner [26].

Theories of Infertility: The Contribution of Ideas About Conception and Spiritual and Social Disharmony

There is little consensus across cultures and even within groups about the relative contributions of males and females to conception and fetal growth [23]. These ideas are dependent to some degree on whether a society is organized according to matrilineal or patrilineal patterns. Education plays a part but even in societies where there is universal schooling, all people do not share a similar model. In one American study, women from a low socio-economic group attending antenatal classes demonstrated a poor knowledge of aspects of bodily function such as menstruation, conception, its timing, the function of contraception and ideas about how STIs might be contracted. Ideas about how infertility might come about also vary greatly ranging from beliefs about the heating or cooling properties of food consumed by a woman, to physical damage occurring to a woman's womb if sexual intercourse takes place at the wrong time in her menstrual cycle [23].

A common theme in theories of conception is that the fetus is made up of semen and maternal blood. The Nayars of Kerala share common South Indian ethnophysiological beliefs about reproduction. These are that male and female alike produce sexual fluids. For fertilization to occur both partners must achieve orgasm so that these fluids can be ejaculated into the uterus, to mix and produce a bubble, (*kumili*) or sprout (*mulai*) that develops into an embryo. The Nayars believe the sexes contribute equally in terms of the fluids that go to make up the embryo. However, women are believed to possess more of the divine procreative force (*śakti*) as personified by Śakti, the feminine aspect of the Sanskritic god, Śiva. This *śakti* is enhanced and harnessed by heat accumulating asceticism (*tapas*), in the form of abstinence, devotion, suffering and sacrifice. Married women focus their *śakti* for their husbands' wellbeing through steadfastness and devotion. This religious belief and the fact that, historically, these groups practised polyandry (which would mask male infertility and highlight female infertility) could be reasons why infertility is still defined amongst them as a woman's failure. It is highly stigmatizing for the afflicted woman but also for her maternal kin, whose duty it is to protect her from dangerous forces that would impede her fertility, such as the wrath of gods and demons, or disharmony within the extended family.

Amongst the Aowin of south-west Ghana, social relationships are seen as a central issue in infertility. This misfortune is seen as a result of troubled relations with the spirit world and said to stem from acts of an individual that have angered the gods. Pollution (*efeya*) can be acquired by not observing traditional purificatory practices, by neglecting to give the gods appropriate offerings or by bearing animosity towards others (such as co-wives, husband or neighbours). This same pollution can prevent a woman from conceiving [22]. Yet other interferences in the procreative process are seen by African peoples as coming from outside themselves. These external agents are most often "witches" and their patrons. As in common with many other African cultures such as the Giriama of East Africa [27] and the Bangangte of Cameroon [24], the Aowin believe that reproductive morbidity of all kinds can be caused by various forms of witchcraft. Not only can a woman be made infertile by the power of witchcraft but also the envy of a barren woman can make her a witch and thus dangerous to other women's fertility.

Mediterranean [26] and Northern Indian ideas [28] use the metaphor of the active, male seed implanted in the inert, female field. This ideology may be driven by the patrilineal structure of these societies. Infertility for them can only result from the barrenness of the soil in which the seed is planted. Women unable to reproduce are seen as inauspicious. In many parts of India, they are barred from taking part in sacred ceremonies. In some parts of India, infertile women are even thought to have the effect of blighting crops and being able to adversely affect the health of other women's children (in common with the African belief about infertile women as harmful witches).

The Pursuit of Treatment

Beliefs about how infertility may occur vary across cultures, but as can be seen from the examples discussed above, there are some common themes in the form of pollution acquired through not observing socio-religious rules. The remedies employed to "cure" infertility are legion and women may take a pluralistic approach to treatment. World-wide, they are as likely to go to spiritual healers and traditional herbalists as they are to biomedical practitioners. This section of the discussion will concentrate on spiritual and traditional healing methods employed in some of the societies mentioned above. Some long-standing, more pragmatic, socially sanctioned alternatives to ART will also be examined briefly, and the discussion of ART in this context will be limited to AID, a technique that is more widely available and perhaps more affordable than IVF and other related, more technically difficult procedures available only in fertility clinics.

Amongst the Nayars of South India *pampin tullal* is a ritual performed daily over 1–3 weeks as a remedy of the curse of the serpent deities (the curse being infertility of one or more members of the group, *taravatu*). The goal of this ritual is fertility and auspicious prosperity achieved through worship of the serpent god by two *taravatu* women who act as proxy for the well-being of the group. In a successful ritual, the deity's presence is achieved when the two women go into a trance and become possessed by the god. During the trance *taravatu* members may pray to and speak to the deity and afterwards receive his blessing. The women who enact the ritual must be unattached so that they can focus their *sakti* for the benefit of the group. More mature women (who are single through being separated, divorced or widowed) are often "chosen" for possession by the deity. In this way, women who are generally disenfranchised are able to highlight grievances or disharmonies within the group that would otherwise remain unaddressed.

The Aowin spirit mediums, again most often women, similarly focus on ritually purifying an infertile woman and restoring harmony to disrupted social relations by acting as informal adjudicators. The woman who has acquired *efeya* will be sent to the forest for a period of time. She will be asked to make offerings to the gods. Her dangerous "red" or "hot" state of pollution is further treated by painting her with white clay or allowing her to only eat "white," "cooling" foods and bathing ritually in the river. If a woman is felt to be infertile as a result of witchcraft, then the medium undertakes to appease the witch. If an Aowin woman goes to a traditional herbalist, he will also give offerings to the spirits, but his emphasis is more on the woman as an individual and he is less likely to look to her social relations for an explanation of her infertility.

Pragmatic solutions to the problem of infertility have long been sanctioned by many societies. In many parts of Africa fostering by close relatives who are childless is common practice. The fostered child will know who his genetic parents are but will carry the name of his foster parents. Legal adoption is less common in many African and Asian settings. Surrogacy is another solution to infertility that has been used throughout history. There is the biblical example of Abraham and his wife Sarah who have a child by Sarah's handmaid (Genesis, Chapter 16, verses 1–4). In some societies, an infertile woman will select a co-wife from amongst her maternal kin or natal village, thus sharing something of the child born to the co-wife. Amongst the Nuer, women unable to have children of their own are allowed to trade in order to collect a bride-wealth and marry another woman. The woman who is the "husband" then chooses men from her kin or neighbours to father children by the woman who is the "wife." Children born of these unions are known by the name of the "woman-husband" and they call her "father" [25].

Surrogacy becomes more of a prickly subject when male infertility is involved. In Africa, as in many other parts of the world, the use of AID in many men's minds is tantamount to their womenfolk committing adultery. For the women, the anonymity of the sperm donor is a major obstacle to the use of AID. They fear they may unwittingly commit incestuous adultery (incest in the African context being broader) and thereby endanger the outcome of the pregnancy. A traditional African alternative to AID is natural insemination by donor. A husband may give unspoken consent for his wife to seek another man from the community to father a child. In some cases, the infertile spouse may choose the donor from amongst his close relatives or friends. The identity of the real genitor is then known to and accepted by the putative genitor and those who share the family secret [20].

The use of natural surrogacy for male infertility problems is also referred to in Indian literature sources. *Niyoga* is the ancient Hindu practice of lawful cohabitation of a childless wife with her husband's brother or a Brahmin of "good character." In the Hindu epic "Mahabharata," the sage Vyasa sires a son by each of his dead brother's wives at the request of his mother [29]. Later in the same source, Pandu, who has been cursed to die if he lies with any of his wives, suggests to them that they have children by the "grace of a Brahmin." These Indian legends have left behind folk myths that in turn have been incorporated into modem literature and film art about India and Pakistan [30–32].

ART is either unavailable or the cost of it is such that it is inaccessible to the majority of infertile couples across the world [18]. Even where it is an option, it is often viewed with suspicion. This is particularly so when there is a need for gamete donation. For many people, men who donate sperm have been seen as somehow deviant and possibly self serving and therefore to be discouraged. On the other hand women who donate eggs, a procedure that has only become possible relatively recently, are felt to be behaving altruistically [33]. It is not surprising therefore that where male infertility is a factor, AID as a form of treatment is often unacceptable. Even in countries where there is a long history of using AID, there can be difficulties. A follow up study in New Zealand that looked at couples up to 10 years after a child had been born revealed there was little consensus between partners as to what they would tell a child about its origins [34]. A study carried out prior to the amendments to the Human Fertilization and Embryology Act (HFEA) in the United Kingdom in 2008 [35] showed that both gamete donors and recipients had significant anxieties about the proposed changes to the Act, which would mean that offspring would be able to access information about their genetic parents, once they reached the age of 18 years.

The descriptions above are not merely a collection of exotica. I have treated White British and European women who have echoed the fears of their African or South Asian peers, as they talked of the envy of female relatives or friends who have fertility problems and how this envy may in some way blight a pregnancy achieved with great difficulty. I have also treated women who have failed to conceive despite repeated interventions with ART, who sadly described the change they observed in female relatives and friends who on conceiving themselves, avoided revealing this news until it was no longer possible to keep it a secret, not out of consideration for the childless woman, but out of some atavistic fear that somehow her lack would become theirs.

In this overview of infertility and attitudes towards it across cultures, I have attempted to demonstrate how stigmatizing and distressing it can be for the individuals affected, especially women, whose identity and position in society is more often impacted on. I have given some diverse examples of the remedies pursued in the treatment of infertility, including some traditional approaches that may still be used as pragmatic alternatives to ART in non-Western cultures as ART may, for some, pose as many difficulties as it solves. Although in the past, couples using biomedical techniques involving donation of gametes would not have been able to give their offspring details about the donor, changes in the HFEA regulations in the United Kingdom [36] will make this information available to a child in future. The first cohort of children who will be able to access this information will reach the age of 18 years in 2023 and it remains to be seen if having information about gamete donors reduces the psychological burden of secrecy on infertile couples who used treatments involving AID or egg donation.

Many societies still value success in an individual's reproductive role above all else. Social attitudes shift at variable rates but what people think of and how they behave towards individuals who are unable to have children of their own is something that must surely change. Perhaps of almost equal importance is the way in which many individuals affected by infertility, especially women, see their personal and social identity as flawed and so devalue themselves, even when they have many other laudable qualities and accomplishments.

Although ART is much more widely available, material cost remains a big issue, especially in low and middle income countries [18]. There will be many who access fertility treatment but for whom it is unsuccessful. If the prevalence of infertility continues to increase worldwide then many ethical and moral issues about what constitutes treatment and how it should be provided may need to be examined. Certainly, more thought will need to be given to psychological interventions before and after ART, whether it is successful or not, as there is a body of evidence now indicating that even when women do not have a pre-existing problem with mental illness, the psychological burden of infertility, the physiological impact of fertility treatment, being pregnant and closely scrutinized, operative interventions in childbirth and expectations around parenting can increase women's vulnerability to acute perinatal mental health problems and severe mental illness [3, 6, 37–39]. It is important to remember that even when a woman does not have a personal history of serious mental illness prior to conception and childbirth, in a small minority, the genetic vulnerability imparted by a family history of serious mental illness, especially mood related psychoses, may result in the first onset of such an illness in late pregnancy or early post-partum [11].

Clinical Scenarios

The following clinical scenarios are based on the experiences of actual patients; personal details have been disguised, to ensure confidentiality, even where permission has been granted to use the clinical material discussed. The purpose of these scenarios is to demonstrate some of the problems facing both patients and fertility specialists when planning ART and during the subsequent pregnancy and peri- and post-partum periods.

Scenario 1: A Woman with a Pre-existing Severe Mood Disorder Who Relapses During Treatment for Sub-fertility and Shows Signs of Recurrence of a Depressive Psychosis

AB is a 39 years-old, professional White British woman established in a stable marriage. She developed a severe depressive illness, with psychotic symptoms, following the birth of her first child, a planned and natural conception. Following her acute presentation to the local Perinatal Psychiatry Service, late in the first post-partum year, she required in-patient treatment on a Psychiatric Mother and Baby Unit (MBU). During the course of the admission, it became apparent that she had suffered from depressive symptoms since the early weeks after giving birth, but had attributed her lack of energy and enjoyment to the demands of breast-feeding and caring for her infant with little in the way of practical support during the day, as her husband worked long hours and they had no family support locally. AB maintained breast-feeding until her return to work at 5 months post-partum and the collateral history provided by her husband indicated that her mood had deteriorated quite markedly after this. However, AB did not seek help for herself at this time, and it was only when her husband noted she had cognitive and motor slowing at 9 months post-partum that she came to the attention of her doctor. Another close relative revealed that AB's father had suffered from severe Bipolar Affective Disorder; AB later revealed that she had become aware of this fact at age 20 and duly informed her community midwife of it at antenatal screening at 12 weeks into her pregnancy. However, as she did not have a personal history of mental illness, the risk related to her family history, 3:100, was judged to be very low.

AB required treatment with a combination of a tricyclic antidepressant in high dose, augmented with an antipsychotic preparation and electro-convulsive therapy (ECT). AB made a full recovery over the next 3 months and complied with follow-up and maintenance treatment with an antidepressant for 2 years after her discharge from hospital. Having been in no particular hurry to plan her first pregnancy ("…I thought I had plenty of time and would get round to it at some point…."), AB said she wanted a sibling for her existing child in the near future. She nevertheless recognised the severity of her illness and the importance of maintaining her recovery before attempting to conceive again. When AB's child was aged 3 years, she sought pre-conceptual advice from the Perinatal Psychiatrist who had treated her previously, with regards conceiving a second pregnancy. Following a discussion of her options for treatment, she decided she would prefer to conceive medication free and recommence a tricyclic antidepressant, if she needed it, once she progressed beyond the first trimester.

Unfortunately, by the time AB halved her usual treatment dose of antidepressant, she developed early signs of recurrence of depressive symptoms. She took her psychiatrist's advice and once more increased the dose of antidepressant to a therapeutic level. AB continued to attempt conception over the course of the next 1 year, whilst using the antidepressant and maintaining out-patient contact with Perinatal Psychiatry. As she failed to conceive during this time, she sought treatment from the local fertility clinic. During the course of preparation for IVF, despite continuing with psychotropic medication, she suffered a brief psychotic illness which required admission to a general adult psychiatric ward. Following her discharge home, AB and her husband decided they could not risk further treatment with ART in case the stress involved, and the drugs/hormones used precipitated another episode of severe illness. They decided to explore the possibility of adopting a child instead, but, although AB has remained well in terms of her mental state for several years now – she has continued on maintenance treatment with an antidepressant – and she is coping well at home and at work, revealing her history of depressive psychosis to the Adoption Agency has made her ineligible to adopt. AB is gradually coming to terms with the fact that she will only raise one child.

Learning Points from Scenario 1

AB is an example of an individual who had no personal history of psychiatric problems prior to giving birth for the first time, but whose family history of severe mood disorder in a first degree relative made her vulnerable to developing a post-partum psychosis. It is possible that the reassurance AB was given in early pregnancy, about the relatively small risk to her of developing a post-partum mood disorder similar to her father's, contributed to her dismissing the symptoms of a biological syndrome of depression in the early weeks and months after delivery as "tiredness" related to caring for a new baby.

AB's symptoms became worse around the time she returned to work, which coincided with her weaning baby off the breast at 5 months post-partum, indicating a sensitivity to changing hormone levels, which is demonstrated again when having treatment with ART, even whilst continuing maintenance treatment with psychotropic medication. AB should therefore be made aware that she may be as sensitive to the changing levels in her hormones approaching the menopause as she was post-partum and whilst receiving treatment with ART, so that she can seek medical advice sooner rather than later, if she experiences further mood-related symptoms.

Several years later, AB has been able to withdraw from her antipsychotic medication; she has successfully made adjustments to a different kind of life than the one she imagined, and has been well enough for long enough to consider whether she can gradually withdraw from her maintenance antidepressant medication. Her good pre-morbid psychological adjustment and a supportive husband and family have helped her in this. For those women who are not so fortunate, psychological interventions, in the form of individual or couple therapy may be necessary.

Scenario 2: A Woman with Pre-existing Severe Mood Disorder Who, with Pre-conceptual Advice and Robust Management of Her Mental Illness During Fertility Treatment, Conceives with IVF and Remains Well During Pregnancy and Postpartum

BC is a 41 years-old woman of South-east Asian extract who suffered her first episode of depressive psychosis aged 31 years, after she came to the United Kingdom to carry out her post-doctoral research. She has since had two further admissions to a psychiatric ward, with psychotic symptoms. Each of her subsequent illnesses has appeared to have a manic flavour and she has therefore been given a diagnosis of Bipolar Affective Disorder. She has used Risperidone, a second generation antipsychotic (SGA) for several years now, and it works well for her, in terms of stabilising her mood and keeping her psychotic symptoms at bay. However, when using the Risperidone at a higher dose, BC has experienced amenorrhoea, secondary to hyperprolactinaemia, a well recognised side effect of this and some other antipsychotic drugs.

BC and her husband first came for pre-conceptual advice when she was aged 38 years. BC stated her preference for attempting to conceive without medication but she also accepted that as she had experienced manic symptoms within the last year, without maintenance treatment, she was at increased risk of relapsing into psychosis. As BC was concerned about ongoing problems with hyperprolactinaemia, it was agreed that she should cautiously reduce her Risperidone to a lower maintenance dose, aiming for 1 mg daily, whilst undergoing fertility treatment. A few months later, BC returned for review. She remained free of psychotic symptoms, but her anxiety was heightened in the context of recent news that her husband had a pituitary tumour, which was impacting on the couple's plans to proceed to IVF using husband's sperm. BC accepted that significant life events and the stress generated by these had previously contributed to her developing mood related symptoms and so it was agreed that she should remain on a moderate dose of Risperidone, as long as she did not become amenorrhoeic again.

Two years later, BC and her husband returned for further discussions about her treatment plan as her husband had been successfully treated for his tumour. Again it was agreed that BC should remain on the lowest dose of Risperidone that kept her well, without impacting on her menstrual cycle, through conception and pregnancy (this information was communicated by letter to the fertility specialist treating BC). Soon afterwards, BC and her husband conceived with the first cycle of IVF. BC engaged well with the Perinatal Psychiatric Service during her pregnancy, which was physically healthy. BC was offered a planned admission to the Psychiatric

MBU in the last two weeks of pregnancy, in order to modify the dose of her medication under supervision, in preparation for delivery. BC preferred to make changes to her treatment at home, with the support of her husband and parents, and the Perinatal Community Psychiatric Nurse (PCPN), who had come to know her well in the preceding months. The nursing team on the Psychiatric MBU was alerted to BC's impending delivery, in case she required telephone advice or out of hours admission. BC had already made a decision that she would not breastfeed, as disruption of her sleep tended to trigger a relapse of her symptoms (her husband and parents planned to support her by carrying out the night-time feeds). A treatment plan was outlined accordingly and shared with all those working with BC (her PCPN, Community Midwife, Obstetrician, Health Visitor and GP).

BC subsequently had an uneventful delivery and a healthy infant. BC's mental state was regularly reviewed at home by her PCPN in the early weeks after delivery, during which time she re-established treatment with her usual dose of Risperidone. Review in outpatient clinic, at 3 months postpartum, showed BC to be well on a moderate maintenance dose of Risperidone. She was therefore advised to continue with this (whilst using a robust contraceptive method), and plans were made for her to be reviewed as an out-patient at regular intervals, with her GP and Health Visitor monitoring her care in-between these appointments.

Learning Points from Scenario 2

BC and her husband accepted that she was at high risk of relapsing into psychosis without maintenance treatment with an antipsychotic preparation. BC was willing to use such medication, as long as the side-effects of this did not impact on her fertility or cause any problems for the child/children she might conceive. Following a discussion of the potential risks and benefits of using psychotropic medication through conception and pregnancy, and gaining BC's consent to continue treatment, adjustments to the dose of her antipsychotic medication allowed BC and her husband to realise their full reproductive potential through ART. Good communication between all the health professionals working with BC and her husband insured that there were plans in place, in case she developed active symptoms of her serious and enduring mental illness.

Scenario 3: A Woman Conceives Through Egg Donation with Husband's Sperm and Subsequently Develops Symptoms Thought to Be Related to the Stress and Anxiety Generated by Repeated Attempts to Conceive

CD is a 37 years-old woman, of South Indian extract, born and raised in the United Kingdom. Although her parents are practising Hindus, and she has some spiritual beliefs, CD has never thought of herself as an orthodox Hindu, or religion an issue in the day to day life she has built with her husband of 7 years, whom she met through work. CD's husband is of North Indian extract and although his family still adhere to traditional Muslim ways of living, he has always thought of himself as a man of liberal ideas and marrying a woman from a different language and faith community, for love, was not a difficult choice to make. CD and her husband were disappointed by their families' response to their marriage, but they hoped that with the arrival of grandchildren, each set of parents would mellow. Sadly, they have been unable to conceive naturally and several cycles of IVF in the NHS, using their own gametes, have failed.

CD has not confided her difficulties to anyone; she rarely sees her parents or siblings and she does not feel able to talk to her friends about her childlessness, as many of them now have young families. When it is suggested that perhaps the next cycle of IVF should be with donor eggs, CD allows her husband to organise a trip to India, in the hope that the money they have raised from downsizing their home, will cover enough cycles of treatment to ensure a pregnancy. CD manages to conceive, with donor eggs and her husband's sperm, and once it is clear that her twin pregnancy is viable, she returns home. CD engages with antenatal care in her home town in the United Kingdom; home and work life is made rather difficult by pregnancy related nausea through to late in the second trimester. Early in the third trimester of pregnancy, just as she feels things may be improving, CD develops tachycardia and breathlessness which are both thought to be driven by her anxiety about the successful outcome of her much longed for pregnancy. CD struggles through the last few weeks of her pregnancy, as she is physically tired and struggles to get about on feet that seem to be perpetually swollen.

CD is relieved to deliver healthy twin girls at 38 weeks gestation, and hopes that her physical health will improve following their birth. CD remains physically tired, despite getting some sleep over the next few nights and a few days after delivery, suffers another prolonged run of tachycardia, accompanied by breathlessness and nausea. Her complaints are initially dismissed as anxiety, related to the practical care of her twins, but when she suffers a physical collapse, it is recognised that she has serious physical problems related to a cardiomyopathy. CD requires care on ICU for the next 2 weeks, but she is eventually re-united with her daughters and goes home, where it is hoped that she will continue to recover with the help and support of her husband and her parents (who have swallowed their anger, in the face of their daughter's severe illness).

Over the course of the next 2 months, CD, who is normally very robust in terms of her psychological health, presents several times to her GP, with complaints of tachycardia and dizziness. She has one brief re-admission to the Medical Assessment Unit but nothing positive is found, in the way of ongoing cardiac pathology, and she is discharged home with a diagnosis of anxiety. The GP requests an assessment from the Perinatal Psychiatric Service, as he feels that CD now has post-natal depression. He feels that antidepressant medication is indicated but CD is not at all keen to use anything that may give her side-effects.

Following assessment in the Perinatal Psychiatric out-patient clinic, it becomes clear that CD does now have symptoms and signs in keeping with mixed anxiety and depression, as well as some features of post-traumatic stress, related to vivid memories of the physical symptoms she had immediately before her collapse (CD said "…. I thought I was going to die"). CD prefers not to use medication as she is aware that some psychotropic drugs can impact on cardiac rhythm and function. As she is willing to engage actively in psychological interventions, the treating Perinatal Psychiatrist is willing to defer the use of an antidepressant. CD is assessed for group psychotherapy, using Compassionate Focused Therapy (CFT) techniques suitable for use in the postpartum period.

CD uses the psycho-educational material and the group process well. It soon becomes apparent to the group leaders that CD's marriage has been strained beyond repair during the course of several years' fertility treatment and a very difficult pregnancy and postpartum period. From CD's description of her husband's behaviour towards her since the twins' birth, it is clear that there is some emotional abuse in the relationship (CD said her husband insists that she has no genetic relationship to the twins, and therefore as their biological father he is the only one who can make decisions about how they will be raised). With the help of other mothers in the group, CD is gradually able to recognise that that although the twins came into being through the kindness of an egg donor and her husband's sperm, they belong equally to her, as it is she who has built every cell in their bodies, nurturing them with her blood via the umbilical cords that attached them to her in-utero. CD is once more able to draw on her family's cultural heritage, especially the notion of *śakti*, the female creative energy in the universe, to tackle her difficult life circumstances. In the months after discharge from the psychotherapy group, CD attempts to work with her husband in couple therapy. When it transpires that CD's husband has asked his female relatives to look for another wife for him, this time from his own community, CD makes the decision to return to her parents with her daughters, with the aim of eventually living independently and making amicable arrangements for sharing custody of her daughters with their father and his new wife.

Learning Points from Scenario 3

CD's story should serve to remind health professionals of all disciplines and backgrounds that although individuals dealing with the stress of infertility, and treatment for this with ART, are struggling with many complex internal, family and social dynamics, this does not preclude them from becoming seriously physically ill. Therefore, persistent complaints of physical ill-health should be taken seriously and if, in the aftermath of a life-threatening illness in the antenatal or post-natal period, a woman does become anxious or depressed, appropriate care and follow-up should be sought for her. The NICE guidelines for antenatal and postnatal mental health (CGs 45 and 192) encourage the provision of psychological interventions for those women who prefer not to use psychotropic medication to tackle their symptoms. As can be seen from the scenario described above, it would have been difficult to treat the complex relationship and social difficulties that grew out of a pregnancy resulting from ART with antidepressant treatment alone; if psychotropic medication had been indicated alongside the psychological interventions used, the potential for adverse effects on cardiac function, certainly during the early stages of recovery from the acute cardiac problem should be kept in mind.

Scenario 4: A Woman Undergoes Fetal Reduction for Triplet Pregnancy and Subsequently Develops a Severe Postpartum Depressive Illness After the Birth of Twins

DE is a 32 years-old professional woman from Ghana, who has come to live in the United Kingdom with her husband of 5 years (DE's husband has a post-graduate scholarship from the Ghanaian government, and is working as a researcher and visiting lecturer at the local university). The couple are devout Christians and hoped for the gift of many children but they were hugely saddened by the fact that DE suffered consecutive miscarriages of three planned pregnancies and subsequently failed to conceive naturally, even though they attempted to do so for over 2 years. DE and her husband recognised that they would not have the same kind of access to fertility treatment in rural Ghana, where DE's husband's work will be based in future and so they sought fertility treatment in the United Kingdom, before DE's husband's contract with the university came to an end. Preliminary investigations had revealed that DE has a large uterine fibroid, and so when she conceived after the first cycle of IVF, and the two embryos implanted were found to have become three, the couple was advised to think about fetal reduction in order to give the pregnancy the best chance of going to term. DE and her husband read around the subject, and after consulting with their fertility specialist, made the painful decision to reduce the number of fetuses to two.

DE managed to get through to 34 weeks gestation, at which time, following signs of early labour, she had an emergency Caesarean section to deliver her twin sons. After an anxious period of 3 weeks, whilst the twins were cared for on the Neonatal Unit, during which it was difficult for DE to maintain breast-feeding as she had hoped to do, the couple took the twins home. In the weeks that followed, DE formed a good attachment with her sons, but as her husband was unable to take much time off from work, she cared for them largely on her own. By the time the twins were 3 months old, DE became aware that her sleep and appetite had deteriorated; she had little energy to do anything other than care for the babies, and even though their arrival had been long-awaited and they were much loved, she felt only guilt when she looked at them. DE was constantly reminded of the third child that would have existed if she and her husband had not made the decision to go ahead with the fetal reduction. Matters were made worse when DE began to have ruminative thoughts that if members of her family or church community knew what she had done, they would be appalled by her actions.

DE began to avoid going to church or inviting people to her home, which increased her social isolation. DE's husband struggled in his own right, but he sought refuge in work. DE's Health Visitor noted the deterioration in her mood and referred her to the GP, who commenced an antidepressant but there was little improvement in DE's mood, even after several weeks of treatment with a therapeutic dose of this. The GP therefore referred DE for further assessment to the Perinatal Psychiatric Service. It was clear to the PCPN who first saw DE that the antidepressant prescribed was not working; DE was clearly suffering from a severe depressive episode, set against a background of loss and grief, not just for the third child DE had carried in the early part of her last pregnancy, but also of the loss of the three pregnancies prior to this.

DE was seen by the Perinatal Psychiatrist for review of her mental state and treatment. An alternative antidepressant was prescribed, and titrated up to a slightly higher than usual treatment dose. DE was offered an admission to the Psychiatric MBU, as there were concerns that with her husband's increasing emotional distance, in the face of his own low mood, and in the absence of support from any other close family members, DE was at risk of deteriorating further whilst waiting for her treatment to take effect. DE preferred to continue with treatment as an outpatient; over the course of the next 9 months, she engaged actively with her PCPN and Perinatal Psychiatrist to work through her grief and guilt, whilst also taking an antidepressant. DE's husband was eventually persuaded to seek help for himself from the couple's GP. At the time of DE's discharge from the Perinatal Psychiatric Service, DE and her husband were beginning to rebuild their relationship with each other and members of the church community who stood in for the family that lived so far away.

Learning Points from Scenario 4

The above case scenario demonstrates how decisions that are much debated and made with the best of intentions can afterwards cause distress and guilt. Also how prolonged periods of stress and anxiety can contribute to pre-existing losses and perpetuate grief that undermines even the strongest of individuals and relationships. DE and her husband would probably have eventually worked through their loss and grief without help from others, but the process would likely have been much longer, and the time taken could potentially have irrevocably damaged the marital relationship, as well as the relationship with their long-awaited children, impacting on their well-being and development. With the combination of supportive psychotherapy and antidepressants, DE recovered enough within 18 months to continue working on her relationship with her husband in another arena: she agreed to reveal the difficulties they had experienced, both in relation to her last pregnancy and afterwards, to their pastor, who is skilled at working with couples and who did not judge them as they had feared. Some 4 years later, the couple are again living relatively contentedly and enjoying their growing sons.

Scenario 5: A Woman in a Same-Sex Relationship with a History of Mental Health Problems Who Struggles with Severe Anxiety in a Pregnancy Conceived with AID

EF is a 29 years-old French woman who has been established in a same-sex relationship with an English woman for 4 years. Following discussion with her partner, it was agreed that she would seek fertility treatment in order to conceive a child for the couple. EF had some pre-existing problems with body image and bulimic eating patterns; she had also engaged in self-harm and substance misuse in the distant past, but as these problems were controlled, she chose not to reveal this history when seen for assessment at the fertility clinic. EF became pregnant after the first round of treatment with AID. The first trimester of her pregnancy was made difficult by hyper emesis and she had to take time off work. The second trimester of her pregnancy was complicated by physical ill-health, related to gallbladder disease, and so she remained on sick leave. The problems with EF's physical health resulted in a decision to induce labour at 37 weeks gestation; EF required a forceps delivery, from which it took her several weeks to recover. EF continued to have bouts of abdominal pain related to inflammation of the gallbladder. As conservative management had not helped the situation, she subsequently had a cholecystectomy and made a good physical recovery.

Despite the improvement in her physical health, EF remained anxious and avoidant around the baby that she had so much wanted. Her partner had to take time off work to care for both EF and the baby. EF began to have intrusive thoughts of harming the child and herself, which she found frightening. This prompted her to seek help from her GP, who prescribed the SSRI antidepressant, Sertraline.

Within 2 weeks of commencing the full dose of Sertraline, EF developed quite marked psychomotor agitation and the intrusive thoughts of harm to her baby and to herself increased in frequency and intensity. EF again visited her GP, who referred her for further assessment and treatment to the Perinatal Psychiatric Service. At assessment, baseline blood investigations revealed abnormal liver function tests and although EF had recently had problems with her liver function, secondary to gallbladder disease, as Sertraline is also known to affect liver function in certain individuals, EF's antidepressant treatment was changed. EF was followed up in the community by a PCPN, who worked with her on managing her distress and anxiety, particularly in relation to the feelings she had about not being safe around her child. During the course of this work, it became apparent that the difficult pregnancy and delivery had re-triggered distressing memories of EF's own childhood; EF also reluctantly acknowledged that although she had actively sought AID to achieve a pregnancy, she felt that she had in some way been "violated" by the clinical procedure of insemination. After working with her PCPN and Perinatal Psychiatrist, for a few months, EF agreed that some of her psychological difficulties predated her pregnancy by many years, and that it might therefore be helpful for her to be referred on to colleagues in the Psychotherapy Department, for a more in-depth assessment for medium to long term psychotherapy.

Learning Points from Scenario 5

The scenario above describes a young woman with long-standing psychological difficulties. Although EF has not been open about it, there is some suggestion of traumas in childhood and adolescence, which may explain some of the unhelpful/maladaptive coping strategies (bulimic eating patterns, substance misuse and self-harm behaviour) used by her to cope with difficult experiences and situations in late adolescence and early adult hood. EF did not reveal this information at assessment for fertility treatment; had she done so, there would have been an opportunity to discuss potential difficulties in her ability to cope with various aspects of the fertility treatment, her pregnancy and postpartum adaptation to parenting. In particular, if there were specific traumatic experiences, in might have been possible to work on the psychological difficulties associated with these, to mitigate the impact of obstetric procedures that might retrigger frightening or unpleasant memories. Although EF describes low mood and there is evidence of moderately severe depressive symptoms, these appear to be secondary to long-standing anxieties and post-traumatic stress, against a background of emotional instability and difficulties in interpersonal relationships; further acquaintance with such individuals may reveal significant problems in personality functioning, which may contribute to significant adjustment to parenting in the longer term.

Scenario 6: A Single, Heterosexual Woman Who Chooses Not to Reveal Her Long-Standing Problems with Severe Anxiety When Embarking on an IVF Pregnancy Because of the Concern That She May Be Refused ART

FG is a 34 years-old single, heterosexual, Black British woman who presents to the Perinatal Psychiatric Service 6 months after the birth of her first child, with symptoms of severe anxiety and obsessive-compulsive behaviour. During the course of the assessment, FG revealed that her son was conceived following AID; FG said she chose this method to conceive as she had experienced many problems over the years in relationships with the opposite sex and therefore did not feel that she could wait to have a child until she found the right man to start a family with. FG said she had not informed anybody other than her parents that her son had been conceived through fertility treatment. As the months had passed, FG said her anxiety had increased and she had begun to ruminate about how "disgusted" people would be, if they ever found out that she, as a single woman, had used AID to conceive.

More recently, FG said she had begun to have frequent "horrible" thoughts that she might be a danger to her child. She had found herself engaging in hand-washing and cleaning routines that were becoming unmanageable, as they took many hours each day. It took several sessions in clinic for FG to overcome her anxiety and reveal that her distressing ruminative thoughts related to a fear that she might behave in a sexually inappropriate manner towards her child. FG said that the troubling thoughts had started after she had heard news reports of enquiries into decades old child abuse cases. Further exploration revealed that FG had long-standing problems with anxiety and obsessive-compulsive behaviour, and that over the years, she had become preoccupied by number of different worries which she managed by developing a obsessive-compulsive hand washing and cleaning routines.

FG had been treated by her GP for many years, with Paroxetine (an antidepressant from the SSRI group); she had withdrawn from this medication with great difficulty in preparation for treatment with ART, as she had read that certain antidepressants used by women through conception could increase the risk of cardiac malformations in their babies. FG said she had not asked for help when her symptoms of anxiety recurred as she feared that she would be refused fertility treatment. Postpartum, it took FG many months to go to her GP, as she feared that if she talked about her distressing thoughts, health professionals would refer her to Children's Social Services and her child would be removed from her care. It was difficult for FG to accept that people did not think of her with disgust or to share the content of her intrusive, ego-dystonic thoughts with others, even her parents. She was initially reluctant to recommence medication but recognised that this had helped to some degree for many years. She agreed to consider further assessment for psychological interventions, so that she could attempt to learn more positive ways of managing her anxiety, ruminative thinking patterns and obsessive-compulsive washing and cleaning rituals.

Learning Points from Scenario 6

FG has long-standing issues with severe anxiety and obsessive-compulsive behaviour, set against a background rather anxious and avoidant personality. She also appeared to have had significant issues in relationships with the opposite sex, although the reasons for this remained unclear at the time of treatment. Had her history of psychological difficulties been elicited prior to commencing treatment with ART, she could have been prepared for some of the difficulties that ensued later on, particularly her beliefs about how others might react to the path she had chosen to parenthood. The great burden of secrecy that she had imposed on herself made it difficult for her to confide in close friends and family; had she been able to work out prior to the birth of her child how she would tackle the situation, she might not have become so very distressed and unwell.

Scenario 7: Cultural and Ethical Issues Arising in the Case of a South Asian Muslim Woman, Married to a Man with Poorly Controlled Schizophrenia, Who Sought Fertility Treatment in Her Home Country Because She Had Not Been Successful in Accessing It in the United Kingdom

GH is a 26 years old Muslim woman, born and raised in Pakistan, who has lived in the United Kingdom since aged 18 years, when she arrived here as a young bride, following an arranged marriage to a first cousin who is 10 years her senior. GH presents to the Perinatal Psychiatric Service clinic at 28 weeks into her first pregnancy, following an urgent referral from her community midwife. It was difficult to get a clear idea of what was going on at first, but following an assessment carried out in her first language, it transpired that GH had become increasingly anxious over the previous few months, about the well-being of the child she was carrying. She had told her midwife, and continued to assert, that some envious person had arranged for a spell to be cast on her; she said she knew this because she had felt something bite her on one of her for arms and move under the skin, along her limb and into her womb. She pointed at the distortions in her abdomen, made by fetal movements, and said "…look, I think it's a snake." GH expressed fears that someone was trying to jeopardise the outcome of her pregnancy, because they were jealous of her good fortune. GH did not think she had any kind of mental illness and she was unwilling to stay in hospital. A Mental Health Act (MHA) assessment was carried out and GH was admitted to the Psychiatric MBU, detained under Section 2 MHA, for further observation and any immediately necessary treatment.

During the course of the admission, it came to light that GH's husband had long-standing problems with serious mental illness; he had been given a diagnosis of Schizophrenia, but his compliance with medication and follow-up was poor. GH's married life had been a difficult one, as her husband's behaviour was rather erratic and much of the time he was not interested in her as a wife. GH's mother-in-law, who was also her paternal aunt, had arranged for the family GP to refer GH to the local fertility clinic, as GH's husband was found to have azospermia. However, following a meeting of the ethics committee attached to the fertility clinic, the couple was not considered suitable for treatment, because of GH's husband's history of poorly controlled mental illness. Following this disappointment, GH's mother-in-law had arranged for her to take a trip to Pakistan, to seek a further opinion and potentially treatment. GH returned from Pakistan, already 16 weeks into her pregnancy, and although the family said that she had been treated by fertility specialists in Pakistan, GH herself remained preoccupied with the possibility that a distant male relative of her husband, on his father's side, had something to do with her pregnancy and that women in this man's family had discovered this, and arranged for a spell to be cast on her.

GH was felt to be suffering from a severe depression, with psychotic features. She was treated accordingly, with a combination of antidepressant and antipsychotic medication, compatible with pregnancy. Her delivery was managed, with the help of obstetric colleagues, to allow adjustment of medication through labour. She returned to the Psychiatric MBU once fit for discharge from the post-natal ward, to continue with treatment of her depressive psychosis. She recovered fully by the time her baby was 8 weeks old and was discharged home on a combination of antidepressant and antipsychotic medication, which she was advised to continue until the end of the postpartum year. Children's Social Services, who were asked to become involved with the family during GH's admission, remained so, in order to assess the ongoing risks to GH and her child, as her husband, who had also been treated more robustly for his psychotic illness whilst GH was an in-patient, remained in the family home, albeit with some improvements in his mental state.

Learning Points from Scenario 7

The local fertility clinic had felt that GH's husband's poorly controlled psychosis would put any child born to the couple at risk of harm. The issue of how GH had conceived her child was never fully elucidated, but it is possible that the family paid for private fertility treatment abroad, without revealing the full picture, with regards to GH's husband's history of serious mental illness.

GH herself had not experienced any symptoms of mental illness prior to her pregnancy, but clearly she had a family history of serious mental illness, as she had at least one first cousin (her husband) with Schizophrenia.

GH had clearly been very anxious all through the first and second trimester of her pregnancy; whether because she was worried about the manner of the conception or the outcome of the longed for pregnancy, or both, remained a moot point. The high levels of stress GH experienced in pregnancy, interacting with her genetic potential for serious mental illness, contributed to a severe depressive illness which remained untreated for many months.

Some of GH's ideas were culturally congruent, even if rather over-valued at this juncture in her life (e.g. the effects of the envious "evil eye" or *nazar* and the use of harmful magic spells, on her pregnancy) but some were frankly psychotic (e.g., the belief that shapes appearing in her abdominal wall, as a result of fetal movements, were actually the movements of a snake, which had entered her body through her arm many months previously). GH therefore required robust treatment of her mood related psychosis in pregnancy, to ensure that she would be as well as could be managed by the time she delivered her child. Treatment was continued postpartum, under supervision on the Psychiatric MBU, to ensure that GH was well enough to engage with and care safely for baby, before discharge home, with further follow-up in the community from the Perinatal Psychiatric Service. Children's Social Services carried out some aspects of their child-safeguarding assessment prior to GH's discharge home, but the core assessment of the family as a whole, for the purpose of planning support for both parents and the "child in need," would take place over a longer period.

Conclusion

The very nature of ART, which results in rapid fluctuations in female reproductive hormone levels, combined with the high levels of stress and anxiety experienced by many individuals after years of infertility, poses a real challenge to the mental health of women undergoing treatment. If there is a pre-existing significant mental illness or there is a family history of such, the burden of treatment for infertility, especially the marked physiological changes that occur, which have an impact on both psychological and physical well-being, can overwhelm some women. It therefore behoves the fertility specialist to pay particular attention to making enquiries about a personal and or family history of serious psychiatric disorder, and any treatments used for this, in both the woman and her partner, so that robust planning for psychological and psychiatric interventions can be put in place before the couple or individual woman embark on ART.

During pregnancy, vulnerable women will require support and forward planning for delivery and after the birth. Therefore, to ensure women remain well, communication at the time of hand-over of care between the fertility and obstetric teams is of paramount importance. Sensitivity, not only to the physical and psychological needs of the individual, but also to the cultural beliefs that may underlie some of their problems, will help clinical teams in caring for all women, and their husbands or partners, effectively.

References

1. Whiteford L, Gonzalez L. Stigma: the hidden burden of infertility. Soc Sci Med. 1995;40(1):27–36.
2. Cousineau TM, Domar AD. Psychological impact of infertility. Best Pract Res Clin Obstet Gynaecol. 2007;21(2):293–308.
3. Hammarberg K, Fisher J, Wynter K. Psychological and social aspects of pregnancy, childbirth and early parenting after assisted conception: a systematic review. Hum Reprod Update. 2008;14(5):395–414.
4. Van den Broeck U, et al. Predictors of psychological distress in patients starting IVF treatment: infertility-specific versus general psychological characteristics'. Hum Reprod. 2010;25(6):1471–80.
5. Boivin J, Griffiths E, Venetis CA. Emotional distress in infertile women and failure of assisted reproductive technologies: meta-analysis of prospective psychosocial studies. BMJ. 2011;342:d223.
6. Burns LH. Psychiatric aspects of infertility and infertility treatments'. Psychiatr Clin North Am. 2007;30:689–716.
7. NICE. Antenatal and postnatal mental health; clinical management and service guidance CG45. London: Department of Health; 2007.
8. NICE. Antenatal and postnatal mental health: clinical management and service guidance CG 192. London: Department of Health; 2014.
9. Doyle JH, et al. The management of bipolar disorder in the perinatal period and risk factors for postpartum relapse. Eur Psychiatry. 2012;27(8):563–9.
10. Di Florio A, et al. Perinatal episodes across the mood disorder spectrum'. JAMA Psychiatry. 2013;70(2):168–75.
11. Di Florio A, et al. Mood disorders and parity – a clue to the aetiology of the postpartum trigger. J Affect Disord. 2014;152–154(100):334–9.
12. Chisolm M, Payne J. Management of psychotropic drugs during pregnancy. BMJ. 2016;352:h5918.
13. Vigod SN, Wilson CA, Howard LM. Depression in pregnancy. BMJ. 2016;352(8050):492–5.
14. Sheard C, et al. Impact of a multiple, IVF birth on post-partum mental health: a composite analysis'. Hum Reprod. 2007;22(7):2058–65.
15. Lessor R. All in the family: social processes in ovarian egg donation between sisters. Sociol Health Illn. 1993;15(3):393–413.
16. Inhorn M. Interpreting infertility: medical anthropological perspectives'. Soc Sci Med. 1994;39(4):459–61.
17. World Health Organization. Infections, pregnancies, and infertility: perspectives on prevention. Fertil Steril. 1987;47:964–8.

18. Cui W. Mother or nothing: the agony of infertility. Bull World Health Organ. 2010;88(12): 877–953.
19. Neff D. The social construction of infertility: the case of the matrilineal Nayars in South India'. Soc Sci Med. 1994;39(4):475–85.
20. Savage O. Artificial donor insemination in Yaounde: some socio-cultural considerations'. Soc Sci Med. 1992;35(7):907–13.
21. Martin E. The woman in the body: a cultural analysis of reproduction. Milton Keynes: Beacon; 1987.
22. Ebin V. Interpretations of infertility: the Aowin People of South-west Ghana. In: MacCormack C, editor. Ethnography of fertility and birth. London: Academic; 1982. p. 141–59.
23. MacCormack C. Biological, cultural and social adaptation in human fertility and birth: a synthesis. In: MacCormack C, editor. Ethnography of fertility and birth. London: Academic; 1982. p. 1–23.
24. Feldman-Savelsberg P. Plundered kitchens and empty wombs: fear of infertility in the in Cameroonian grassfields. Soc Sci Med. 1994;39(4):463–74.
25. Evans-Pritchard E. Kinship and marriage among the Nuer. Oxford: Clarendon; 1990.
26. Delaney C. Seeds of honour, fields of shame. In: Gilmore D, editor. Honour and Shame and the unity of the Mediterranean. Washington, DC: American Anthropology Association; 1987.
27. Parkin D. Alternative authorities: incest and fertility. In: The sacred void. Cambridge: Cambridge University Press; 1991.
28. Manu. The laws of Manu (trans: G. Buhler). Oxford: Clarendon Press; 1886.
29. Anon. Mahabharata. (trans: C. V. Narasimhan). Columbia: Columbia University Press; 1965.
30. Tully M. The barren woman of Balramgaon. In: The heart of India. London: Penguin Books Limited (Viking); 1995. p. 1–21.
31. Moggach D. Hot water man. 1999th ed. London: Arrow Books Limited; 1982.
32. Immaculate conception. Film. Directed by Jamil Dehlavi. UK: Dehlavi Films; 1992.
33. Haines E. Issues of gender in gamete donation'. Soc Sci Med. 1993;36(1):85–93.
34. Daniels KR, Lewis GM, Gillett W. Telling donor insemination offspring about their conception: the nature of couples' decision-making. Soc Sci Med. 1995;40(9):1213–20.
35. Frith L, Blyth E, Farrand A. UK gamete donors' reflections on the removal of anonymity: implications for recruitment. Hum Reprod. 2007;22(6):1675–80.
36. Department of Health; United Kingdom. Human Fertilization and Embryology Act. 2008.
37. Reis S, Xavier MR, Coelho R, Montenegro N. Psychological impact of single and multiple courses of assisted reproductive treatments in couples: a comparative study. Eur J Obstet Gynecol Reprod Biol. 2013;171(1):61–6.
38. Smorti M, Smorti A. Medical success and couples' psychological problems in assisted reproduction treatment: a narrative based medicine approach'. J Mater Fetal Neonatal Med. 2013;26(2):169–72.
39. Listijono DR, Mooney S, Chapman M. A comparative analysis of postpartum maternal mental health in women following spontaneous or ART conception'. Psychosom Obstet Gynaecol. 2014;35(2):51–4.

Bibliography

Lawson AK, et al. Prospective study of depression and anxiety in female fertility preservation and infertility patients'. Fertil Steril. 2014;102(5):1377–84.

Morreale M, Balon R, Tancer M, Diamond M. The impact of stress and psychosocial interventions on assisted reproductive technology outcome. J Sex Marital Ther. 2011;37:56–69.

Van den Broeck U, et al. Reasons for dropout in infertility treatment. Gynecol Obstet Invest. 2009;68:58–64.

Chapter 4
Preconceptual Diagnosis

Deivanayagam Maruthini, Colleen Lynch, and Maha Ragunath

Introduction

Assisted reproductive technology (ART) has advanced tremendously in the last 10 years making preconceptual diagnosis possible with more precision than ever before. Preconceptual diagnosis includes two main categories of embryo screening prior to implantation, namely, preimplantation genetic diagnosis (PGD) and preimplantation genetic screening (PGS).

Preimplantation genetic diagnosis (PGD) is defined as "testing for deleterious, heritable genetic conditions which are known to be present in the family of those seeking treatment and from which the embryos are known to be at risk." Since its first introduction in humans in 1990 for X linked monogenic disorders such as adenoleukodystrophy and X-linked mental retardation, PGD has advanced tremendously [1, 2]. In addition to extending the scope of PGD to detection of chromosomal rearrangements [3, 4], achieving a HLA matched sibling through PGD to save an affected child was another breakthrough in ART [5, 6].

Preimplantation genetic screening means "testing for chromosomal abnormalities where there is perceived to be a higher than average risk of conceiving abnormal embryos." The age related decline in natural and IVF birth rates is linked to increased aneuploidy rates, which contribute to failed implantation, miscarriage and increased

D. Maruthini, MBBS, DGO, MS (OG), MRCOG, MD (✉)
M. Ragunath, MB BS, DGO, MSc, FRCOG
Department of Medicine and Gynaecology, CARE Fertility, Nottingham, UK
e-mail: maruthini@yahoo.co.uk; Maha.ragunath@carefertility.com

C. Lynch, BSc, MSc
Department of Embryology, Genesis Genetics Europe, CARE Fertility, Nottingham, UK

School of Biosciences, University of Kent, Canterbury, UK
e-mail: colleenalynch@hotmail.com

K. Jayaprakasan, L. Kean (eds.), *Clinical Management of Pregnancies following ART*, DOI 10.1007/978-3-319-42858-1_4

rates of Downs, Edwards and Patau syndromes. Theoretically, the identification and selection of chromosomally abnormal embryos should mitigate the effect of age on IVF and increase implantation and reduce miscarriage rates in patients of advanced maternal age. Thus, PGS was generally indicated in patients with advanced maternal age, recurrent miscarriage and recurrent implantation failure and was reported to improve success rates [7, 8]. Initially, there were concerns that PGS using fluorescent *in situ* hybridization (FISH) technique reduced the overall pregnancy rates [9]. However, studies on PGS using comparative genomic hybridization (CGH) have subsequently shown a significant improvement in detection of aneuploidy in embryos [10].

The objectives of this chapter are to enable the clinicians to identify patients with positive genetic history and organise multi-specialty management using PGD. The aim is also to provide the readers an up-to-date knowledge on PGS of embryos for chromosomal aneuploidy. The scope for achieving healthy live births has been greatly improved by using recent advances in molecular and bioinformatics technology for PGD and PGS.

Preimplantation Genetic Diagnosis

Parents at risk of an inheritable condition have several reproductive options such as avoiding a pregnancy altogether, getting pregnant with or without prenatal testing for the genetic mutation, using donor gametes and adoption. Preimplantation diagnosis is another revolutionary option, especially for those who do not wish to undergo prenatal testing or termination of an affected pregnancy.

PGD has found its place in those with monogenic disorders, chromosomal rearrangements, medically indicated gender selection – where a genetic condition only affects one gender, or affects one gender more severely, and in those requiring a Human Leucocyte Antigen (HLA) – matched sibling to save a sick child. Prior to undertaking PGD, patients should have undertaken detailed genetic counselling explaining the probabilities of inheriting the condition, effects of the condition on the offspring and various options to achieve an unaffected child.

When the mutation causing a genetic condition is located on the X chromosome, a male with the X chromosome with the mutation is affected by the condition, while a female with this X chromosome is considered a carrier. However, it is important to note that female carriers of X linked recessive conditions can sometimes show mild symptoms, or in rare case, be affected by the condition. In the case where an X linked condition is considered dominant, males and females with the X chromosome with the mutation will be considered affected. Therefore, in couples undergoing PGD for X linked conditions, the geneticist must discuss the implications of using carrier embryos in treatment as the carriers may themselves be affected by the condition to a varying degree.

In Vitro Fertilisation for PGD

Couples at risk of transmitting a genetic mutation have the option of choosing IVF with PGD to create embryos for genetic analysis. Prior to accepting patients for PGD, affected women in particular, must be assessed for their disease prognosis, fitness to carry a pregnancy, effect of pregnancy on their condition and *vice versa*. Their fitness to undergo sedation for egg recovery must also be determined by the anaesthetist with the help of the medical experts monitoring the patient. For example, Becker muscular dystrophy may affect the cardiac muscles in 5 % of carriers requiring cardiac screening every 5 years. In certain forms of muscular dystrophies, women may already have difficulties in swallowing and breathing. Additionally, the degree of symptoms may not be predictive of the risk of respiratory distress after sedation. Therefore, caution is needed in monitoring such women during and after egg recovery.

Men suffering from cystic fibrosis wanting PGD often present with azoospermia due to congenital absence of vas deferens as do some male carriers. Assessment of their ability to go through surgical sperm retrieval, especially in terms of their respiratory function is vital, before deciding the form and route of anaesthesia necessary.

Men with adult polycystic kidneys (APKD) frequently show severe oligo-astheno-teratozoospermia and also a high degree of necrospermia (dead sperm) in their semen sample [11, 12]. Ejaculatory duct cysts have also been reported to cause an obstruction to the sperm passage in some men with APKD. In these men, surgical sperm retrieval from the testicles may form the sole source of live sperm for PGD treatment [11].

It is equally important that these patients undergo an assessment of the welfare of unborn child prior to treatment. If there are concerns, these are best discussed at multidisciplinary clinical meetings prior to offering treatment. A suitable IVF protocol is chosen based on the woman's ovarian reserve and her individual risk of hyperstimulation. Controlled ovarian stimulation is achieved using urinary or recombinant gonadotropins. Following adequate follicular development, egg collection is usually performed under sedation, transvaginally under ultrasound guidance. Each mature metaphase II egg is injected with a single sperm, using the ICSI procedure, as standard IVF insemination is liable to cause sperm contamination from the several sperm that may remain attached to the egg post fertilisation.

The popular source of DNA for genetic testing is either from cleavage stage or blastocyst embryos [13]. For cleavage stage biopsy, a single blastomere is removed from a day-3 embryo. Sometimes two cells need removing, but it is not advisable in terms of embryo viability. Conventionally, the practice involves processing the results within 48 h to enable the transfer of a single blastocyst embryo on day 5. More recently, there has been a shift towards trophectoderm biopsy on day 5, followed by freezing of the embryos and transfer in a subsequent frozen embryo replacement cycle [14, 15]. On achieving a pregnancy, prenatal diagnosis is strongly recommended given the small risk of misdiagnosis (less than 3 %) associated with

PGD [16]. Most of the PGD centres have the policy of transferring a single embryo not only to reduce the risk of multiple pregnancy with its attendant obstetric risks, but also that the prenatal diagnosis will prove to be more difficult in such a situation [17].

PGD for Single Gene Mutations

More than 200 diseases with single gene mutations can now be diagnosed through PGD. They can be autosomal dominant in which the risk of inheritance is 1 in 2, e.g., Huntington's, Neurofibromatosis and some types of breast cancer. Autosomal recessive conditions carry a 1 in 4 risk of inheritance as in cystic fibrosis, sickle cell anaemia, thalassemia. X linked conditions carry a risk of inheritance of 25 % in carriers and 50 % in X linked dominant conditions. Haemophilia is an example of a condition considered as X linked recessive, while Incontinentia Pigmenti is considered dominant. However, as mentioned previously, there is a grey area with many X linked recessive conditions showing incomplete penetrance and a range of clinical symptoms in female carriers, possibly due to patterns of X inactivation.

When first introduced in 1990, sexing of the embryo was the only available method of PGD and allowed gender selection for conditions such as X linked Duchene muscular dystrophy and X linked mental retardation [2]. For this, embryo biopsy was carried out on day 3 and the analysis was performed by amplification of a Y chromosome-specific repeat sequence detected via gel electrophoresis. In the absence of amplification, the embryo was inferred to be female. The testing was made possible by the development of polymerase chain reaction (PCR), allowing exponential amplification of specific DNA targets. The short amount of time required for the analysis protocol meant that embryos could be transferred on the same day, as biopsy blastocyst culture would not be robust or routine for a number of years. Later, the technique was improved by amplification of both X and Y linked sequences and then by the use of FISH, allowing for the visualisation of both sex chromosomes, XX or XY, and reducing the possibility of misdiagnosis. See Fig. 4.1.

In 1992, the molecular techniques that first allowed the gender determination of embryos were extended to look at specific disease causing genetic mutations. While the majority of groups continued to focus on blastomere biopsy, some undertook a combination of polar body and blastomere analysis – a position that was as much to do with legal implications as science. Cystic fibrosis was the first monogenic condition for which PGD was undertaken on human embryos to detect a specific disease causing mutation [18]. Much research had taken place on mouse embryos prior to this. The deltaF508 mutation is the highest frequency CFTR mutation and is a 3 base pair deletion. Thus a nested PCR of the region and gel electrophoresis allowed the detection of DNA homo- and heteroduplexes and the identification of affected, unaffected and carrier embryos. However, this technique was vulnerable to failed amplification of a specific allele, as the first gender selection cases had been. The introduction of multiplexing protocols allowed multiple linked markers to be used

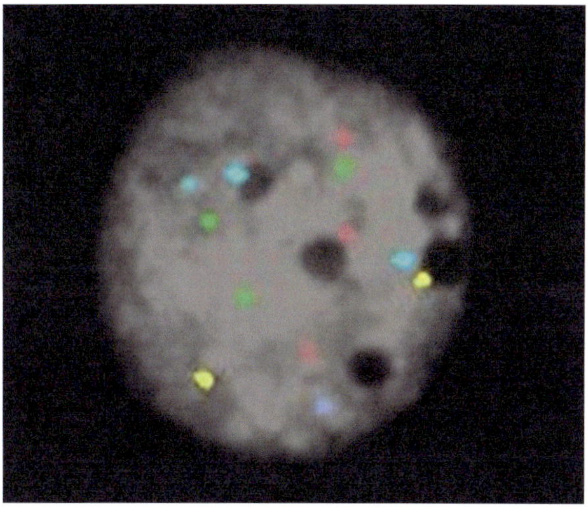

Fig. 4.1 Fluorescence in situ hybridization of the nucleus from a single blastomere for chromosomes 13 (*green*), 16 (*aqua*), 18 (*blue*), 21 (*red*) and 22 (*yellow*), displaying trisomy 13 and trisomy 21 (Image courtesy of Professor Darren K Griffin, PhD, DSc, FIBiol, FRCPath, FRSA, School of Biosciences, University of Kent, UK)

to follow disease inheritance. Subsequently, robust and accurate methods of whole genome amplification negated the need for multiplexing and greatly increased the number of linked markers that could be run and the reliability of testing [19, 20]. This also allowed more than one genetic condition to be tested for, or more commonly, to test for both disease and HLA type in embryos. These technologies were employed with little change to the diagnosis of monogenic disorders for many years. However, the advent of single nucleotide polymorphism (SNP) arrays promises to be the biggest paradigm shift in the field since its introduction and will ultimately allow parallel PGD and PGS in tandem via parallel test [21].

PGD for "De Novo" Mutations

PGD for "de novo" genetic mutations is a challenge, as the person affected and liable to transfer the genetic changes to the child, maybe the only person in the family affected by the mutation. This makes it difficult to test for the abnormality, as the genetic test will normally need other affected or carrier individuals in the family to establish inheritance and increase the robustness of the test used. Hence, PGD for 'de novo' mutations is available only in some IVF centres, and several different strategies such as, polymorphic marker evaluation, whole and single sperm testing to establish the normal and mutant haplotypes and PGD by polar body and/or embryo analysis, have been used by PGD providers [22]. Yet another successful strategy is to use the embryos created in an IVF cycle as another generation, allowing the genetic test to follow the mutation [23]. However, this may imply that more embryos have to be tested over more than one IVF cycle, before the diagnosis can be made.

PGD for Sex Selection

According to ESHRE consortium data collection from 2010, PGD for social sex selection was reported in 48 out of 5780 cycles [24]. Some parents undertake PGD to "balance" their family or to satisfy their gender preference [25], a practice that is deemed illegal in Europe, China and Australia. In the UK sex selection may only be performed where one gender is at risk of a genetic condition.

PGD for Chromosomal Rearrangement

Parents carrying a balanced translocation, whether it is reciprocal, Robertsonian or inversion, generally have no clinical symptoms, but carry a higher risk of recurrent miscarriages, recurrent implantation failure with IVF having children born with disability and sometimes infertility [26]. See Fig. 4.2.

Preimplantation genetic diagnosis for chromosomal rearrangements was first applied in the mid 1990s, using FISH probes specific to the chromosomal breakpoints that enabled the detection of unbalanced segregation patterns [3, 8]. However, FISH was unable to identify other aneuploidies leading to poor PGD outcome. This compromised the faith in using FISH for PGD in chromosomal rearrangements. Whilst there was a reasonable argument for natural conception being more successful in the same time frame as multiple PGD cycles [27], it failed to consider the impact of recurrent miscarriages.

The advent of array comparative genomic hybridisation (CGH) or single nucleotide polymorphism array (SNP) not only allowed the identification of unbalanced segregants but also allowed the identification of aneuploidy [4]. This has significantly contributed to higher pregnancy rates with lowered miscarriage rates. Whilst array based testing is expensive and relatively prohibits its wider usage, the latest technology called Next Generation Sequencing (NGS) is proving cost effective and accurate [28].

PGD for HLA Tissue Typing

The short arm of chromosome 6 holds a cluster of genes that encode the major histocompatibility complex (MHC) comprising the HLA family of genes. HLA genes encode cell surface proteins that play a crucial role in the immune response.

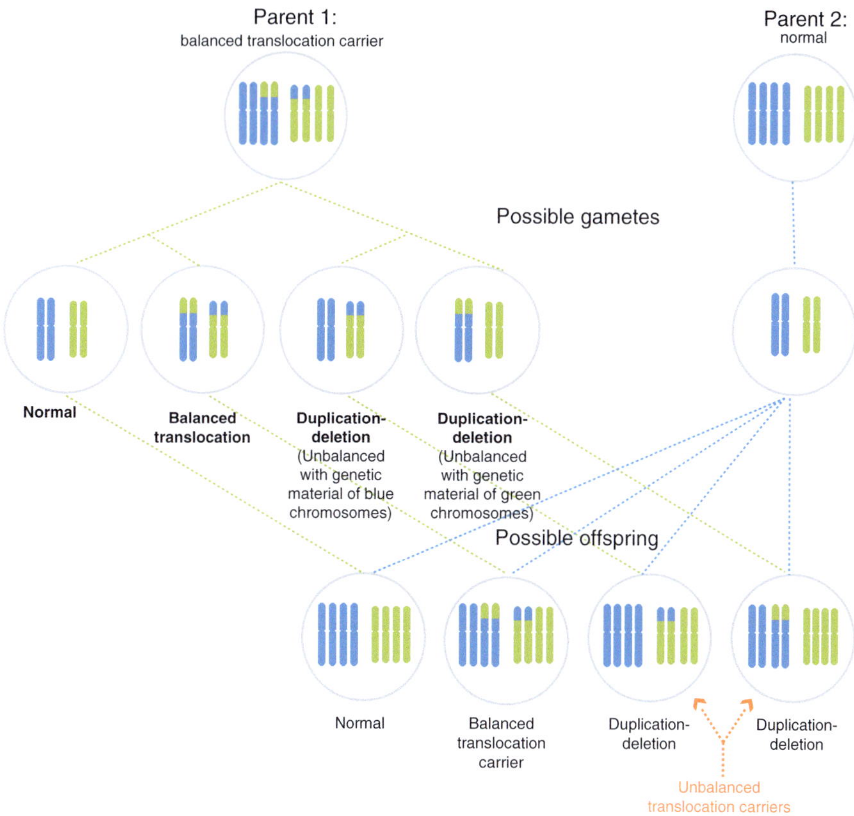

Fig. 4.2 Diagrammatic representation of the possible inheritance patterns of a chromosomal rearrangement from a parent with a balanced translocation (Image courtesy of Illumina, Inc.)

Pre-implantation genetic diagnosis for HLA tissue typing enables the conception of a child who is HLA compatible with a disease-affected existing child. The baby's cord blood is then used for stem cell transplantation or bone marrow transplant. The term "saviour sibling" is frequently used for such PGD treatment. HLA typing is often performed in conjunction with testing for a recessive monogenic disorder [29, 30]. Conditions such as β-thalassemia and Fanconi's anaemia have been treated with HLA tissue typing [6] with a 3 in 16 chance of finding an unaffected and HLA matched embryo for transfer via PGD [30].

Preimplantation Genetic Screening

Chromosome anomalies are the major cause of unsuccessful IVF or pregnancy loss after IVF. The age related decline in natural and IVF birth rates is linked to increased aneuploidy rates, which contribute to, failed implantation, miscarriage and increased rates of Downs, Edwards and Patau syndromes. Whilst the rate of aneuploidy in women under the age of 36 years is around 55 %, this increases to around 90 % in women aged 43 years. Theoretically, then, the identification and negative selection of chromosomally abnormal embryos should mitigate the age effect in IVF and increase implantation and reduce miscarriage rates in patients of advanced maternal age [31]. Thus, PGS in patients with advanced maternal age, recurrent miscarriage and recurrent implantation failure was reported to improve success rates [32].

The introduction of FISH to single cell PGD was expanded to chromosome screening – PGS – in 1993. However, there were a number of issues with this strategy. Firstly, FISH could only test a limited number of chromosomes – generally between 5 and 8. The chromosomes tested were those associated with miscarriage and live birth, meaning many abnormalities, which would result in failed implantation, were undetected. Secondly, there were a number of technical artefacts affecting the reliability of the testing – loss of micronuclei during cell fixing, split signals, and overlapping signals. Thirdly, the incidence and impact of mosaicism was not fully understood. Published RCTs, 10 years after its clinical introduction showed no advantage from PGS, and even reduced success rates [33]. This was controversial at the time and hotly contended by initial pioneers of the treatment who continued to evidence improved success rates [34]. However, the controversy did lead to many changes in practice, most notably the introduction of comprehensive chromosome screening (CCS). Despite more recent RCTs and systematic reviews supporting the use of PGS when CCS is employed [35], the majority of the scientific community seem to remain sceptical, and, professional bodies including American Society of Reproductive Medicine the European Society of Human Reproduction and Embryology, and British Fertility Society have not changed their guidance to reflect this.

For some reason, human reproduction, among mammalian species, is characterised by a high rate of chromosomally abnormal gametes and embryos produced. Around 10–15 % of clinically recognised pregnancies end in first trimester miscarriage, which does not include occult or missed abortions. Transient implantation may occur with minimal disruption to the menstrual cycle and an individual might never realise it has occurred. More than half of these events, 60–80 %, are a result of aneuploidy in the embryo. Additionally, an even higher rate of aneuploidy exists at the embryo stage than detected in pregnancy given many chromosomally abnormal embryos will simply fail to implant. Thus, the rationale behind PGS remains sound and the advent of CCS has led to evidence that PGS is suitable to be employed as a method of embryo selection in good prognosis patients [35].

Potential Risks of PGD and PGS

There are general risks of IVF treatment namely, suboptimal or excessive ovarian response resulting in either low egg numbers or ovarian hyperstimulation syndrome, respectively. If there are fewer eggs, there is a lower chance of finding suitable embryos from a genetic and developmental perspective. Fertilisation and embryo development during IVF may be poorer than expected thereby limiting the number of blastocysts available on day 5 or 6 for biopsy and freezing.

In terms of risks that are specific for PGD, the risk of accidental damage to the embryo is quoted as less than 0.6 %. When an embryo does not yield a result, this is usually due to the embryo having been of poorer quality when biopsied or not having developed correctly. Embryos with a clear genetic result are deemed suitable for transfer. Couples should understand that there may not be a genetically or developmentally suitable embryo for transfer after IVF/PGD.

The misdiagnosis rate of PGD testing for a genetic disease is less than 3 % [36]. Several intrinsic, extrinsic and human factors have been reported to cause misdiagnosis. These include unprotected sex during treatment, mislabelled tube, misidentified embryo/slide/tube, misinterpreted report, transfer of wrong embryo, chromosomal mosaicism, parental/operator contamination, and allele drop-outs. Allele drop-outs may cause erroneous results owing to the failure of all genetic material to be amplified during PCR.

The error rate after PGS using CCS has been reported as low [37]. Adhering to robust quality control measures can reduce the misdiagnosis arising from the IVF and genetics laboratories. Additionally, it is vital that the couples are advised to use an effective form of contraception during treatment to avoid a natural conception. Couples are also strongly advised to undergo prenatal testing by chorionic villus sampling or amniocentesis on achieving a pregnancy though clinical experience shows few do proceed to invasive testing. Non-invasive prenatal testing is often preferred by couples in these circumstances as providing reassurance that the fetus is not affected by the common trisomies.

Uniparental disomy (UPD) is a condition in which both chromosome pairs in an embryo are derived from the same parent. Such an inheritance may disrupt the imprinting mechanism in the embryo thereby leading to the development of imprinting disorders such as Prader-Willi and Angelman syndrome [38]. The occurrence of UPD in human blastocysts is random and rare [39]. Couples undertaking PGD for chromosomal rearrangements should be counselled that UPD cannot be routinely diagnosed via PGD.

The Future of PGD and PGS: Karyomapping and Next Generation Sequencing

PGS has seen vast and regular changes in the technologies employed – from the advent of PGS via FISH, looking at a single data point on a limited number of chromosomes, to quantitative PCR looking at two to four data points per chromosome, array-based comparative hybridisation looking at hundreds of points per chromosome and NGS, looking at tens of thousands of data points per chromosomes. A large amount of sequence data can be generated using high-throughput NGS tools such as Illumina MiSeq DNA sequencing platform. Diagnosis of chromosomal

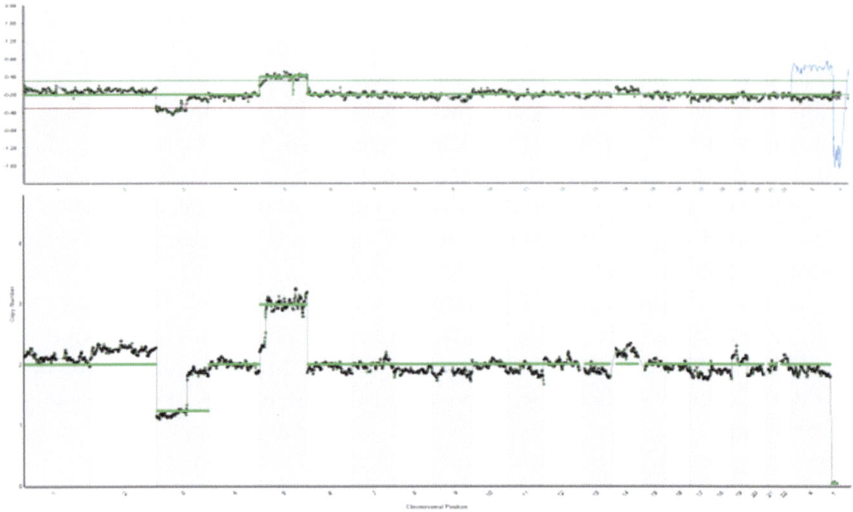

Fig. 4.3 Results of chromosomal aneuploidy screening in an embryo by Next Generation Sequencing (NGS) – *bottom image*, compared to array Comparative Genomic Hybridization (aCGH) – *top image*. Values on the Y axis represent chromosome copy number, the image shown displaying a deletion on chromosome 3 and trisomy 5. The changes are more apparent in NGS as it is a quantitative method based on copy number counting, whereas aCGH qualitatively looks at relative fluorescence of sample and reference (Image courtesy of Genesis Genetics Europe)

rearrangements using NGS has been shown to improve the accuracy of detection of chromosomal abnormalities [28]. Additionally, reports have shown that both single gene disorder and chromosomal testing can be performed simultaneously on the same sequencing platform without the need for the pre-test workup of single gene disorders [40]. See Fig. 4.3.

Karyomapping is another new technology that has revolutionized PGD for monogenic disorders. Karyomapping, which uses SNP genetic haplotyping, works by identifying the differences in genetic markers between the couples. The aim is to differentiate the four parental copies of the gene an embryo may inherit and identify which are associated with the genetic mutation/disease. This is known as genetic linkage. However, the genetic information is "shuffled" as it is inherited. See Fig. 4.4.

Karyomapping examines the chromosomes at approximately 300,000 different points and finds a DNA fingerprint unique to the chromosome that carries the affected gene. It is then possible to test the fingerprint in the embryos produced by the parents, revealing those that have inherited the affected gene. If the fingerprint characteristic of the chromosome carrying the affected gene is not detected, then it can be inferred that the embryo has inherited normal copies of the gene and is therefore likely to be free of the disorder. The test will tell which copies of a gene, an embryo has inherited from each parent, rather than identifying genetic mistakes or mutations. As a bonus by-product, karyomapping also identifies any anomalies present in other chromosomes. Karyomapping will also identify some chromosome anomalies where, rather than seeing a maternal and paternal SNP at each point on a

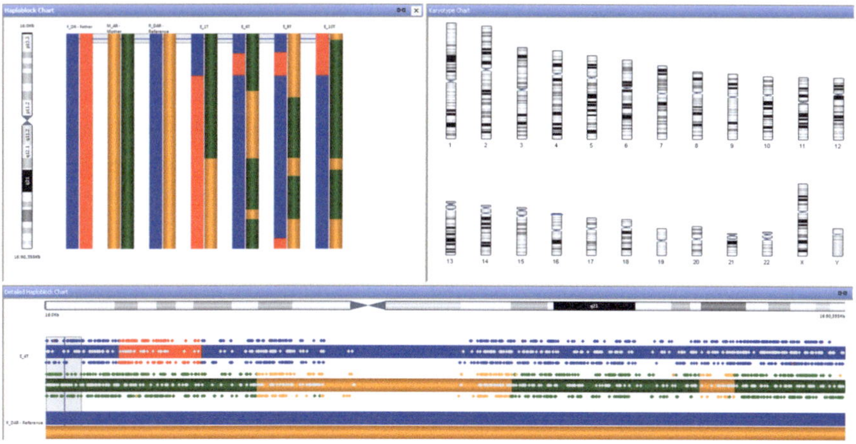

Fig. 4.4 Using a reference of known genetic status, Karyomapping assigns maternal and paternal haplotypes – M1(*yellow*)/M2(*green*) and P1(*blue*)/P2(*red*). The figure represents a family with a father and child affected by a dominant genetic condition on chromosome 16p. Thus P1 can be identified as the affected allele and embryos 1, 4, and 8 diagnosed as affected and embryo 10 diagnosed as unaffected. The detailed haploblock chart show the whole of chromosome 16 for embryo 4 T. Along the top of the chromosome are the informative (key) SNPs and along the bottom are the non informative (non key) SNPS (Image courtesy of Genesis Genetics Europe)

chromosome, or region of chromosome, only one, or three, SNPs are detected, indicating a monosomy or trisomy respectively.

Details of gene mutation analysis of the affected parent or parents are required to determine if PGD could be offered for the specific genetic condition. Genetic samples are required from the affected family members and the partner for the initial work-up for the test. While the initial work up takes up to 16 weeks for conventional PGD by short tandem repeat (STR) analysis, it takes 2–4 weeks for karyomapping.

Outcome of Children Born Following PGD/PGS

The European Society of Human Reproduction and Embryology Preimplantation Genetic Diagnosis (ESHRE-PGD) Consortium, established in 1997, attempts to track PGD treatment on an international scale. According to its most recent report, there were a total of 6160 preimplantation genetic testing cycles from December 2009 to October 2010, of which 3551 (58 %) were for screening and 2609 (42 %) for diagnosis [24]. This is a substantial increase from the previous report for the 10 years between January 1997 and December 2007.

Reassuringly, a pilot study on neuropsychological outcome at the age of 4–5 years in children born following PGD has shown normal development [41]. Similarly, cognitive and motor developments have also been reported to be normal in 5–6 years old children born though PGD [42]. The data capture is an ongoing process with ESHRE and other national/international organisations.

PGD for Mitochondrial DNA Diseases

Unlike the nuclear DNA which is inherited from both parents, mitochondrial DNA (mtDNA) is inherited from the oocyte [43]. Mitochondrial DNA is present in multiple copies within the cell and each copy carries 37 genes that are responsible for energy production by cells. Mutations in mtDNA, when occurs over a threshold, will lead to metabolic diseases that can be life threatening. Cleavage stage biopsy of embryos followed by PGD has been shown to reliably predict the mutation load and disease. However, some women may not produce eggs and embryos with a high mutation load. Currently, new reproductive technologies such as meiotic nuclear transplantation are being researched under strict regulations.

Regulations of PGD

Preimplantation genetic diagnosis is a prescribed treatment option to those with a genetic condition sufficiently serious to lead to the development of lethal abnormalities or handicap in the offspring. In the UK, both, the condition and the centre offering PGD should be licensed for the purpose.

Currently, the HFEA has licensed over 200 monogenic conditions for PGD. The full list of genetic conditions is available on HFEA website. When an IVF clinic wishes to offer PGD for a condition not yet licensed, they must submit an application to the HFEA providing details of the condition. The HFEA must ensure legal criteria are met when considering new conditions, mainly that there is a significant risk of a serious medical condition in any children. They take into account:

- Penetrance and variability
- Age of onset
- Symptoms

Their decision is based on the most severe presentation on the condition and IVF centres are then required to satisfy themselves that their patients fit the legal requirements for treatment.

In 2000, the HFEA added PGD for HLA to the expanding indications of PGD. Licensing for HLA matching is done on a named patient basis and requires the support of a clinician treating the child requiring bone marrow or stem cell transplant, for example a paediatric haematologist or oncologist. The HFEA will additionally take into account:

- The degree of suffering associated with the existing child's condition
- The speed of degeneration in progressive disorders
- The extent of any intellectual impairment
- The prognosis of the existing child, considering all treatment options available
- The availability of alternative sources of tissue for treating the existing child, now and in the future
- The availability of effective therapy for the existing child, now and in the future

Gender selection may be licensed for conditions only affecting one gender, or affecting one gender more severely. This is normally only required where the genetic basis is not fully understood, as in many cases of X-linked mental retardation (XLMR). Social sex selection, or family balancing, is not allowed in the UK. The HFEA is also cautious with respect to sperm sorting to create, or maximise the chance of creating, embryos of specific gender, and specifically prohibit the use of sperm sorted via gradient methods in PGD due to concerns as to its reliability.

Conclusions

Preimplantation genetic diagnosis and screening are entering a new era due to the recent advances in DNA sequencing technology. Whole genome sequencing opens up a huge potential to extensively screen the embryos for genetic diseases. However, unless strict legal regulations and ethical definitions are applied, PGD and PGS may be overused injudiciously including for those variants of unknown significance.

Author Declaration The authors declare no conflict of interest.

References

1. Harper JC, Sengupta SB. Preimplantation genetic diagnosis: state of the art 2011. Hum Genet. 2012;131(2):175–86.
2. Handyside AH, Kontogianni EH, Hardy K, Winston RM. Pregnancies from biopsied human preimplantation embryos sexed by Y-specific DNA amplification. Nature. 1990;344(6268): 768–70.
3. Munne S, Scott R, Sable D, Cohen J. First pregnancies after preconception diagnosis of translocations of maternal origin. Fertil Steril. 1998;69(4):675–81.
4. Fiorentino F, Caiazzo F, Napolitano S, Spizzichino L, Bono S, Sessa M, et al. Introducing array comparative genomic hybridization into routine prenatal diagnosis practice: a prospective study on over 1000 consecutive clinical cases. Prenat Diagn. 2011;31(13):1270–82.
5. Alby N. The child conceived to give life. Bone Marrow Transplant. 1992;9 Suppl 1:95–6.
6. Fernandez RM, Pecina A, Lozano-Arana MD, Sanchez B, Guardiola J, Garcia-Lozano JC, et al. Experience of preimplantation genetic diagnosis with HLA matching at the University Hospital Virgen del Rocio in Spain: technical and clinical overview. Biomed Res Int. 2014;2014:560160.
7. Simon C, Rubio C, Vidal F, Gimenez C, Moreno C, Parrilla JJ, et al. Increased chromosome abnormalities in human preimplantation embryos after in-vitro fertilization in patients with recurrent miscarriage. Reprod Fertil Dev. 1998;10(1):87–92.
8. Munne S, Marquez C, Reing A, Garrisi J, Alikani M. Chromosome abnormalities in embryos obtained after conventional in vitro fertilization and intracytoplasmic sperm injection. Fertil Steril. 1998;69(5):904–8.
9. Checa MA, Alonso-Coello P, Sola I, Robles A, Carreras R, Balasch J. IVF/ICSI with or without preimplantation genetic screening for aneuploidy in couples without genetic disorders: a systematic review and meta-analysis. J Assist Reprod Genet. 2009;26(5):273–83.
10. Wells D, Alfarawati S, Fragouli E. Use of comprehensive chromosomal screening for embryo assessment: microarrays and CGH. Mol Hum Reprod. 2008;14(12):703–10.

11. Manno M, Marchesan E, Tomei F, Cicutto D, Maruzzi D, Maieron A, et al. Polycystic kidney disease and infertility: case report and literature review. Arch Ital Urol Androl. 2005;77(1): 25–8.
12. Vora N, Perrone R, Bianchi DW. Reproductive issues for adults with autosomal dominant polycystic kidney disease. Am J Kidney Dis. 2008;51(2):307–18.
13. Kuliev A, Rechitsky S. Polar body-based preimplantation genetic diagnosis for Mendelian disorders. Mol Hum Reprod. 2011;17(5):275–85.
14. Magli MC, Gianaroli L, Grieco N, Cefalu E, Ruvolo G, Ferraretti AP. Cryopreservation of biopsied embryos at the blastocyst stage. Hum Reprod. 2006;21(10):2656–60.
15. McArthur SJ, Leigh D, Marshall JT, de Boer KA, Jansen RP. Pregnancies and live births after trophectoderm biopsy and preimplantation genetic testing of human blastocysts. Fertil Steril. 2005;84(6):1628–36.
16. Amagwula T, Chang PL, Hossain A, Tyner J, Rivers AL, Phelps JY. Preimplantation genetic diagnosis: a systematic review of litigation in the face of new technology. Fertil Steril. 2012;98(5):1277–82.
17. Gagnon A, Audibert F. Prenatal screening and diagnosis of aneuploidy in multiple pregnancies. Best Pract Res Clin Obstet Gynaecol. 2014;28(2):285–94.
18. Handyside AH, Lesko JG, Tarin JJ, Winston RM, Hughes MR. Birth of a normal girl after in vitro fertilization and preimplantation diagnostic testing for cystic fibrosis. N Engl J Med. 1992;327(13):905–9.
19. Dreesen JC, Jacobs LJ, Bras M, Herbergs J, Dumoulin JC, Geraedts JP, et al. Multiplex PCR of polymorphic markers flanking the CFTR gene; a general approach for preimplantation genetic diagnosis of cystic fibrosis. Mol Hum Reprod. 2000;6(5):391–6.
20. Spits C, Le Caignec C, De Rycke M, Van Haute L, Van Steirteghem A, Liebaers I, et al. Optimization and evaluation of single-cell whole-genome multiple displacement amplification. Hum Mutat. 2006;27(5):496–503.
21. Natesan SA, Handyside AH, Thornhill AR, Ottolini CS, Sage K, Summers MC, et al. Live birth after PGD with confirmation by a comprehensive approach (karyomapping) for simultaneous detection of monogenic and chromosomal disorders. Reprod Biomed Online. 2014;29(5):600–5.
22. Rechitsky S, Pomerantseva E, Pakhalchuk T, Pauling D, Verlinsky O, Kuliev A. First systematic experience of preimplantation genetic diagnosis for de-novo mutations. Reprod Biomed Online. 2011;22(4):350–61.
23. Peters BA, Kermani BG, Alferov O, Agarwal MR, McElwain MA, Gulbahce N, et al. Detection and phasing of single base de novo mutations in biopsies from human in vitro fertilized embryos by advanced whole-genome sequencing. Genome Res. 2015;25(3):426–34.
24. De Rycke M, Belva F, Goossens V, Moutou C, SenGupta SB, Traeger-Synodinos J, et al. ESHRE PGD Consortium data collection XIII: cycles from January to December 2010 with pregnancy follow-up to October 2011 dagger. Hum Reprod. 2015;30(8):1763–89.
25. Stern HJ. Preimplantation genetic diagnosis: prenatal testing for embryos finally achieving its potential. J Clin Med. 2014;3(1):280–309.
26. Hofherr SE, Wiktor AE, Kipp BR, Dawson DB, Van Dyke DL. Clinical diagnostic testing for the cytogenetic and molecular causes of male infertility: the Mayo Clinic experience. J Assist Reprod Genet. 2011;28(11):1091–8.
27. Scriven PN, Flinter FA, Khalaf Y, Lashwood A, Mackie OC. Benefits and drawbacks of preimplantation genetic diagnosis (PGD) for reciprocal translocations: lessons from a prospective cohort study. Eur J Hum Genet. 2013;21:1035–41.
28. Tan Y, Yin X, Zhang S, Jiang H, Tan K, Li J, et al. Clinical outcome of preimplantation genetic diagnosis and screening using next generation sequencing. Gigascience. 2014;3(1):30.
29. Fernandez RM, Pecina A, Lozano-Arana MD, Garcia-Lozano JC, Borrego S, Antinolo G. Novel one-step multiplex PCR-based method for HLA typing and preimplantational genetic diagnosis of beta-Thalassemia. Biomed Res Int. 2013;2013:585106.
30. Kakourou G, Destouni A, Vrettou C, Traeger-Synodinos J, Kanavakis E. A generic, flexible protocol for preimplantation human leukocyte antigen typing alone or in combination with a monogenic disease, for rapid case work-up and application. Hemoglobin. 2014;38(1):49–55.

31. Munne S, Lee A, Rosenwaks Z, Grifo J, Cohen J. Diagnosis of major chromosome aneuploidies in human preimplantation embryos. Hum Reprod. 1993;8(12):2185–91.
32. Munne S. Preimplantation genetic diagnosis of numerical and structural chromosome abnormalities. Reprod Biomed Online. 2002;4(2):183–96.
33. Mastenbroek S, Twisk M, van der Veen F, Repping S. Preimplantation genetic screening: a systematic review and meta-analysis of RCTs. Hum Reprod Update. 2011;17(4):454–66.
34. Munne S, Cohen J, Simpson JL. In vitro fertilization with preimplantation genetic screening. N Engl J Med. 2007;357(17):1769–70; author reply 70–1.
35. Lee E, Illingworth P, Wilton L, Chambers GM. The clinical effectiveness of preimplantation genetic diagnosis for aneuploidy in all 24 chromosomes (PGD-A): systematic review. Hum Reprod. 2015;30(2):473–83.
36. Wilton L, Thornhill A, Traeger-Synodinos J, Sermon KD, Harper JC. The causes of misdiagnosis and adverse outcomes in PGD. Hum Reprod. 2009;24(5):1221–8.
37. Werner MD, Leondires MP, Schoolcraft WB, Miller BT, Copperman AB, Robins ED, et al. Clinically recognizable error rate after the transfer of comprehensive chromosomal screened euploid embryos is low. Fertil Steril. 2014;102(6):1613–8.
38. Liu W, Zhang R, Wei J, Zhang H, Yu G, Li Z, et al. Rapid diagnosis of imprinting disorders involving copy number variation and uniparental disomy using genome-wide SNP microarrays. Cytogenet Genome Res. 2015;146(1):9–18.
39. Gueye NA, Devkota B, Taylor D, Pfundt R, Scott Jr RT, Treff NR. Uniparental disomy in the human blastocyst is exceedingly rare. Fertil Steril. 2014;101(1):232–6.
40. Treff NR, Fedick A, Tao X, Devkota B, Taylor D, Scott Jr RT. Evaluation of targeted next-generation sequencing-based preimplantation genetic diagnosis of monogenic disease. Fertil Steril. 2013;99(5):1377–84.e6.
41. Sacks GC, Altarescu G, Guedalia J, Varshaver I, Gilboa T, Levy-Lahad E, et al. Developmental neuropsychological assessment of 4- to 5-year-old children born following Preimplantation Genetic Diagnosis (PGD): a pilot study. Child Neuropsychol. 2016;22(4):458–71.
42. Winter C, Van Acker F, Bonduelle M, Desmyttere S, De Schrijver F, Nekkebroeck J. Cognitive and psychomotor development of 5- to 6-year-old singletons born after PGD: a prospective case-controlled matched study. Hum Reprod. 2014;29(9):1968–77.
43. Richardson J, Irving L, Hyslop LA, Choudhary M, Murdoch A, Turnbull DM, et al. Concise reviews: assisted reproductive technologies to prevent transmission of mitochondrial DNA disease. Stem Cells. 2015;33(3):639–45.

Chapter 5
Complications of ART and Associated Early Pregnancy Problems

Lukasz T. Polanski and Miriam N. Baumgarten

Introduction

Assisted reproductive techniques (ART) have become the only hope for biologically own progeny for numerous infertile couples. In the developed world, 1.7–4.0 % of all children born are the result of assisted conception [1, 2]. The interventions, though common and well established, are not without complications. To these, the couples are often oblivious, as the hope of having a child might diminish one of the most significant and basic human instincts of self-preservation.

It is estimated, that complications during the ART process occur in approximately 2 % of cases. When discussing the complications of ART, a division into procedure related and pregnancy related can be made. The procedure related complications include bleeding and infection following transvaginal ultrasound guided oocyte retrievals (TVOR) with associated comorbidities and ovarian hyperstimulation syndrome (OHSS).

If a pregnancy is achieved, the first trimester is a perilous period for the conceptus, with the risk of ectopic pregnancy and miscarriage being the most common complications. Failure of treatment is an emotional and financial burden for the couples and can have significant emotional and social implications, such as depression and relationship breakdown, to quote just a few. ART pregnancies are at an increased risk of congenital anomalies, preterm birth, low birth weight, gestational diabetes and pre-eclampsia [3, 4]. The exact cause of the increase in the adverse outcomes can be sought in the technology or underlying maternal factors [5].

In this chapter we will cover the clinical aspects of the procedure and pregnancy related complications of ART.

L.T. Polanski, MD, PhD • M.N. Baumgarten, MD (✉)
Department of Obstetrics and Gynaecology, Addenbrooke's Hospital, Cambridge, UK
e-mail: Lucas.polanski@hotmail.com; Miriam.baumgarten@addenbrookes.nhs.uk

K. Jayaprakasan, L. Kean (eds.), *Clinical Management of Pregnancies following ART*, DOI 10.1007/978-3-319-42858-1_5

Ovarian Hyperstimulation Syndrome (OHSS)

This iatrogenic complication of ovarian stimulation is a potentially fatal condition related to ovarian enlargement with systemic increase in vascular permeability. The condition can occur following any form of ovarian stimulation, including clomiphene citrate and gonadotropins, with the latter being responsible for majority of the cases. Spontaneous, non-related to ovulation induction, OHSS has been reported but is a rare event [6].

The reported incidence of OHSS is 2–10 % of IVF cycles. Varying classification systems and potential underreporting contribute to lack of definite knowledge of the accurate prevalence of the condition [6]. The severe form of OHSS can complicate 0.1–2 % of all IVF cycles, with a mild form occurring in up to 23 % of IVF cycles [7]. The reported mortality rate related directly to OHSS or indirectly (due to arising complications) is estimated at 1 in 400,000 to 1 in 500,000 ovarian stimulation cycles [8]. Though low, it is still unacceptably high as it is related to infertility treatment – a non-lifesaving therapy.

The shifts in fluid from the intravascular to the extravascular compartment are the main pathogenetic changes in OHSS leading to relative hypovolaemia, hypotension, tachycardia, haemoconcentration with increasing haematocrit, renal hypoperfusion with associated renal failure, and acute respiratory failure. Electrolyte disturbances ensue and are the result of renal failure. Albumin rich ascites and pleural effusions are a common finding causing abdominal girth distension and discomfort. Shortness of breath can be related to a combination of ascites and hydrothorax. Pericardial effusions can be present in the more severe forms of the syndrome [9]. Increased intraabdominal pressure impairs the renal blood flow further and can lead to compression of the low pressure abdominal vessels supplying intraabdominal organs (liver, intestines) causing derangement in liver function tests and gastro-intestinal symptoms in the form of diarrhoea and vomiting [10]. The altered thrombotic state related to hyperoestrogenaemia and haemoconcentration can lead to venous thrombotic events (VTE), which can complicate the course of the disease. The release of vascular endothelial growth factor (VEGF) from the ovaries and associated activation of the renin-angiotensin system (RAS) is the pathway responsible for the increase in the global vascular permeability [6]. The exact mechanism of this process is still under debate and oestrogens, progestogens, interleukins, angiogenins, endothelins, prostaglandins, histamine, prolactin and kinins are thought to play a role in this [11].

OHSS can be divided into early and late onset, and mild, moderate, severe and critical. Most often quoted classification is based on ultrasound findings of ovarian enlargement and ascites [7]. Modifications to the basic classification aim to distinguish between the severe and life-threatening, or critical, forms of the syndrome [12]. A recent new classification combines the ultrasound findings, clinical signs and symptoms, and laboratory investigations [6, 13, 14]. The resolution of symptoms is expected by the 6th week of gestation. Mild OHSS is associated with mild clinical symptoms of abdominal distension, associated discomfort and nausea. Ultrasound assessment demonstrates mildly enlarged ovaries (<8 cm) with no ascites (Fig. 5.1a–f). The critical form is associated with respiratory distress, tense

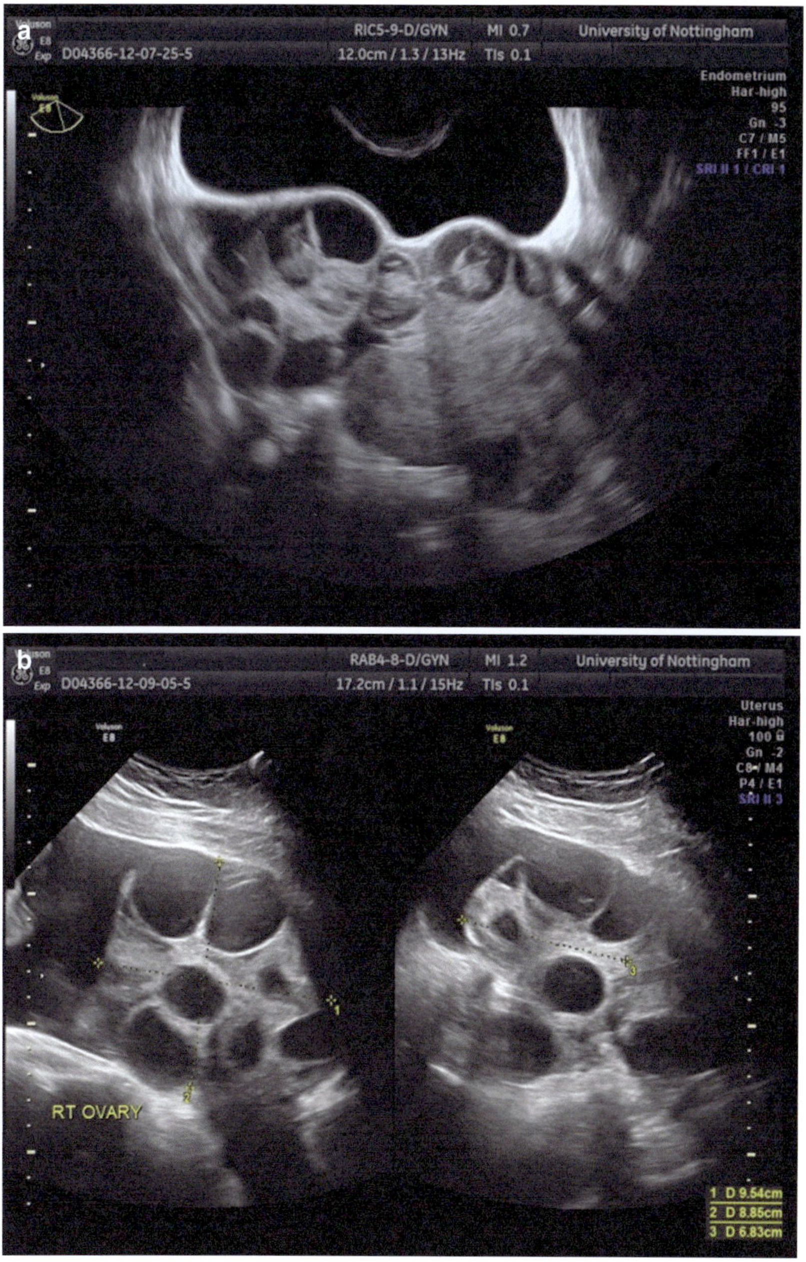

Fig. 5.1 (**a**) Bilaterally enlarged ovaries following ART. Both ovaries are displaced superiorly above the uterus and are meeting in the midline ('kissing ovaries'). (**b**, **c**) Moderately enlarged ovaries following ART with post-oocyte collection follicles of varying size. Some of the follicles contain clotted blood (*arrow*). (**d**) Post-oocyte collection ovary. Note enlarged follicle with re-accumulated fluid and significantly increased vascularity as demonstrated by power Doppler modality. (**e**, **f**) Trans-abdominal scan of the right upper quadrant demonstrating the liver and right kidney (**e**). I cases of severe OHSS, free fluid can be seen in the pouch of Morrison (*arrow*). The left upper quadrant can also be filled with free fluid in severe cases of OHSS (**f**). Note free floating loops of bowel (*arrow*)

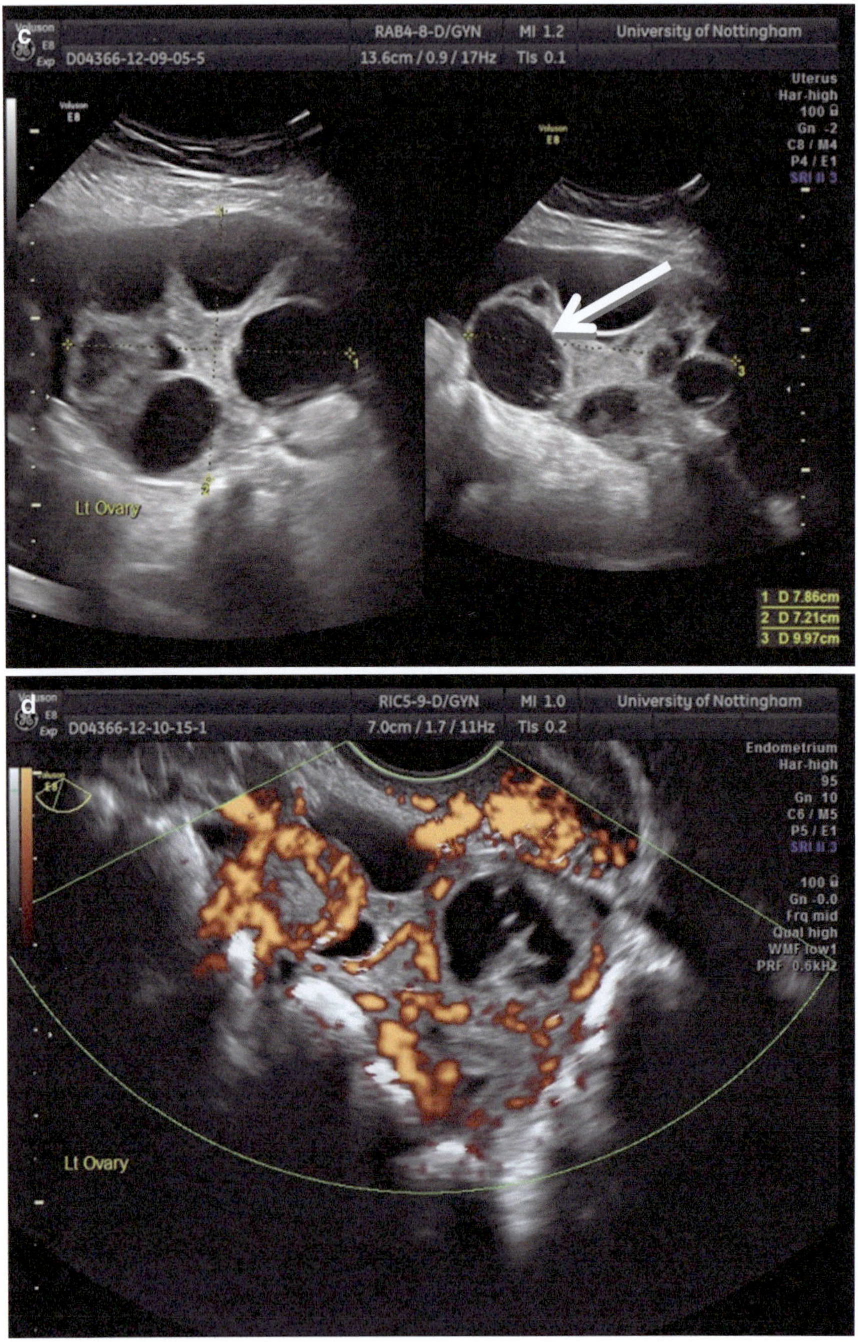

Fig. 5.1 (continued)

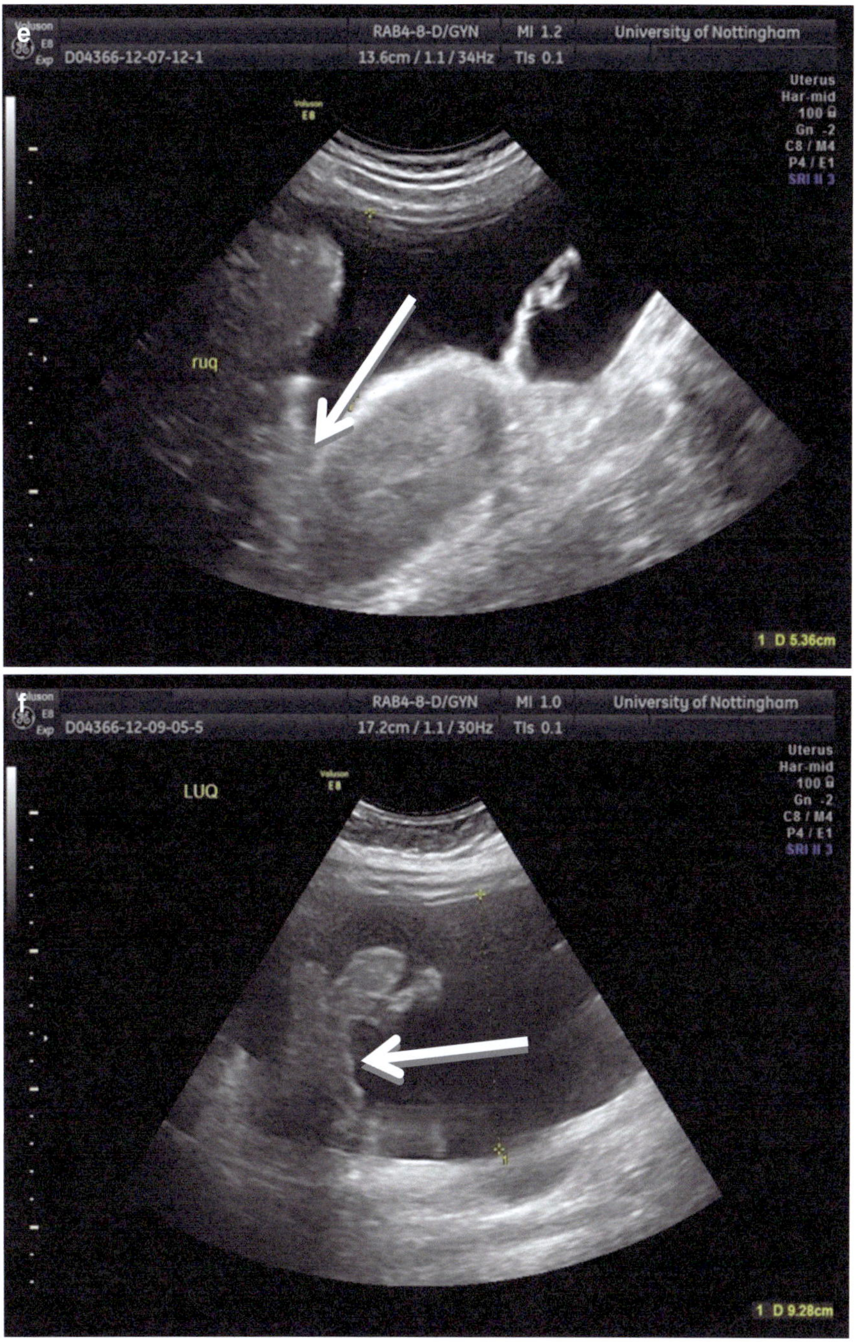

Fig. 5.1 (continued)

Table 5.1 Leuven University Fertility Centre classification system of OHSS

Grade of OHSS	Symptoms	Management
Mild OHSS	Mild abdominal bloating and pain No weight gain Ovarian size <8 cm	Conservative, outpatient based If symptoms deteriorate, advice to seek medical help
Moderate OHSS	Moderate abdominal pain controlled with rest and simple analgesia Nausea Weight gain up to 1 kg Ultrasound evidence of ascites (deepest pool <3 cm) Ovarian size 8–10 cm	Conservative, outpatient based
Severe OHSS	Uncontrolled abdominal pain Weight gain >1 kg Clinical ascites (with occasional hydrothorax) Oliguria Haematocrit >45 % Ultrasound evidence of significant ascites (deepest pool >3 cm) Ovarian size >10 cm	Hospital based
Critical OHSS	Tense ascites or large hydrothorax Haematocrit >55 % White cell count >25,000/ml Oligo/anuria Venous-thromboembolic events Adult respiratory distress syndrome	Admission to critical care unit

Used with permission of Elsevier from Vloeberghs et al. [6]

ascites, renal failure, and venous thrombo-embolic events. Marked leucocytosis (>25,000/mL), ovarian size >12 cm, hydrothorax and ascites are common features. The detailed description of each clinical form is contained in Table 5.1. The early onset OHSS is usually a milder and self-limiting form that develops within 10 days of oocyte maturation triggering. OHSS developing after this initial period is usually associated with pregnancy and tends to have a more protracted and severe clinical course [15].

The recognised OHSS risk factors, according to the ESHRE special interest group for quality and safety in ART, can be divided into primary and secondary [9]. The primary risk factors include polycystic ovarian syndrome (PCOS) [16], high number of antral follicles (≥10 in each ovary), LH/FHS ratio >2, hyperandrogenism, previous OHSS, young age, and low body mass index (BMI) [6]. Anti-Müllerian (AMH) hormone levels of ≥40 pmol/L put a patient at approximately a 33 % risk of developing moderate to severe OHSS (a fivefold increase from when AMH levels are <40 pmol/L) [17]. Similarly, a fourfold increase (to 8.6 %) in mild to moderate OHSS risk can be observed in women with and AFC of >23 [18]. Recognised secondary risk factors include high serum oestradiol levels (>9000 pmol/L; >3000 pg/mL) with rapidly increasing levels being of more clinical importance, use of human chorionic gonadotropin (hCG) as a final oocyte maturation trigger, >20–25 follicles in both ovaries, over 20 oocytes retrieved, and multiple pregnancy [6, 9].

Prevention of development of the condition, similarly to risk factors, can be categorised into primary and secondary. Recognition of potential risk factors is essential to minimise the chances of development of OHSS, with subsequent individual-tailored protocols using the lowest dose and shortest stimulation regimens. Antagonist protocol with agonist trigger is generally considered as the best approach in minimising or eliminating the risk of OHSS in high-risk women [14]. Ovarian drilling and metformin administration prior to ART have also been suggested as alternative methods of OHSS prevention. *In vitro* maturation is a novel, however not fully assessed, method of minimising OHSS prevalence [19].

Secondary prevention can be achieved by cycle cancellation and withholding hCG triggering [13], coasting – discontinuation of gonadotrophins with continuing GnRH agonist until oestradiol falls below 3500 pg/mL [6], cryopreservation of all embryos [20], albumin administration at the time of oocyte retrieval [21], cabergoline [22], in vitro maturation or GnRH antagonist cycles [23]. If the secondary precautions are taken, there is still no guarantee that OHSS will not develop, as even when hCG is withheld and the cycle cancelled, spontaneous LH surge can occur leading to symptom development [13]. Early stage research indicates that the use of kisspeptin-54 as a final oocyte maturation trigger can produce very acceptable oocyte yields with minimal or no risk of developing OHSS, even in a group of highly susceptible individuals [24].

Management of OHSS

OHSS management depends on the severity of the condition, and can be performed on an out-patient basis in the mild forms, or in the hospital setting in the intensive therapy unit in the severe cases. VTE events, renal failure not responding to treatment and pulmonary compromise are indications for ITU care [6]. As the condition is most often self-limiting, reassurance has to be given to the woman and her partner. In extremely severe and protracted cases, when supportive treatment is not sufficient, termination of the pregnancy in order to decrease the circulating hCG levels may be necessary.

According to the RCOG, mild to moderate OHSS can be managed on an outpatient basis, with paracetamol and codeine used for pain control. Drinking to thirst is encouraged [25] and avoidance of strenuous exercise and intercourse is advised. Clinical assessment including body weight recording, abdominal girth measurement and pelvic ultrasound should be carried out every 2–3 days in order to determine deterioration of condition [14]. In more severe cases, multidisciplinary inpatient approach to treatment should be considered. When abdominal distension due to ascites causes severe discomfort or impedes respiration, ultrasound guided paracentesis should be considered [26, 27]. Similarly, women with inadequate urine output despite appropriate parenteral rehydration and ascites could benefit from decreased intra-abdominal pressure, as this might improve renal circulation and restore urine production [28]. Cardiovascular collapse due to rapid fluid shifts can be avoided by gradual drainage of ascites and the use of pigtail catheters [29]. Thromboprophylaxis should be considered in all women admitted to hospital due to OHSS in order to minimize the incidence of VTE [14].

TVOR Related Complications

Transvaginal ultrasound guided oocyte retrieval (TVOR) is currently the procedure of choice for oocyte collection in most IVF centres worldwide [30]. Though the procedure is deemed safe, there are associated risks related to bleeding and intraabdominal sepsis.

Bleeding

Vaginal bleeding can be limited by minimizing the number of vaginal punctures and is the most common form of haemorrhagic complications occurring in 0.5–8.6 % of oocyte retrievals. Significant vaginal blood loss of >100 ml has been reported to occur in 0.8 % of cases [31]. Application of pressure, or occasionally suturing of the bleeding site, is sufficient to stop the loss [32]. A more severe complication – intraabdominal haemorrhage – has a reported incidence between 0 and 0.35 %. This complication is related to direct injury to the ovary, bleeding from the ruptured follicle or injury to large pelvic vessels [33]. Coagulation disorders, inherited or iatrogenic, increase the risk of haemorrhagic complications.

Careful visualization of the follicle and neighbouring iliac vessels and application of modality Doppler if doubt as to the nature of the structure exists, allows for unequivocal identification of follicles and avoidance of puncturing the blood vessels.

In the event of an uncomplicated TVOR, the expected blood loss should not exceed 250 ml with a haematocrit drop of approximately 5 %. Larger blood loss, or unexpectedly low haemoglobin values following TVOR, should warrant investigations to identify possible bleeding site [34]. Abdominal ultrasound scan should suffice to identify free fluid in the abdomen (Fig. 5.2a–e). Organised blood collections or retroperitoneal haematomas might not be immediately visible and may necessitate employment of other imaging modalities such as computer tomography (CT) imaging.

Visceral Injury

Injury to the bowel, bladder and ureters is an uncommon complication. Two case reports of repeated perforations of the appendix following TVOR exist [35, 36]. It is thought that bowel injury is relatively common; however, most cases resolve

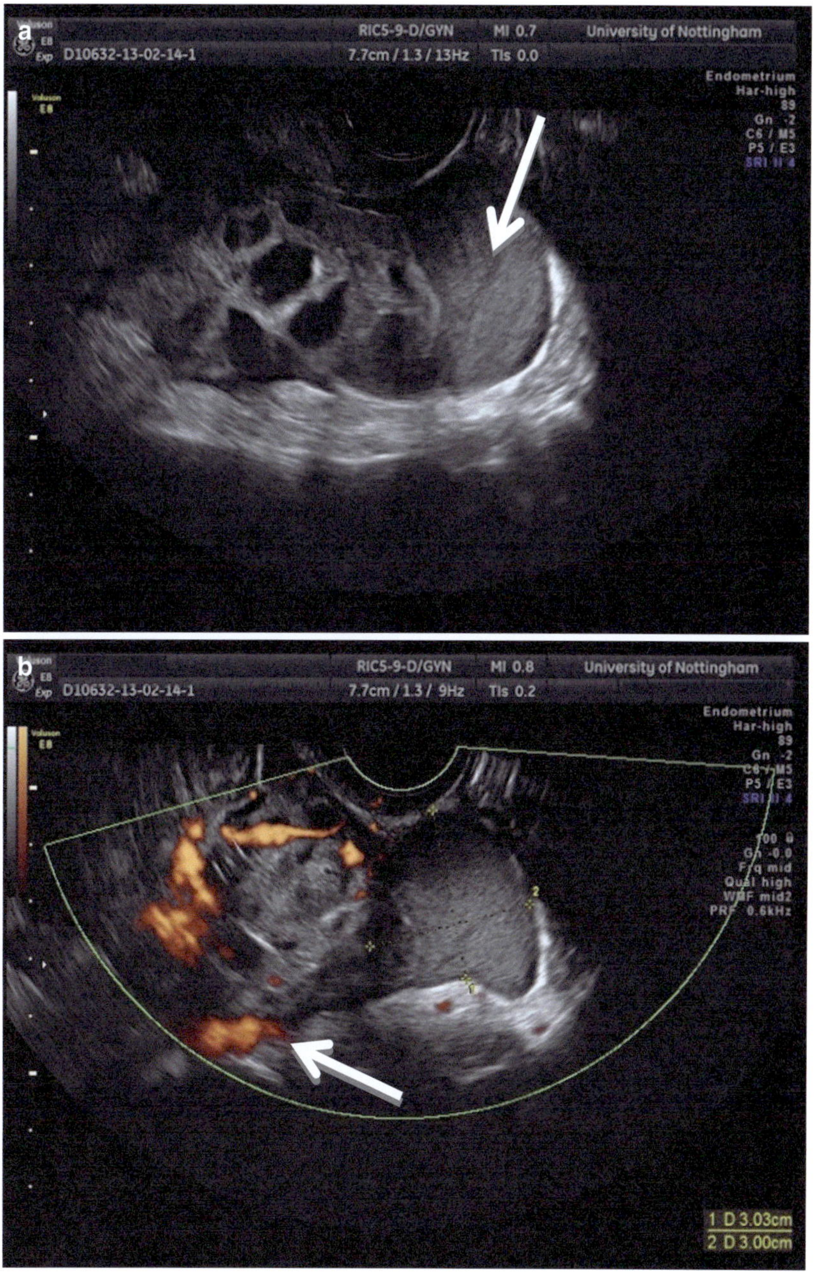

Fig. 5.2 (**a**) Fresh bleeding into pouch of Douglas following TVOR. Note the difference in echogenicity of the free fluid (*arrow*). Live scanning would reveal movement of the particles. (**b**, **c**) Blood in pouch of Douglas. The fluid appears homogenous. This patient was monitored and treated conservatively with this examination performed 2 days after TVOR. The ovary is enlarged with active Doppler signal (*arrow*). (**d**, **e**) Haemorrhagic follicular cyst following TVOR. Note the extensive fibrin deposits within the cysts (*arrow*) and lack of Doppler signal within the cyst (**e**)

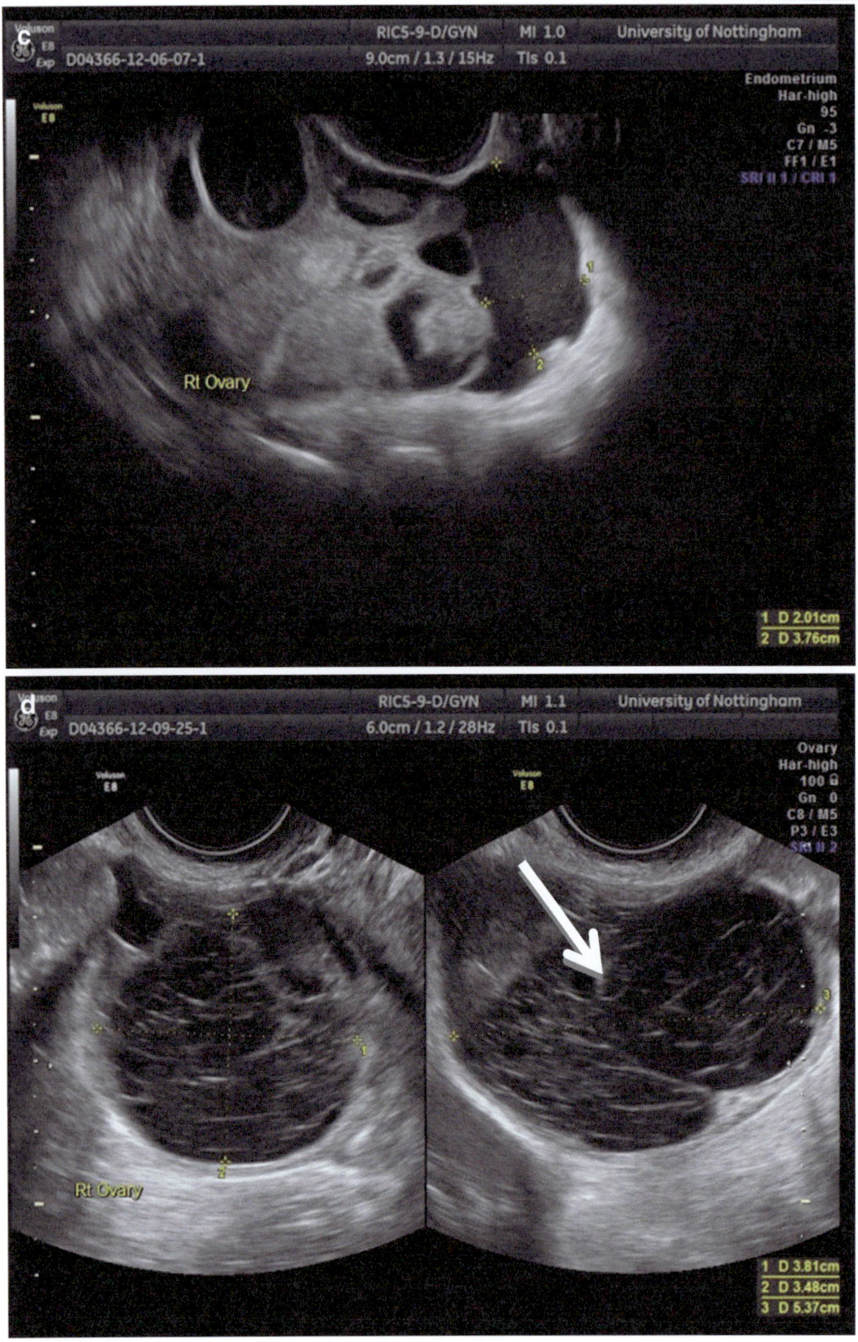

Fig. 5.2 (continued)

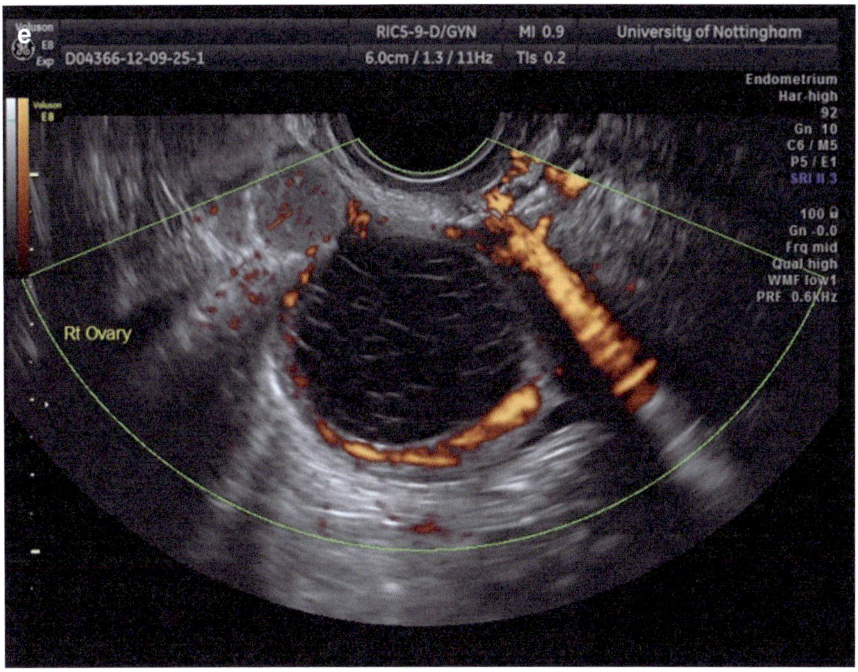

Fig. 5.2 (continued)

spontaneously with no clinical manifestations [32]. Urinary retention and/or haematuria should raise the suspicion of bladder injury [37]. Ureteric obstruction related to TVOR has also been reported but is a very rare complication [32, 38].

Infections

Pelvic infection is another serious complication of TVOR occurring in 0–1.3 % of women following oocyte retrieval procedures [6]. Bowel injury, reactivation of quiescent pelvic inflammatory disease or introduction of pathogens from the vagina are the possible mechanisms of TVOR related infections [39]. Abdominal pain, pyrexia and elevated laboratory markers of infection should aid in making the diagnosis. Treatment should be prompt with parenteral antibiotics, rehydration, appropriate imaging including ultrasound or CT scans, and surgical intervention as guided by the clinical picture and suspected cause. Routine use of antibiotic prophylaxis prior to TVOR is not widely practiced; however, in high risk patients (active or recent PID, endometriosis and associated adhesions, ovarian endometriomas, hydrosalpinx and previous pelvic surgery) it should be considered [40].

Other Complications

Ovarian pedicle torsion is a rare but serious complication of ART with a reported incidence of 0.08–0.2 % of women undergoing fertility treatment [6, 33, 36, 41]. Diagnosis is not always clear, but presence of risk factors such as pre-existing ovarian cysts, pregnancy, ovarian hyperstimulation or just history of ovulation induction raises the suspicion of this event [42, 43]. Worsening unilateral pain with leucocytosis, nausea and vomiting form the classical presentation. The differential diagnosis should always include ectopic pregnancy, with transvaginal or abdominal ultrasound used to diagnose the condition. Blurred ovarian margins and enlargement of the ovary with absent Doppler signal signifying stromal oedema and absent or decreased blood flow, respectively, indicate ovarian torsion. A vortex pattern of blood flow in the region of the ovarian pedicle can be another helpful sign to diagnose adnexal torsion. Presence of blood flow does not exclude torsion and diagnosis should be made on clinical grounds [6, 44]. Reversion of torsion with ovarian sparing via the laparoscopic route is the treatment of choice with favourable subsequent reproductive outcomes [6, 42].

First Trimester Miscarriage

Loss of pregnancy before the arbitrary gestation of viability (24 completed weeks) is defined as a miscarriage. Multiple studies have reported an increased risk of miscarriage in the ART population with the prevalence of 17–32.6 % [4, 45]. When analysing these reports in the context of miscarrige, it is important to differentiate the causes of underlying subfertility and the risk of ART *per se*. Infertile couples are more likely to be older (5 years on average) than their fertile counterparts, are more likely to have endocrine disorders (thyroid dysfunction and PCOS) and/or structural uterine anomalies [46–49]. The intense surveillance of ART pregnancies and very early serum testing for implantation, might also contribute to the relatively high prevalence of very early ART pregnancy losses, when compared to less monitored spontaneous conceptions.

A retrospective study by Pezeshki et al. in 2000 has demonstrated a miscarriage rate of 21.3 % in the ovulation induction population, 19.8 % in the IVF population and 26.2 % after spontaneous conception. Maternal age was the most significant predictor of miscarriage, but the cause of infertility did not play an important role in the miscarriage risk [50]. Comparison of ART pregnancies with historical data on spontaneous conceptions has revealed that the unadjusted relative risk of miscarriage following ART was 1.33–1.49 (95 % CI 1.08–1.68), with maternal age being a significant contributor. Intense stimulation protocols and high estradiol levels (>8 nmol/L) were associated with an increased risk of miscarriage (23 % versus 10 % when estradiol was <2 nmol/L) [51]. In the above-mentioned study, the authors have reported a significant difference in the first and second trimester miscarriage rates between the ART and historical control cohorts. The authors concluded that maternal age, history of previous miscarriage and ‘some’ treatment related factors might be responsible for the observed increase in miscarriage rates, with further studies required to validate the statement [51]. Overall, miscarriage rates in ART pregnancies are similar or marginally higher when compared to spontaneous conceptions.

Ectopic Pregnancy

Development of a pregnancy outside of the endometrial cavity can be broadly termed as an ectopic pregnancy (EP). Multiple implantation sites of an early pregnancy are possible, including the Fallopian tubes, ovaries, the cervix, cesarean section scar, interstitial portions of the tube, and the abdominal cavity, with Fallopian tubes being the most frequent site. Contemporaneous existence of an ectopic and an intrauterine gestation is termed a heterotopic pregnancy. Approximately 1 % of all spontaneously conceived pregnancies develop as an ectopic pregnancy. The incidence of heterotopic pregnancies in the general population is estimated to be 1 in 20,000 to 1 in 50,000 pregnancies. In the ART setting, this can be as frequent as 1 in 100 [52].

The overall trend of ectopic gestations is on the increase. This is thought to be related to an increasing prevalence of pelvic infections caused by such pathogens as *Chlamydia trachomatis* and *Neisseria gonorrhea*, as well as the wide spread use of ART. The incidence of ectopic pregnancies associated with ART with an embryo transfer performed is approximately 1–5 % [53]. In view of the high frequency of occurrence of this potentially fatal condition, an early transvaginal scan is recommended in all women undergoing IVF or ICSI. This should be routinely performed between 6 and 8 weeks gestation [53]. The clinical manifestations of an ectopic pregnancy can vary greatly, with the initial symptoms developing as early as the 5th week of gestation, or as late as the 12th week [54]. Asymptomatic patients are diagnosed during and ultrasound scan; however, symptomatic cases can present with a significant intra-abdominal haemorrhage and signs of hypovolaemic shock requiring immediate surgery (Fig. 5.3).

In the case of ART, when patients present with abdominal pain and a positive pregnancy test, the differential diagnoses need to include ovarian hyperstimulation syndrome with possible adnexal torsion and ectopic pregnancy. The timing of presentation in relation to the ART procedures might aid in making one or the other diagnosis likely. It is also worth remembering, that the hCG used to trigger final oocyte maturation might produce a positive pregnancy test result if performed within 12 days of administration of 5000 units of hCG [55].

Multiple Pregnancies

Multifetal pregnancy rates following ART range from 5 to 40 % [56]. Dichorionic twin pregnancies are the most common form of multiple gestation following ART; however, monozygotic and monochorionic pregnancy rate in the IVF population is estimated at 0.9–2 %, compared to 0.4 % of spontaneous conceptions [57–59].

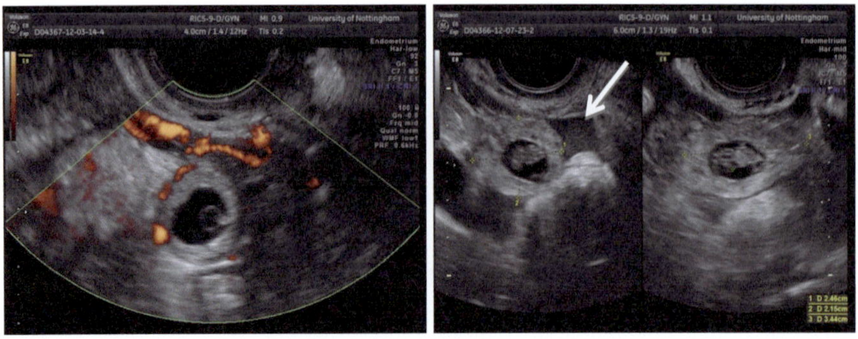

Fig. 5.3 Tubal ectopic pregnancy following IVF. Hyperechoic trophoblastic tissue encompasses the gestation sac in both cases containing fetal poles. Particulate free fluid (*arrow*) surrounding the ectopic pregnancy signifies intraabdominal bleeding

Higher order pregnancies (triplet or more) in approximately two-third of cases are the result of ovulation induction without the use of IVF or any similar procedure [60]. See Fig. 5.4a–d.

Blastocyst transfers contribute to the increase of multiple gestations, as embryo splitting at this stage can occur in 6 % of cases [61]. During IVF treatment, irrespective of age, transfer of a single blastocyst stage embryo carries a less than 2 % multiple gestation risk. For a double blastocyst embryo transfer, the risk approximates 39 %, whereas a double cleavage stage embryo transfer carries a 27 % risk of multiple gestation [62]. Preterm birth associated with multiple gestations is deemed as one of the most important adverse outcomes following ART. Care for such neonates incurs significant costs to the healthcare systems with the long-term outcomes of such babies being difficult to predict. Neonatal intensive care unit (NICU) admissions in 12–17 % of cases are related to multiple pregnancies, with up to 91 % of these related to IVF, where two to six embryos were transferred [63]. Most systematic reviews on outcomes of ART pregnancies indicate statistically better pregnancy outcomes for ART twins compared to spontaneous conceptions. This is in contrast to singleton pregnancies, where natural singletons perform better compared to ART conceived infants [5]. However, depending on the study and populations assessed, preterm birth, low birth weight and congenital anomalies can be either similar or worse in the ART population compared to spontaneously conceived multiple gestations [64, 65]. A systematic review of a total of 4385 ART twin pregnancies and 11,793 spontaneous twin gestations indicates an increased risk of preterm birth and low birth weight of <2500 g in ART pregnancies (RR 1.23, 95 % CI 1.09–1.41 and RR 1.14, 95 % CI 1.06–1.22, respectively) [66]. Maternal anaemia, pregnancy associated hypertensive disorders, gestational diabetes, caesarean section rates and post partum haemorrhage are a well-known risk of multiple gestations. With increasing prevalence of multiple pregnancies, these complications are a more frequent event on the current labour ward.

Parental mental health is more negatively affected by multiple pregnancies, irrespective of the mode of conception [67], with economic costs adding extra strain on

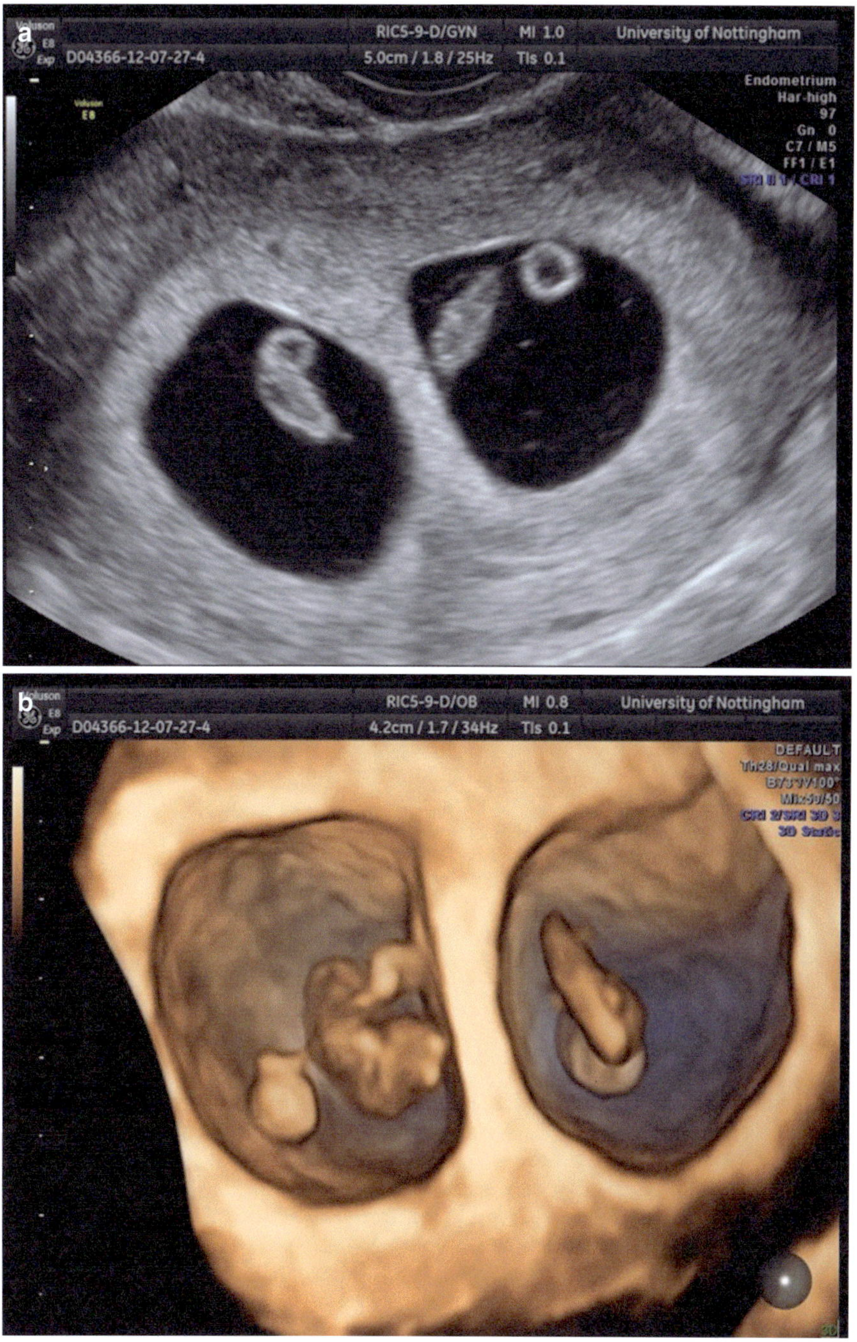

Fig. 5.4 (**a–d**) Multiple pregnancies following ART. (**a**, **b**) Dichorionic diamniotic (DCDA) twin pregnancy at approximately 8 weeks gestation (**b**: 3D rendering). (**c**) Monochorionic diamniotic (MCDA) twin pregnancy. Note the thin separating membrane representing two fused amnions (*arrow*). (**d**) Triplet pregnancy with two gestation sacs, one of which contains two fetuses (*arrow*)

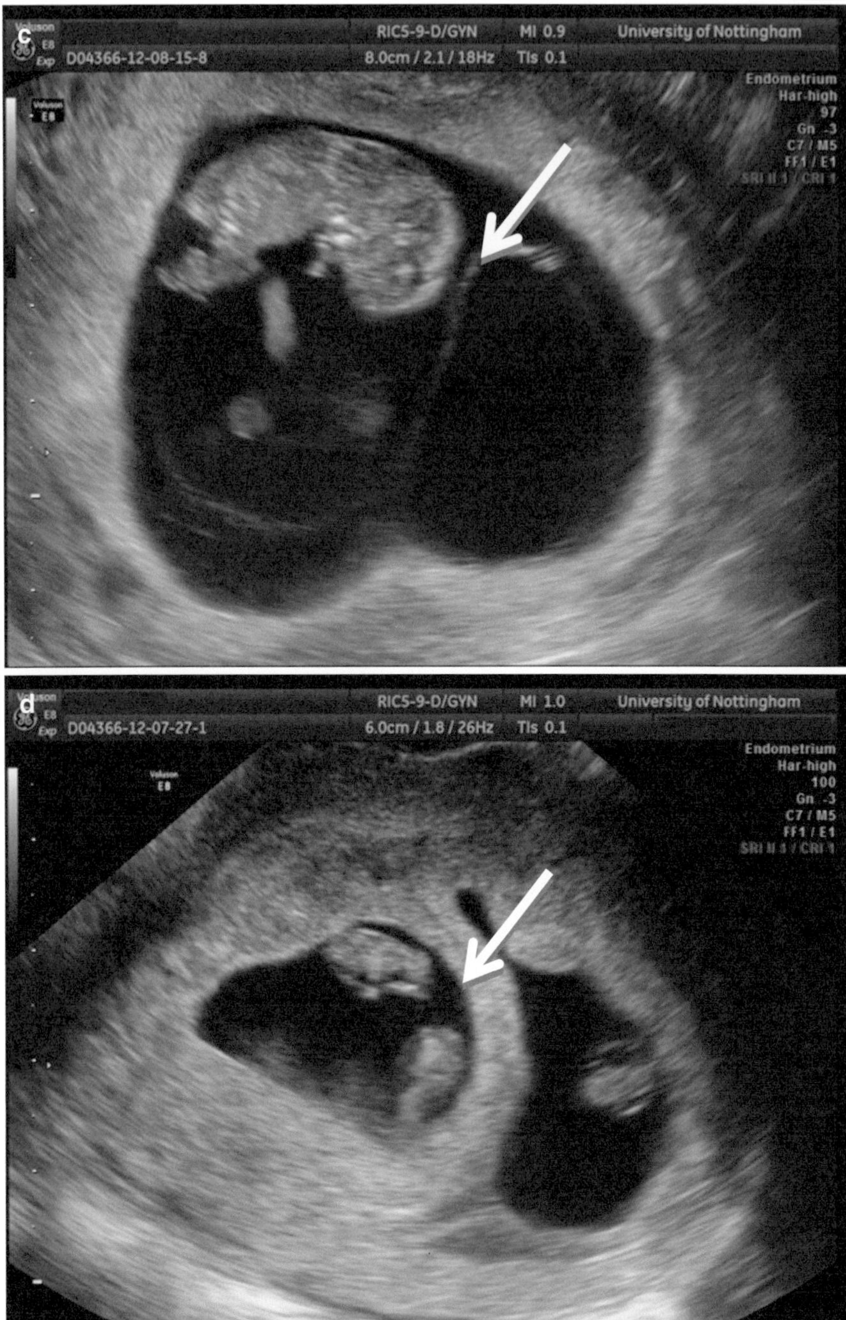

Fig. 5.4 (continued)

the relationship [68]. When considering multiple pregnancies following ART, selective feto-reduction should be discussed with the couple as one of the means to overcome complications related to higher order multiple pregnancies. This should be done tactfully and in a multi-disciplinary setting, with emotional and psychological support, as not all couples that have achieved a precious ART pregnancy will be willing to accept the small but present chance of miscarriage associated with feto-reduction. Nevertheless, current evidence supports the reduction of higher order multiple gestations to twins in order to improve all obstetric outcomes [69, 70].

Conclusions

Apart from the early and procedure related complications of ART, evidence also indicates that ART pregnancies are more likely to be complicated by placental problems, mainly pre-eclampsia [71], antepartum haemorrhage or placenta *praevia* [72], which are discussed specifically in other relevant chapters (see Chaps. 9 and 10, on maternal complications and fetal complications, respectively). An association between ART and congenital anomalies (including septal heart defects, oesophageal atresia, anorectal atresia) [73] and genital organ malformations (hazards ratio 2.32; 95% CI 1.24–4.35) has also been reported [74]. Reassuringly, long term behavioural and neurodevelopmental child outcomes seem to be little different in the ART conceptions compared to naturally conceived pregnancies [75]. As ART is becoming increasingly more common and affordable, we can expect an increase in the procedure related complications. Awareness of what these are, will aid in early recognition, prompt and appropriate management aiming to minimise any potential physical and psychological impact on the individual and the couple.

When embarking on assisted reproduction, the couple should be counselled not just about the unit's success rates, what the treatment process involves, but also about the complication rates. Though majority of the serious ART complications are rare, a balance must always be sought between the individualised risks and benefits of treatment. Patient choice and will to start a family should be respected. However, if the burden of treatment or subsequent pregnancy is deemed too significant for the coupe to bear, as medical professionals, we have a duty of care and in selected cases should not shy away from declining the non-life saving assisted reproductive treatment.

References

1. Klemetti R, Gissler M, Hemminki E. Comparison of perinatal health of children born from IVF in Finland in the early and late 1990s. Hum Reprod. 2002;17(8):2192–8.
2. Williams C, Sutcliffe A. Infant outcomes of assisted reproduction. Early Hum Dev. 2009;85(11):673–7.
3. Isaksson R, Gissler M, Tiitinen A. Obstetric outcome among women with unexplained infertility after IVF: a matched case–control study. Hum Reprod. 2002;17(7):1755–61.

4. Talaulikar VS, Arulkumaran S. Reproductive outcomes after assisted conception. Obstet Gynecol Surv. 2012;67(9):566–83.
5. Talaulikar VS, Arulkumaran S. Maternal, perinatal and long-term outcomes after assisted reproductive techniques (ART): implications for clinical practice. Eur J Obstet Gynecol Reprod Biol. 2013;170(1):13–9.
6. Vloeberghs V, et al. Ovarian hyperstimulation syndrome and complications of ART. Best Pract Res Clin Obstet Gynaecol. 2009;23(5):691–709.
7. Golan A, et al. Ovarian hyperstimulation syndrome: an update review. Obstet Gynecol Surv. 1989;44(6):430–40.
8. Brinsden PR, et al. Diagnosis, prevention and management of ovarian hyperstimulation syndrome. Br J Obstet Gynaecol. 1995;102(10):767–72.
9. European Society of Human Reproduction (ESHRE). Special Interest Group (SIG) guidelines on ovarian hyperstimulation syndrome (OHSS). 2005. Available from: http://www.eshre.com/emc.
10. Vlahos NF, Gregoriou O. Prevention and management of ovarian hyperstimulation syndrome. Ann N Y Acad Sci. 2006;1092:247–64.
11. Soares SR, et al. Targeting the vascular endothelial growth factor system to prevent ovarian hyperstimulation syndrome. Hum Reprod Update. 2008;14(4):321–33.
12. Navot D, Bergh PA, Laufer N. Ovarian hyperstimulation syndrome in novel reproductive technologies: prevention and treatment. Fertil Steril. 1992;58(2):249–61.
13. Aboulghar MA, Mansour RT. Ovarian hyperstimulation syndrome: classifications and critical analysis of preventive measures. Hum Reprod Update. 2003;9(3):275–89.
14. Royal College of Obstetricians and Gynaecologists (RCOG). The management of ovarian hyperstimulation syndrome. Green-top Guideline. 2006;5:1–11.
15. Mathur RS, et al. Distinction between early and late ovarian hyperstimulation syndrome. Fertil Steril. 2000;73(5):901–7.
16. Delvigne A, Rozenberg S. Epidemiology and prevention of ovarian hyperstimulation syndrome (OHSS): a review. Hum Reprod Update. 2002;8(6):559–77.
17. Lee TH, et al. Serum anti-Mullerian hormone and estradiol levels as predictors of ovarian hyperstimulation syndrome in assisted reproduction technology cycles. Hum Reprod. 2008;23(1):160–7.
18. Jayaprakasan K, et al. Prediction of in vitro fertilization outcome at different antral follicle count thresholds in a prospective cohort of 1,012 women. Fertil Steril. 2012;98(3):657–63.
19. Zhao JZ, et al. In vitro maturation and fertilization of oocytes from unstimulated ovaries in infertile women with polycystic ovary syndrome. Fertil Steril. 2009;91(6):2568–71.
20. D'Angelo A, Amso N. Embryo freezing for preventing ovarian hyperstimulation syndrome. Cochrane Database Syst Rev. 2007;3, CD002806.
21. Aboulghar M, Evers JH, Al-Inany H. Intravenous albumin for preventing severe ovarian hyperstimulation syndrome: a Cochrane review. Hum Reprod. 2002;17(12):3027–32.
22. Baumgarten M, et al. Do dopamine agonists prevent or reduce the severity of ovarian hyperstimulation syndrome in women undergoing assisted reproduction? A systematic review and meta-analysis. Hum Fertil (Camb). 2013;16(3):168–74.
23. Al-Inany HG, Abou-Setta AM, Aboulghar M. Gonadotrophin-releasing hormone antagonists for assisted conception: a Cochrane review. Reprod Biomed Online. 2007;14(5):640–9.
24. Abbara A, et al. Efficacy of Kisspeptin-54 to trigger oocyte maturation in women at high risk of ovarian hyperstimulation syndrome (OHSS) during in vitro fertilization (IVF) therapy. J Clin Endocrinol Metab. 2015;100(9):3322–31.
25. Evbuomwan IO, Davison JM, Murdoch AP. Coexistent hemoconcentration and hypoosmolality during superovulation and in severe ovarian hyperstimulation syndrome: a volume homeostasis paradox. Fertil Steril. 2000;74(1):67–72.
26. Maslovitz S, et al. Renal blood flow alteration after paracentesis in women with ovarian hyperstimulation. Obstet Gynecol. 2004;104(2):321–6.
27. Levin I, et al. Effect of paracentesis of ascitic fluids on urinary output and blood indices in patients with severe ovarian hyperstimulation syndrome. Fertil Steril. 2002;77(5):986–8.

28. Meldrum DR, et al. Prospective characterization and selective management of the abdominal compartment syndrome. Am J Surg. 1997;174(6):667–72; discussion 672–3.
29. Abuzeid MI, et al. Pigtail catheter for the treatment of ascites associated with ovarian hyperstimulation syndrome. Hum Reprod. 2003;18(2):370–3.
30. Wikland M, Enk L, Hamberger L. Transvesical and transvaginal approaches for the aspiration of follicles by use of ultrasound. Ann N Y Acad Sci. 1985;442:182–94.
31. Bennett SJ, et al. Complications of transvaginal ultrasound-directed follicle aspiration: a review of 2670 consecutive procedures. J Assist Reprod Genet. 1993;10(1):72–7.
32. Ludwig AK, et al. Perioperative and post-operative complications of transvaginal ultrasound-guided oocyte retrieval: prospective study of >1000 oocyte retrievals. Hum Reprod. 2006;21(12):3235–40.
33. Bodri D, et al. Complications related to ovarian stimulation and oocyte retrieval in 4052 oocyte donor cycles. Reprod Biomed Online. 2008;17(2):237–43.
34. Dessole S, et al. Blood loss following noncomplicated transvaginal oocyte retrieval for in vitro fertilization. Fertil Steril. 2001;76(1):205–6.
35. Akman MA, et al. Perforated appendicitis and ectopic pregnancy following in-vitro fertilization. Hum Reprod. 1995;10(12):3325–6.
36. Roest J, et al. The incidence of major clinical complications in a Dutch transport IVF programme. Hum Reprod Update. 1996;2(4):345–53.
37. Sauer MV. Defining the incidence of serious complications experienced by oocyte donors: a review of 1000 cases. Am J Obstet Gynecol. 2001;184(3):277–8.
38. Fugita OE, Kavoussi L. Laparoscopic ureteral reimplantation for ureteral lesion secondary to transvaginal ultrasonography for oocyte retrieval. Urology. 2001;58(2):281.
39. Sharpe K, et al. Transvaginal oocyte retrieval for in vitro fertilization complicated by ovarian abscess during pregnancy. Fertil Steril. 2006;86(1):219.e11–3.
40. Kelada E, Ghani R. Bilateral ovarian abscesses following transvaginal oocyte retrieval for IVF: a case report and review of literature. J Assist Reprod Genet. 2007;24(4):143–5.
41. Serour GI, et al. Complications of medically assisted conception in 3,500 cycles. Fertil Steril. 1998;70(4):638–42.
42. Gorkemli H, Camus M, Clasen K. Adnexal torsion after gonadotrophin ovulation induction for IVF or ICSI and its conservative treatment. Arch Gynecol Obstet. 2002;267(1):4–6.
43. Mashiach S, et al. Adnexal torsion of hyperstimulated ovaries in pregnancies after gonadotropin therapy. Fertil Steril. 1990;53(1):76–80.
44. Fleischer AC, Brader KR. Sonographic depiction of ovarian vascularity and flow: current improvements and future applications. J Ultrasound Med. 2001;20(3):241–50.
45. Grady R, et al. Elective single embryo transfer and perinatal outcomes: a systematic review and meta-analysis. Fertil Steril. 2012;97(2):324–31.
46. Katalinic A, et al. Pregnancy course and outcome after intracytoplasmic sperm injection: a controlled, prospective cohort study. Fertil Steril. 2004;81(6):1604–16.
47. Raber W, et al. Thyroxine treatment modified in infertile women according to thyroxine-releasing hormone testing: 5 year follow-up of 283 women referred after exclusion of absolute causes of infertility. Hum Reprod. 2003;18(4):707–14.
48. Ehrmann DA. Polycystic ovary syndrome. N Engl J Med. 2005;352(12):1223–36.
49. Sutcliffe AG, Ludwig M. Outcome of assisted reproduction. Lancet. 2007;370(9584):351–9.
50. Pezeshki K, et al. Bleeding and spontaneous abortion after therapy for infertility. Fertil Steril. 2000;74(3):504–8.
51. Wang JX, Norman RJ, Wilcox AJ. Incidence of spontaneous abortion among pregnancies produced by assisted reproductive technology. Hum Reprod. 2004;19(2):272–7.
52. Ludwig M, et al. Heterotopic pregnancy in a spontaneous cycle: do not forget about it! Eur J Obstet Gynecol Reprod Biol. 1999;87(1):91–3.
53. Kennedy, R. Risks and complications of assisted conception. British Fertility Society Factsheet 2005 [cited 2012 01.10.2012]. Available from: http://www.britishfertilitysociety.org.uk/public/factsheets/docs/BFS-risksandcomplicationsofassistedconception.pdf.
54. Winder S, Reid S, Condous G. Ultrasound diagnosis of ectopic pregnancy. Australas J Ultrasound Med. 2011;14(2):29–33.

55. Noci I, et al. Interference of exogenous HCG on pregnancy tests. Acta Eur Fertil. 1987;18(6):391–3.
56. Fauser BC, Devroey P, Macklon NS. Multiple birth resulting from ovarian stimulation for subfertility treatment. Lancet. 2005;365(9473):1807–16.
57. Blickstein I. Estimation of iatrogenic monozygotic twinning rate following assisted reproduction: pitfalls and caveats. Am J Obstet Gynecol. 2005;192(2):365–8.
58. Vela G, et al. Monozygotic pregnancies conceived by in vitro fertilization: understanding their prognosis. Fertil Steril. 2011;95(2):606–10.
59. Vitthala S, et al. The risk of monozygotic twins after assisted reproductive technology: a systematic review and meta-analysis. Hum Reprod Update. 2009;15(1):45–55.
60. Wilcox L, et al. Assisted reproductive technologies: estimates of their contribution to multiple births and newborn hospital days in the United States. Fertil Steril. 1996;65(2):361–6.
61. Milki AA, et al. Incidence of monozygotic twinning with blastocyst transfer compared to cleavage-stage transfer. Fertil Steril. 2003;79(3):503–6.
62. HFEA. Improving outcomes for fertility patients: multiple births. 2011 [cited 2012 15.10.2012]. Available from: http://www.hfea.gov.uk/docs/2011-12-01_-_Multiple_Births_Publication_2011_-_Rationalising_Register_Data_-_FINAL_1.2.DOC.pdf.
63. Janvier A, Spelke B, Barrington KJ. The epidemic of multiple gestations and neonatal intensive care unit use: the cost of irresponsibility. J Pediatr. 2011;159(3):409–13.
64. Joy J, McClure N, Cooke IE. A comparison of spontaneously conceived twins and twins conceived by artificial reproductive technologies. J Obstet Gynaecol. 2008;28(6):580–5.
65. Morcel K, et al. Perinatal morbidity and mortality in twin pregnancies with dichorionic placentas following assisted reproductive techniques or ovarian induction alone: a comparative study. Eur J Obstet Gynecol Reprod Biol. 2010;153(2):138–42.
66. McDonald SD, et al. Preterm birth and low birth weight among in vitro fertilization singletons: a systematic review and meta-analyses. Eur J Obstet Gynecol Reprod Biol. 2009;146(2):138–48.
67. Vilska S, et al. Mental health of mothers and fathers of twins conceived via assisted reproduction treatment: a 1-year prospective study. Hum Reprod. 2009;24(2):367–77.
68. Society of Obstetricians annd Gynaecologists of Canada, Okun N, Sierra S. Pregnancy outcomes after assisted human reproduction. J Obstet Gynaecol Can. 2014;36(1):64–83.
69. Skiadas CC, et al. Spontaneous reduction before 12 weeks' gestation and selective reduction similarly extend time to delivery in in vitro fertilization of trichorionic-triamniotic triplets. Fertil Steril. 2011;95(2):596–9.
70. Stone J, et al. Contemporary outcomes with the latest 1000 cases of multifetal pregnancy reduction (MPR). Am J Obstet Gynecol. 2008;199(4):406.e1–4.
71. Calhoun KC, et al. Evaluating the association between assisted conception and the severity of preeclampsia. ISRN Obstet Gynecol. 2011;2011:928592.
72. Healy DL, et al. Prevalence and risk factors for obstetric haemorrhage in 6730 singleton births after assisted reproductive technology in Victoria Australia. Hum Reprod. 2010;25(1):265–74.
73. Reefhuis J, et al. Assisted reproductive technology and major structural birth defects in the United States. Hum Reprod. 2009;24(2):360–6.
74. Basso O, Olsen J. Subfecundity and neonatal mortality: longitudinal study within the Danish national birth cohort. BMJ. 2005;330(7488):393–4.
75. Leunens L, et al. Follow-up of cognitive and motor development of 10-year-old singleton children born after ICSI compared with spontaneously conceived children. Hum Reprod. 2008;23(1):105–11.

Chapter 6
Early Pregnancy Support: Evidence-Based Management

Valarmathy Kandavel and Siobhan Quenby

Introduction

The physiology of very early pregnancy is a complex mechanism that happens over a narrow window of opportunity against a background of synchronised hormonal and immune factors that lead up to the adequate preparation of the endometrium for the implanting embryo. The peak of the LH surge precedes ovulation by 10–12 h initiated by the raise in the levels of oestrogen. The endometrium transforms into a highly modified endometrium referred as decidua. The decidualisation is dependent on oestrogen, progesterone and other factors secreted by the implanting blastocyst and are complete with the implantation.

The endometrial glands exhibit extensive coiling and luminal secretions become visible. Epithelial cells show decreased microvilli and cilia along with appearances of luminal protrusions of the apical cell surface, referred to as the pinopodes, which are important in preparation for the blastocyst to implant. The crucial steps of successful implantation are detailed in Table 6.1.

Failure of implantation can present as subfertility or miscarriage. Despite advances in understanding the biological and immunological mechanisms underpinning early pregnancy there is a lack of good quality evidence detailing optimal early pregnancy support. We will detail the evidence for the advice that does exist to improve early pregnancy outcomes once pregnancy is achieved. The discussion focuses on the four key elements (Fig. 6.1) throughout the chapter: life style advice

V. Kandavel, MBBS, MRCOG, DGO (✉)
Department of Obstetrics and Gynaecology, University Hospitals of Coventry and Warwickshire NHS Trust, Coventry, UK
e-mail: drvalar2001@yahoo.com

S. Quenby, BSc, MD, FRCOG
Department of Reproductive Health, University of Warwick, University Hospitals Coventry and Warwickshire NHS Trust, Coventry, UK
e-mail: s.quenby@warwick.ac.uk

K. Jayaprakasan, L. Kean (eds.), *Clinical Management of Pregnancies following ART*, DOI 10.1007/978-3-319-42858-1_6

Table 6.1 Crucial initial steps for successful implantation

Apposition – initial embryo contact with the endometrium
Adhesion – further contact of embryo and endometrium
Invasion – of the developing embryo to the endometrium and inner third of the myometrium

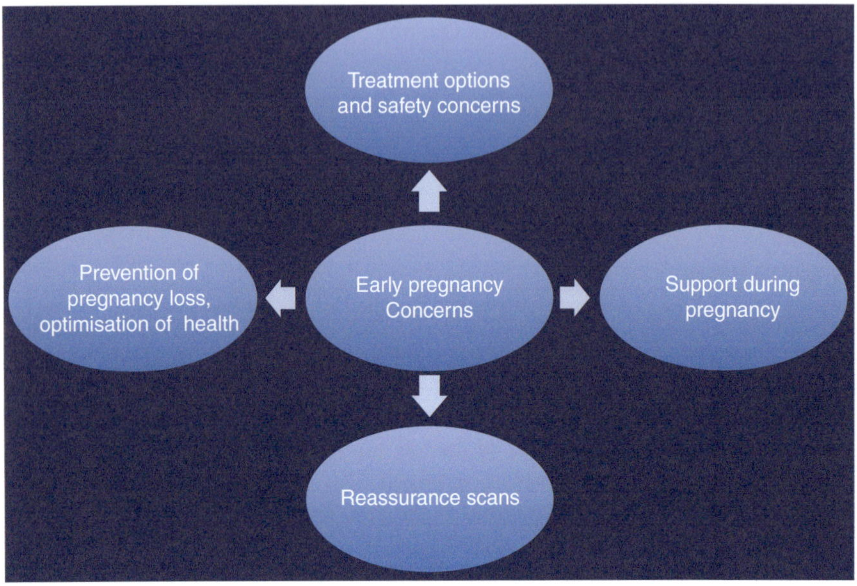

Fig. 6.1 Outline of the expectations of pregnant women from the healthcare professionals [1–7]

to optimise health, pharmacological interventions and safety, ultrasound for reassurance and supportive care during pregnancy.

Life Style Advice

There is information overload regarding life style choices and advice with conflicting headline grabbing evidence presented to women and their partners. The role of clinical staff supporting women is to present the current evidence in relation to those options which enables the women to choose effectively. The most common choices are included in the discussion that follows.

Smoking

There is a dose dependent association between smoking and outcomes such as abruption, stillbirth, recurrent pregnancy loss, decline in ovarian reserve and fertility, intrauterine growth restriction and placental insufficiency. The evidence is particularly strong with smoking > 20 cigarettes per day. The recommendation is that women stop smoking in pregnancy and evidence suggests that those that do are likely to permanently quit smoking. A review comparing different options of nicotine replacement to help women to stop suggests that after the exclusion of studies with bias, there is no difference in the fetal outcomes between the treatment and the placebo group [8]. The SNAP trial of nicotine replacement reported that there was survival without developmental disorder at the 2 year follow up for babies, making this a safe option for women, but no more likely to be successful than placebo [9].

Use of E-Cigarettes

There is heavy public advertising and marketing of e-cigarettes as a safe alternative to smoking. Though e-cigarettes reduce the harm from carbon monoxide, carcinogens and toxins that contribute to lung cancer, e-cigarettes are still addictive secondary to nicotine release. A published article from 2016 confirms the positive effect of reduction of harm secondary to the carcinogens and toxins in the smoke [10]. There is no published evidence of benefit of use in pregnant women. Until more evidence is available, the advice would be not to recommend e-cigarettes due to variable amounts of caffeine and absorption of inhalational agents of unproven safety.

Alcohol

Alcohol affects fertility and pregnancy outcomes in a dose dependent manner with the well recognised fetal alcohol syndrome relating to excessive alcohol consumption in pregnancy. Consumption of greater than 7 units of alcohol/week is associated with growth restriction and can lead to increased risk of behavioural problems and learning difficulties in children [11]. The current national guidelines also comments that there is no health benefit related to alcohol [12]. Standard advice should be to stop alcohol consumption ideally prior to a planned pregnancy and that there is no safe limit in pregnancy.

Exercise

There is no published evidence to suggest an adverse pregnancy outcome secondary to excessive exercise. Due to the detrimental effects of obesity in pregnancy the advice is to continue with moderate exercise during pregnancy. The review of the effect of aerobic exercise on pregnancy is that it improves maternal fitness [13].

Vitamin Supplementation

Folic Acid

Folic acid is recommended as a pre-conception vitamin supplementation from the time of trying for a pregnancy up to the end of the first trimester in order to prevent neural tube defects. Folic acid deficiency can also contribute to anaemia in the mother.

The Cochrane review of Folic acid supplementation in pregnancy (2013) [14] looked into the evidence from 31 trials (involving 17,771 women) regarding folic acid supplements during pregnancy and the effect on the baby. Whilst there was beneficial improvement in folate indicators in the mother, there was no reduction in the risk of preterm births, low birth weight, stillbirth and neonatal death. The review also did not show any impact of folate supplementation on improving mean birth weight and the mother's mean hemoglobin levels during pregnancy compared with taking a placebo.

The Cochrane review of the effects of folic acid supplementation pre-pregnancy to 12 weeks of pregnancy (2015) [15] found evidence of reduction of the occurrence of both first and second time occurrence of neural tube defects (NTDs). However, there was insufficient evidence to determine if it prevents other defects such as cleft lip with or without cleft palate and congenital cardiovascular disorders.

There were insufficient data to evaluate the effects of folic acid supplementation in prevention of miscarriage, though the quality of evidence was rated as moderate. The data from the Folic acid supplementation during pregnancy [14] review also did not find any conclusive evidence regarding the benefit of folic acid in the prevention of pregnancy loss.

High dose folate is indicated certain condition such as previous NTDs, epilepsy, obesity, MHTFR mutation, sickle cell disease and for women living in areas of high prevalence of malaria. In the absence of these specific factors there are no beneficial effects of high dose folic acid supplementation and concern in some women that this may be harmful by masking vitamin b12 deficiency.

Vitamin D

There is an association between vitamin D deficiency and miscarriage, but no causality has been established. A recent study has established that up to 50 % of the population in the UK has vitamin D deficiency with a higher prevalence in obese women. Routine calcium and vitamin D supplementation is recommended for pregnant women due to the prevalence and the increased demand of calcium metabolism during pregnancy. Vitamin D is essential for calcium homeostasis and calcium metabolism [16].

A Cochrane review [16] included 15 randomised controlled trials involving 2833 women. Nine trials compared the effects of vitamin D alone with no supplementation or a placebo and six trials compared the effects of vitamin D and calcium with no supplementation.

With vitamin D supplementation, the 25-hydroxyvitamin D concentrations at term improve. This reduces the risk of a low birth weight baby (less than 2500 g) and of both preterm delivery less than 37 weeks and developing high blood pressure.

Data on adverse effects for the mother were not well reported. The authors conclude that further randomised trials are required to confirm the effects of vitamin D supplementation and effects on birth weight and blood pressure.

It is unclear if routine supplementation should be recommended during pregnancy.

Caffeine Intake

There is a dose related effect on pregnancy with an increased risk of miscarriage at higher levels. Women should be advised to limit the amount of caffeine to 150 mg/day; equivalent to two cups of normal coffee or three cups of black tea. One study has shown an adverse profile if levels are greater than 300 mg/day [17]. However, the Cochrane review concluded that there was insufficient evidence to correlate the fetal outcomes with maternal caffeine consumption due to the low quality of the studies [18].

Complimentary Therapy

Acupuncture is a well-established mode of complimentary therapy that aims at helping women cope with the stress of subfertility, miscarriage and pregnancy. There are well-established studies that have shown improvements in coping with stress after acupuncture but not in the prevention of miscarriage [19].

Weight

Reproductive outcomes are worse in both underweight (BMI < 18) and obese women (BMI > 30). Any further excessive weight gain in obese women accentuates the adverse perinatal and neonatal outcomes. There is an increased risk of intra-uterine growth restriction, stillbirth, operative deliveries and increased morbidity secondary to infection and thromboembolism. Unfortunately diet and exercise interventions in pregnancy have not shown an impact on neonatal outcome (Cochrane meta-analysis 2015) [20].

However, lifestyle interventions do reduce excessive maternal weight gain and development of maternal hypertension and possibly reduce the risk of caesarean section. Therefore pre-pregnancy advice on diet and exercise to women with high BMI should be routine.

There is no established safety profile for appetite suppressants in pregnancy. The recently published EMPOWAR study [21] did not show any benefit in terms neonatal outcomes for metformin supplementation in women with obesity. The study published in *NEJM* randomised women with BMI > 35 to metformin supplementation or placebo showed a reduction in maternal weight gain but no difference in the neonatal weight in the treatment arm [22].

Pharmacological Interventions to Support Pregnancy

There is a wealth of information and treatment options available to women who undergo ART preconception and during their pregnancy. The only ones of proven benefits are for the following:

- Luteal phase support with progesterone during IVF
- Use of heparin in pregnancy for women with acquired thrombophilia
- Thyroxine in women with clinical hypothyroidism

Progesterone

The Cochrane review suggests that luteal phase progesterone during assisted reproduction improves pregnancy and live birth rates [23]. However, once pregnancy is achieved it is less clear when to discontinue the treatment. Offering luteal phase support for an extended period of time do not appear to result in more clinical benefits, or to cause more harm, than a short period of luteal phase support. While the evidence on this is limited, NICE suggests that it is biologically plausibile for luteal phase support to be effective for up to 8 weeks after embryo transfer, after which time the pregnancy is self supporting.

A review of 14 randomized controlled trials (2158 women) found no evidence that routine use of progestogens can prevent miscarriages [24]. No difference in the incidence of adverse effects on either the mother or baby was apparent. There was evidence that women who have suffered three or more miscarriages may benefit from progestogen during pregnancy. Four trials showed a decrease in miscarriage compared with placebo or no treatment in these women; however, the trials were of poorer methodological quality so these findings should be interpreted with caution. The recently published robust large multicentre double blinded randomised controlled trial (PROMISE trial) [25] did not show any reduction in the miscarriage rates or improvement in live birth rates in women who suffered from recurrent miscarriages and randomised to progesterone support or placebo in early pregnancy

In the case of threatened miscarriage, a systematic review of trials located four randomised studies involving 421 women that compared the use of progestogens in the treatment of threatened miscarriage with either placebo or no treatment [26]. The limited evidence suggests that the use of a progestogen does reduce the rate of spontaneous miscarriage. Two trials reported that treatment with progestogens did not increase the occurrence of congenital abnormalities in the newborns and the women did not have any significant difference in incidence of pregnancy-induced hypertension and antepartum haemorrhage. Further larger studies are warranted for firmer conclusions. The on-going PRISM trial is powered to definitively answer the question as to whether there is a role for progesterone in early pregnancy bleeding [27].

Heparin

The Cochrane database suggests that in antiphospholipid syndrome and recurrent miscarriage, unfractionated heparin is effective at preventing miscarriage but this was not confirmed in the one trial using low molecular weight heparin (LMWH) [28]. However, the evidence from unfractionated heparin was of such a large magnitude that it is now routine practice to give LMWH to women with antiphospholipid syndrome and recurrent miscarriage. There is a dearth of evidence as to the management of women with inherited thrombophilia with conflicting results from the published studies. The on-going multicentre randomised controlled trial (ALIFE2) [29] will shed light on the treatment of women with inherited thrombophilia especially with recurrent pregnancy loss. Peri-implantation LMWH may improve implantation in IVF but the trials are of insufficient quality to draw firm conclusions [30]. LMWH has been demonstrated to have no effect at preventing miscarriage during pregnancy in idiopathic recurrent miscarriage in several trials [31].

Aspirin

Low dose aspirin is indicated for women who are considered high risk for developing pre-eclampsia. In the United Kingdom low dose aspirin is recommended to be commenced from 12 weeks of pregnancy until labour in women at high risk of hypertensive disease in pregnancy [32]. A systematic review showed no benefit from low dose aspirin in preventing miscarriage in unexplained recurrent miscarriage. In one large randomised controlled trial there was a lower live birth rate in women with unexplained recurrent miscarriage in women taking aspirin than placebo and so should not be used for this indication [33].

Steroids

One small study suggested an improvement in pregnancy outcomes in women treated with prednisolone with raised uterine natural killer cells and recurrent miscarriage [34]. Prednisolone in early pregnancy has been associated with gestational diabetes, preterm birth. Until large randomised controlled trails have established the efficacy of prednisolone, its use as a treatment option remains in research settings only.

Immunotherapy

The immune mechanisms of recurrent implantation failure and recurrent pregnancy loss postulate the rejection of the embryo by the mother. Injection of paternal leucocytes in early pregnancy was done initially to overcome the postulated rejection phenomenon. Intravenous immunoglobulin has been subject to a series of randomised controlled trials and has potential side effects including anaphylaxis. Paternal cell immunization, third-party donor leukocytes, trophoblast membranes, and intravenous immunoglobulin provide no significant beneficial effect over placebo in improving the live birth rate. TNF-Alpha use is associated with severe reactions such as immunosuppression and granulomatous disease.

However, current meta-analysis of evidence has shown no benefits from the immunotherapy approaches in preventing miscarriage [35].

Use of Granulocyte Colony Stimulating Factor (G-CSF)

Has shown promising results from the use in women with recurrent implantation failure; persistent thin endometrium and recurrent miscarriage [36]. However, there have been no published randomised control trial evidence and therefore there is currently no role in early pregnancy support.

Use of Human Chorionic Gonadotropin

Improved pregnancy outcomes in women with oligomenorrhoea and suspected luteal phase deficiency have been reported [37] but the studies are not large enough to support the routine use of HCG for pregnancy support, outside of a research setting. A Cochrane review of HCG in recurrent miscarriage included five studies (involving 596 women) and suggested a statistically significant reduction in miscarriage rate using HCG. The number of women needed to treat to prevent subsequent pregnancy loss was seven. However, when two studies of weaker methodological quality were removed, there was no longer a statistically significant benefit (risk ratio 0.74; 95 % confidence interval 0.44–1.23). There were no documented adverse effects of using HCG. The evidence supporting HCG supplementation to prevent RM remains equivocal. A well-designed randomised controlled trial of adequate power and methodological quality is required to determine whether HCG is beneficial in RM [38].

A Cochrane review of HCG for threatened miscarriage included three trials (with a total of 312 participants), found no evidence that HCG is effective as treatment for threatened miscarriage. There was no report on adverse effects of HCG on the mother or baby. More good-quality research is needed to study the impact of HCG on miscarriage [39].

Ultrasound in Early Pregnancy for Reassurance

The waiting period between the embryo transfer and pregnancy test is a period of uncertainty and anxiety and is stressful for the couple. The evidence for supportive care is predominantly from the management of women with recurrent miscarriage and pregnancy loss. Women who undergo ART experience emotional, physical and physiological stress associated with the burden of expectations and the impending fear of failure and anxiety surrounding the outcomes. This heightened sense of anxiety is worse during the waiting time between embryo transfer and pregnancy test.

The IVF protocol of units will accommodate a viability scan for all patients who underwent embryo transfer between 6 and 7 weeks of gestation. The positive information given is important and begins with a pregnancy test signalling the implantation and possible selective selection of an embryo. The ultrasound identification of an intra uterine pregnancy rules out ectopic sites of implantation. The ultrasound identification of the presence of cardiac activity adds additional reassurance as the risk of miscarriage falls significantly to 9 % at 6 weeks and further down to 0.5 % at 9 weeks. Further pregnancy care and scan will be arranged as offered routinely for any pregnancy.

While this approach is suitable for most patients, the expectations of patients with previous repeated failed IVF cycles or previous pregnancy loss would be for earlier access to ultrasound assessment of pregnancy and repeated reassurance scans. Musters et al, who conducted a qualitative research study examining the supportive care options for women who suffered from recurrent pregnancy loss, further confirmed this [1]. This was an explorative semi-structured in depth interview of 20 different options that were presented to the 17 participating women. Data were published from the interviews of 15 women excluding the two pilot study entrants. Sixteen options were preferred for the next pregnancy and four options were rejected. Examples of the preferred supportive care were early and frequently repeated ultrasounds, βHCG monitoring, practical advice concerning life style and diet, emotional support in the form of counselling, a clear formulated plan including medications for the upcoming 12 weeks of pregnancy. Though the women acknowledged the heightened anxiety in the lead up to the scans, they still wanted the scans for reassurance and certainty that the pregnancy was ongoing.

The setting for the delivery of such services would be in a specialist clinic such as early pregnancy unit or recurrent miscarriage clinics, which are generally staffed by permanent team members. This would ensure continuity of care for the patients, familiarity with the team and the patient preference of avoiding meeting and recounting the history to several clinicians. This helps the patient and partner to build rapport with the clinician, adhere to advice, and have an agreed discussion based on the expectations with the individual couple. The setting should ideally have published protocols and adherence to the emerging evidence. Practise and outcomes should be monitored regularly against the guidelines. The research evidence must be updated and the management changed accordingly when new evidence emerges as the field is moving quickly.

Li recommends having a specialist clinic for a population of two million to adequately counsel, manage and support couples using the early pregnancy clinic service [2]. Dedicated specialist clinics should reduce the variation of practise among the clinicians and reduce the widespread use of empirical unproven treatments. The published evidence from the recurrent miscarriage/one stop clinics suggests that the scans can be offered fortnightly from 6 weeks until 12 weeks [3, 4]. Further scans can be offered for on-going support based on the anxiety of the individual patient. The one stop clinic set up in Leicester [5] significantly reduced the waiting times to access a specialist with reported live birth rate of around 67 % in women who have previously suffered from three or more miscarriages. This was possibly due to the extensive work up by investigations and tailored treatment along with supportive care.

Supportive Care

Women are routinely offered an early pregnancy scan at the fertility clinic where they are having ART. For women, who have had recurrent pregnancy losses or adverse reproductive outcome, a tailored approach is suggested to offer women support, advice and reassurance ultrasound in a dedicated setting such as Early pregnancy unit or Recurrent miscarriage clinic with a multi disciplinary team of doctors, midwives, nurses and/or psychologists.

Women who suffer from negative reproductive outcomes suffer from guilt, depression, anxiety, and psychological trauma similar to bereavement. Patients undergoing treatment for subfertility and patients with recurrent miscarriage suffer the most. There is widespread published evidence supporting the distress suffered by women with failed outcomes. 1:5 women who experience miscarriage have anxiety levels similar to people attending the psychiatric outpatient services. One-third of the women attending specialist clinics as a result of miscarriage are clinically depressed [40].

A small prospective study of 45 women evaluating the psychological component of pregnancy loss was done after two first trimester miscarriages, with other causes eliminated. Self report questionnaires and interviews before their next pregnancy showed that ten pregnancies (22.2 %) resulted in a miscarriage. The degree of baseline depressive symptoms predicted the rate of miscarriage [41]. Recurrent pregnancy loss patients are prone to heightened anger, depression, anxiety and feelings of guilt and grief.

A study from Japan showed statistically significant higher scores of mental distress as assessed by the Kesler score in women with recurrent unexplained pregnancy loss. The study acknowledged that the significance of mental state and the cardiovascular risk factors in women with unexplained recurrent pregnancy loss needs to be clarified [42]. Kolte et al. also encountered indices suggestive of high levels of stress on the PSS (perceived stress scale) among women who attended their specialist clinic [43]. Feelings of guilt and self-blame typical of depressive disorders, were highly prevalent in women with recurrent pregnancy loss. Whilst patients scored high on the MDI (Major Depressive Inventory) there was no association with lower chance of on-going pregnancy and live birth rate. A successful outcome lowered the scores in a follow up assessment. This study is useful to counsel women regarding the emotional affects of negative reproductive outcomes but can be reassured that they do not adversely affect the future pregnancy outcomes [44].

Treatment for subfertility and pregnancy loss places huge stress and strain in the marital relationship. This is due to the differing methods of coping mechanisms adopted by men and women. This can sometimes lead to the woman feeling isolated with lack of acknowledgement. Hence any support or therapy should ideally be directed to the couple rather than just the woman. Men usually feel that they are not spoken to or in the periphery of the decision making process. The acknowledgement and support from friends and family contributes positively to the emotional wellbeing of the pregnant mother. A clinical nurse with training in counselling skills or a professional psychologist can offer counselling. The women in the study by Kolte et al. rejected the option of counselling by their family doctor. Acknowledgement of the anxiety and support by the caring clinician helps women cope with the pregnancy and the outcomes even if negative.

The evidence for the use and efficacy of supportive care in early pregnancy is derived from management of patients with recurrent miscarriage or pregnancy loss. The earliest evidence is from Pedersen and Pedersen 1984 who managed women with unexplained recurrent pregnancy loss [6]. In the 85 women with the diagnosis there were 61 conceptions that were either assigned to tailored supportive antenatal care or no specific care. The outcomes in the two groups were statistically significantly different. Whilst 86 % of the pregnancies in the supportive group reached term gestation in the supportive group, the outcomes in the other group of patients was 67 % (p value <0.001). Though the study was offered to only patients who lived close to the hospital it nevertheless paved way for more studies to evaluate the novel concept of supportive care in pregnancy. A subsequent study by Clifford et al. from UK confirmed that the rates of miscarriage was significantly lower in women who attended the early pregnancy clinic at 26 % vs. the 51 % repeat miscarriage in women who did not attend the specialist clinic [7]. The exact mechanism by which supportive care improves outcomes is not understood. Not all women with the supportive care package will have a successful outcome. However, the support that they received in the pregnancy will equip them to face and prepare for the pregnancy with confidence.

The evidence for the supportive care comes from the participation of Caucasian women in the developed countries. The participation and representation of ethnic minority women and as a couple should be encouraged. The small number of ethnic minority women in the study by Musters et al. chose a different set of options to the native Dutch women. The limited evidence suggests that they are less likely to depend on family members and peer group support and would rely on the support and treatment from clinicians [1].

Research Participation

Management of women in dedicated clinics provides the opportunity for women to participate in clinical trials to guide evidence-based management. There is still ambiguity and variation in the management of early pregnancy issues. The study by Musters et al. from the Netherlands also reported the willingness of women to participate in scientific research. The reasons behind the participation were twofold-contribution to the greater good and personal gains for themselves [1]. The Miscarriage Association Patient Information Leaflet acknowledges that taking part in a clinical trial can be helpful, even if the treatment does not turn out to be effective. It states that "patients taking part in the trial tend to get additional care and monitoring and there is some evidence that enhanced care can have a positive impact in reducing miscarriage rates." A review by Tang and Quenby concluded that women should be encouraged to participate in studies with robust questions and methodology so as to optimise investigations and treatment modalities [45]. Li et al. discuss the difficulties surrounding the set up, planning and statistical considerations required in research studies involving a sensitive and multifactorial early pregnancy issue such as recurrent miscarriage [2]. There is a current feasibility study to assess the efficacy of PCRI (Positive Reinforcement and Coping Intervention) for women who are in the waiting period of their next pregnancy. The PRCI is a novel self-administered supportive technique, which has been shown to be effective in patients awaiting the outcome of in vitro fertilisation treatment [46].

Conclusion

Early pregnancy care to women undergoing ART should be tailored specific to her pregnancy. While progesterone luteal support following IVF, heparin in acquired thrombophilia, and thyroxin in hypothyroidism are proven to be the beneficial pharmacological interventions, most of the other interventions commonly employed to support early pregnancy are not evidence based and are to be tested in robust randomised controlled trials. Women and couples undergoing ART experience emotional, physical and physiological stress associated with the burden of expectations and the impending fear of failure and anxiety surrounding the outcomes. Ultrasound and supportive care along with provision of counselling service in a specialist clinic offers the best choice for these patients.

References

1. Musters AM, Taminiau-Bloem EF, van den Boogaard E, van der Veen F, Goddijn M. Supportive care for women with unexplained recurrent miscarriage: patient's perspectives. Hum Reprod. 2011;26(4):873–7.
2. Li TC. Recurrent miscarriage: principles of management. Hum Reprod. 1998;13(2):478–82.
3. Van den Berg MM, Vissenberg R, Goddijn M. Recurrent miscarriage clinics. Obstet Gynecol Clin N Am. 2014;41:145–55.
4. Nikcevic DAV, Tunkel SA, Nicolaides KH. psychological outcomes following missed abortions and provision of follow-up care. Ultrasound Obstet Gynecol. 1998;11(2):123–8.
5. Habayeb OM, Konje JC. The one-stop recurrent miscarriage clinic: an evaluation of its effectiveness and outcome. Hum Reprod. 2004;19(12):2952–8.
6. Stray-Pedersen B, Stray-Pedersen A. Etiologic factors and subsequent reproductive performance in 195 couples with a prior history of habitual abortion. Am J Obstet Gynecol. 1984;148.
7. Clifford K, Rai R, Regan L. Future pregnancy outcome in unexplained recurrent first trimester miscarriage. Hum Reprod. 1997;12(2):387–9.
8. Coleman T, Chamberlain C, Davey M, Cooper SE, Leonardi-Bee J. Pharmacological interventions for promoting smoking cessation during pregnancy. Cochrane Database Syst Rev. 2015;(12):CD010078.
9. Cooper S, Lewis S, Thornton JG, Marlow N, Watts K, Britton J, Grainge MJ, Taggar J, Essex H, Parrott S, Dickinson A, Whitemore R, Coleman T. The SNAP trial: a randomised placebo-controlled trial of nicotine replacement therapy in pregnancy—clinical effectiveness and safety until 2 years after delivery, with economic evaluation; Smoking, Nicotine and Pregnancy Trial Team. Health Technol Assess. 2014;18(54):1–128.
10. Britton J, McNeill A, Hopkinson N. Nicotine without smoke: putting electronic cigarettes in context. BMJ. 2016;353:i1745.
11. Stade BC, Bailey C, Dzendoletas D, Sgro M, Dowswell T, Bennett D. Psychological and/or educational interventions for reducing alcohol consumption in pregnant women and women planning pregnancy. Cochrane Database Syst Rev. 2009;(2):CD004228.
12. Department of Health. Health risks from alcohol: new guidelines. 8 Jan 2016.
13. Kramer MS, McDonald SW. Aerobic exercise for women during pregnancy. Cochrane Database Syst Rev. 2006;(3):CD000180.
14. Lassi ZS, Salam RA, Haider BA, Bhutta ZA. Folic acid supplementation during pregnancy for maternal health and pregnancy outcomes. Cochrane Database Syst Rev. 2013;(3):CD006896.
15. De-Regil L, Peña-Rosas J, Fernández-Gaxiola AC, Rayco-Solon P. Effects and safety of periconceptional oral folate supplementation for preventing birth defects. Cochrane Database Syst Rev. 2015;(12):CD007950.
16. De-Regil L, Palacios C, Lombardo LK, Peña-Rosas J. Vitamin D supplementation for women during pregnancy. Cochrane Database Syst Rev. 2016;(1):CD008873.
17. Martin TR, Bracken MB. The association between low birth weight and caffeine consumption during pregnancy. Am J Epidemiol. 1987;126(5):813–21.

18. Jahanfar S, Jaafar S. Effects of restricted caffeine intake by mother on fetal, neonatal and pregnancy outcomes. Cochrane Database Syst Rev. 2015;(6):CD006965.
19. Wing Sze E, Hung Yu Ng E. Acupuncture in reproductive medicine. Womens Health. 2010;6(4):551–63.
20. Furber CM, McGowan L, Bower P, Kontopantelis E, Quenby S, Lavender T. Antenatal interventions for reducing weight in obese women for improving pregnancy outcome. Cochrane Database Syst Rev. 2013;(1):CD009334.
21. Chiswick C, Reynolds RM, Denison F, et al. Effect of metformin on maternal and fetal outcomes in obese pregnant women (EMPOWaR): a randomised, double-blind, placebo-controlled trial. Lancet Diabet Endocrinol. 2015;3(10):778–86.
22. Syngelaki A, Nicolaides KH, Balani J, Hyer S, Akolekar R, Kotecha R, Pastides A, Shehata H. Metformin versus placebo in obese pregnant women without diabetes mellitus. N Engl J Med. 2016;374:434–43.
23. van der Linden M, Buckingham K, Farquhar C, Kremer JAM, Metwally M. Luteal phase support for assisted reproduction cycles. Cochrane Database Syst Rev. 2015;(7):CD009154.
24. Coomarasamy A, Williams H, Truchanowicz E, Seed PT, Small R, Quenby S, Gupta P, Dawood F, Koot Y, Atik RB, Bloemenkamp KWM, Brady R, Briley AL, Cavallaro R, Cheong YC, Chu JJ, Eapen A, Ewies A, Hoek A, Kaaijk EM, Koks CAM, Li T-C, MacLean M, Mol BW, Moore J, Ross JA, Sharpe L, Stewart J, Vaithilingam N, Farquharson RG, Kilby MD, Khalaf Y, Goddijn M, Regan L, Rai R. A randomized trial of progesterone in women with recurrent miscarriages. N Engl J Med. 2015;373:2141–8.
25. Haas DM, Ramsey PS. Progestogen for preventing miscarriage. Cochrane Database Syst Rev. 2013;(10):CD003511.
26. Wahabi HA, Fayed AA, Esmaeil SA, Al Zeidan RA. Progestogen for treating threatened miscarriage. Cochrane Database Syst Rev. 2011;(12):CD005943.
27. The PRISM study is a large randomised, double-blind and placebo-controlled multi-centre trial of the effectiveness of progesterone in reducing miscarriage rates in women with early pregnancy bleeding. The PRISM trial is funded solely by NIHR-HTA (UK). http://www.birmingham.ac.uk/research/activity/mds/trials/bctu.
28. de Jong PG, Kaandorp S, Di Nisio M, Goddijn M, Middeldorp S. Aspirin and/or heparin for women with unexplained recurrent miscarriage with or without inherited thrombophilia. Cochrane Database Syst Rev. 2014;(7):CD004734.
29. de Jong PG, Quenby S, Bloemenkamp KWM, Braams-Lisman BAM, de Bruin JP, Coomarasamy A, David M, DeSancho MT, van der Heijden OWH, Hoek A, Hutten BA, Jochmans K, Koks CAM, Kuchenbecker WH, Mol BWJ, Torrance HL, Scheepers HCJ, Stephenson MD, Verhoeve HR, Visser JV, de Vries JIP, Goddijn M, Middeldorp S. ALIFE2 study: low-molecular-weight heparin for women with recurrent miscarriage and inherited thrombophilia – study protocol for a randomized controlled trial. Trials. 2015;16:208.
30. Akhtar MA, Sur S, Raine-Fenning N, Jayaprakasan K, Thornton JG, Quenby S. Heparin for assisted reproduction. Cochrane Database Syst Rev. 2013;(8):CD009452.
31. Check JH. The use of heparin for preventing miscarriage. Am J Reprod Immunol. 2012;67(4):326–33.
32. Hypertension in pregnancy: diagnosis and management NICE guidelines [CG107]. Published date: Aug 2010. Last updated: Jan 2011.
33. Kaandorp SP, Goddijn M, van der Post JA, Hutten BA, Verhoeve HR, Hamulyák K, Mol BW, Folkeringa N, Nahuis M, Papatsonis DN, Büller HR, van der Veen F, Middeldorp S. Aspirin plus heparin or aspirin alone in women with recurrent miscarriage. N Engl J Med. 2010;362(17):1586–96.
34. Tang AW, Alfirevic Z, Turner MA, Drury JA, Small R, Quenby S. A feasibility trial of screening women with idiopathic recurrent miscarriage for high uterine natural killer cell density and randomizing to prednisolone or placebo when pregnant. Hum Reprod. 2013;28(7):1743–52.
35. Wong LF, Porter T, Scott JR. Immunotherapy for recurrent miscarriage. Cochrane Database Syst Rev. 2014;(10):CD000112.

36. Zeyneloglu HB, Onalan G. Remedies for recurrent implantation failure. Semin Reprod Med. 2014;32(4):297–305.
37. Quenby S, Farquharson RG. Human chorionic gonadotropin supplementation in recurring pregnancy loss: a controlled trial. Fertility Sterility. 1994;62(4):708–10.
38. Morley LC, Simpson N, Tang T. Human chorionic gonadotrophin (hCG) for preventing miscarriage. Cochrane Database Syst Rev. 2013;(1):CD008611.
39. Devaseelan P, Fogarty PP, Regan L. Human chorionic gonadotrophin for threatened miscarriage. Cochrane Database Syst Rev. 2010;(5):CD007422.
40. Rai L, Regan L. Recurrent miscarriage. Lancet. 2006;601–11.
41. American Society for Reproductive Medicine. Evaluation and treatment of recurrent pregnancy loss: a committee opinion. Fertil Steril. 2012;98:1103–11.
42. Kataoka K, Tomiya Y, Sakamoto A, Kamada Y, Hiramatsu Y, Nakatsuka M. Altered autonomic nervous system activity in women with unexplained recurrent pregnancy loss. J Obstet Gynaecol Res. 2015;41(6):912–8.
43. Kolte AM, Olsen LR, Mikkelsen EM, Christiansen OB, Nielsen HS. Depression and emotional stress is highly prevalent among women with recurrent pregnancy loss. Hum Reprod. 2015;4:777–82.
44. Kolte AM, Olsen LR, Christiansen OB, Nielsen HS. Stress and depression at referral do not entail a lower chance of live birth/ongoing pregnancy for women with recurrent pregnancy loss. Copenhagen University Hospital Rigshospitalet, Recurrent Pregnancy Loss Unit Fertility Clinic Section 4071, Copenhagen, ESHRE 2015 abstract O-168.
45. Tang AW, Quenby S. Recent thoughts on management and prevention of recurrent early pregnancy loss. Curr Opin Obstet Gynecol. 2010;22(6):446–51.
46. Bailey S, Bailey C, Boivin J, Cheong Y, Reading I, Macklon N. A feasibility study for a randomised controlled trial of the positive reappraisal coping intervention, a novel supportive technique for recurrent miscarriage. BMJ Open. 2015;5, e007322.

Chapter 7
Screening for Fetal Abnormalities

Alec McEwan

Introduction

The UK NSC defines screening as "*a process of identifying apparently healthy people who may be at increased risk of a disease or condition. They can then be offered information, further tests and appropriate treatment to reduce their risk and/or any complications arising from the disease or condition.*" A screening test is usually offered to a specific larger population and identifies individuals who are at much higher risk than background of the condition which is being screened for. This smaller group can then be offered *diagnostic tests*, which are usually highly accurate. In the context of pregnancy, this of course means offering tests which will identify women at increased risk of fetal problems such as congenital anomalies (chromosomal and structural) but also fetal growth restriction, gestational diabetes and pre-eclampsia. This chapter focuses on the screening tests available to women aimed at detecting fetal anomalies, with an emphasis on how this screening might be influenced by preceding assisted reproduction.

Before examining these screening tests in detail, it is helpful to revise some of general characteristics of a screening test so that we might better understand what makes a screening test a "good" one and how one screening test compares with another.

The *sensitivity* of a test measures its performance, or its detection rate (DR). If, in a given screened population, there are 100 individuals affected by condition X, and the screening test identifies 85 of these people as being at particularly high risk of X, then the sensitivity is 85 %. Unfortunately, all screening tests will identify some of the unaffected population as high risk, even when they do not actually have

A. McEwan, BA, BM, BCh, MRCOG
Department of Obstetrics and Gynaecology (Queens Medical Centre Campus),
Nottingham University Hospitals NHS Trust, Nottingham, UK
e-mail: Alec.mcewan@nuh.nhs.uk

K. Jayaprakasan, L. Kean (eds.), *Clinical Management of Pregnancies following ART*, DOI 10.1007/978-3-319-42858-1_7

the condition. These are the "*false positives*" and they will be exposed to anxiety and the risks of the subsequent diagnostic tests only to discover later that they were unaffected.

Some screening tests quote the "*screen positive rate*." This totals all of the positives together (true positives plus false positives). It is clear that a "good" screening test should have a high sensitivity and low false positive and screen positive rates. The *positive predictive value* of a screening test (PPV) indicates how likely an individual is to actually have the condition if their screening result is positive (i.e., high risk). This depends very much on the prevalence of the condition in the screened population. A high PPV is ideal for a screening test. However, if the prevalence of the condition is low, then the PPV will be limited because of the high proportion of positive results being "false" positives. Furthermore, the value of these parameters achieved by a screening test is highly dependent on where the threshold is set for a screening result to be deemed positive. The lower this threshold is made, the more cases will be deemed high risk and the higher the detection rate will be. However, this comes at the cost of a higher false positive rate (FPR) and lower PPV. Increasing the threshold reduces the FPR and increases the PPV, but causes a fall in detection rate (sensitivity).

Screening tests should not only be judged by their statistical outcomes. A screening test will inevitably be offered to a large subpopulation (e.g., all pregnant women), so it must be acceptable to those being screened, cost effective, safe and most importantly there must be value in screening for the specific condition. Those deemed "high risk" following screening will then be offered a diagnostic test and this is usually more expensive and hazardous to undertake than the screening test. Whilst waiting for these second line tests, patients will usually be very anxious about the test itself, the potential result and all its implications. It is clear that keeping the false positive rate of a screening test low is of vital importance.

The background incidence of major congenital anomalies (including chromosomal abnormalities) is usually quoted as 2–3 %. Worldwide, many countries now offer all pregnant women screening for the common trisomies (principally Down syndrome) and fetal structural abnormalities. In the UK, screening regimens for fetal anomalies were initially varied, haphazard and poorly standardised until the Fetal Anomaly Screening Programme (FASP) was established by the Department of Health in 2003. It is now overseen by the UK NSC, within Public Health England (PHE), and it has the following aims:

- To provide information so that women can exercise informed choice
- Identify abnormalities inconsistent with life
- Identify abnormalities which may benefit from antenatal treatment
- Identify abnormalities which require early intervention

FASP have systematically defined and monitored screening standards and have supervised a stepwise improvement in Down syndrome screening and the recent introduction of screening for trisomies 18 and 13 (Edward's syndrome and Patau's syndrome). The UK Fetal Anomaly Ultrasound Screening Programme is also working to standardise the aims and outcomes from the second trimester detailed scan so that it also fulfils its role as a screening test. It is clear that where these tests are offered outside of a formal national screening programme, standards fall, detection rates slide and false positives increase.

Screening for Trisomies

It is still the case that a definitive prenatal diagnosis of a chromosomal disorder can only be made by invasive testing with amniocentesis or chorionic villus sampling. These carry a 0.5–1.0 % risk of causing a miscarriage, and it is this fact which prevents some women from choosing screening or diagnostic testing for these conditions. The UK screening programme offers screening for T21, 18 and 13, with opt out for T21 available to mothers. The discussion here will focus mostly on screening for Down syndrome, with a mention of these other autosomal trisomies later.

The subject of Down syndrome screening is a complex and confusing one. Biochemical and ultrasound variables in the first and second trimester can be combined with a maternal age "*a priori*" risk to give an individualised risk for Down syndrome in each pregnancy. These variables are mostly continuous and independent of one another and can be used to increase or decrease the *a priori* risk depending on how far they deviate from the median value for a normal pregnancy. Women with a final adjusted risk above a predetermined threshold are offered invasive testing. Exciting new molecular approaches using cell free DNA have recently transformed the landscape and a review of these will follow.

Biochemical Variables

It has been known since the 1980s that the maternal serum levels of certain pregnancy-derived proteins are shifted away from the median in pregnancies affected by Down syndrome. In the second trimester (14–20 weeks), for example, hCG values in a pregnancy affected by T21 are approximately twice those of a normal pregnancy, and the maternal serum AFP is approximately half. The higher the hCG, and the lower the AFP, the higher the risk for Down syndrome becomes. Low hCG and high AFP levels are conversely associated with a lower risk of Down syndrome. Computer algorithms combine maternal serum levels with the maternal age at conception and compute an adjusted risk value for T21, which is usually expressed as the chance of a livebirth of a baby with Down syndrome. In the 1980s and early 1990s in the UK, if this risk was higher than 1 in 250, the result was described as "screen positive" and an amniocentesis was offered. This was called the double test, and it carried a false positive rate (FPR) of 5 %, with a sensitivity of only approximately 60–65 %. The later addition of oestriol, and then inhibin A, described as the triple and quadruple tests, respectively, has helped to improve the sensitivity. The quadruple test remains the *second* trimester screening test recommended in the UK by FASP [1], where the standard to be reached is a DR of 80 % for a FPR of between 2.5 and 3.5 %. Only women with a risk of 1 in 150, or greater, are now offered invasive testing with amniocentesis. This detection rate of 80 % means that 1 in 5 affected pregnancies will be deemed "low risk" by the screening test (so the diagnosis will be missed) and approximately 1 in 30 women will have a false positive screening result. Furthermore, not all screening programmes using the quadruple test have been able to reach these standards.

There is an understandable desire for Down syndrome screening to occur as early in pregnancy as possible. The levels of pregnancy associated plasma protein A (PAPP-A) tend to be lower in Down syndrome pregnancies in the first trimester (9–13 weeks), and those of human chorionic gonadotrophin (hCG) and free β-hCG tend to be higher. Even when used together, these first trimester biochemical markers have insufficient sensitivity to constitute a viable screening test, but they have been very successfully combined with nuchal translucency scanning (see below – the combined test) resulting in a much higher sensitivity despite lower false positive rates. The addition of first trimester maternal serum levels of AFP and placental growth factor (PlGF) may further benefit the performance of first trimester Down syndrome screening protocols in the future.

Ultrasound Variables

As the quality of ultrasound images improved in the 1980s and 1990s it became clear that the collection of fluid in the skin at the back of the fetal neck between 11 and 13+6 weeks gestation, the "nuchal translucency" (NT), could also be used to adjust the *a priori* risk for T21. The greater the measurement of the NT, the more likely Down syndrome would be. The fluid of the nuchal translucency accumulates during this time whilst the fetal lymphatics are still developing and vascular resistance in the placenta is still relatively high. The maturation of the fetal lymphatics tends to occur later in the fetus with a chromosomal anomaly, and the amount of fluid collecting tends to be greater. NT scanning was introduced in 1990 and although it lead to risk estimates being performed significantly earlier in pregnancy, used in isolation it failed to significantly raise the detection rate much above that of the triple test, reaching a DR of approximately 70 % for a FPR of 5 %. Chorionic villus sampling was required if the couple chose immediate invasive testing, with concerns that the miscarriage risk was slightly higher than that of amniocentesis. The Fetal Medicine Foundation and, more recently, the Fetal Anomaly Screening Programme have invested hugely in the education and audit of sonographers performing these technically demanding scans, pushing up the quality of nuchal translucency scanning country wide, and subsequently increasing its contribution to screening performance.

There are also additional first trimester ultrasound features that can be used to further refine the risk for Down syndrome. Tricuspid regurgitation, reversal of the "a" wave in the ductus venosus, and absence or hypoplasia of the nasal bone are all more common in the fetus with trisomy 21. These are perhaps even more demanding to perform than a nuchal translucency measurement and their use tends to be confined to private services, and fetal medicine units.

Second trimester scanning can also be used to adjust the risk for Down syndrome [2], although opinions vary significantly with regard to the value of the "genetic sonogram" in this regard [3]. Finding a congenital heart defect will significantly increase the risk of Down syndrome, with approximately 40 % of fetuses with major septal defects having aneuploidy, very commonly T21 [4]. However, short femur, increased nuchal fold, echogenic cardiac foci, mild renal pelvic dilatation, echogenic bowel, mild cerebral ventriculomegaly and absent or hypoplastic nasal bone have all been found more commonly in pregnancies affected by T21. Some of these ultrasound features carry a greater likelihood ratio of T21 than do others, and the more of these features that are present, the higher the risk becomes. Absence of any of these features on ultrasound at 18–23 weeks probably does reduce the prior screening or age related risk for Down syndrome and Agathokleous et al [5] have calculated that the combined negative likelihood ratio is 0.13.

The UKNSC issued a Programme Statement in 2009 following review of the available evidence. This stated that women who were found to be at low risk of DS following a formal first or second trimester screening test should *not* have this chance value recalculated in the presence of the following findings on the second trimester scan:

- Choroid plexus cysts
- Dilated cisterna magna
- Cardiac echogenic foci
- Two vessel cord

These "soft markers" were considered to have too weak an association with T21 to be of value. The statement went on to say that there are other findings which should be reported and should prompt referral for further assessment. These are;

- A nuchal fold >6 mm
- Ventriculomegaly (ventricular atrium >10 mm)
- Echogenic bowel
- Renal pelvic dilatation >7 mm
- Small measurements compared to dating scan (significantly <5th centile)

It is not clear from the statement what effect, if any, these should have on the quoted Down syndrome risk. Most fetal medicine specialists will offer amniocentesis if there is cerebral ventriculomegaly, a significantly small baby or an enlarged nuchal fold. Some still also offer invasive testing for a finding of echogenic bowel.

Combining the Variables

It is clear then that there are a plethora of variables, accessible to prenatal scrutiny, which can be used to refine a risk for Down syndrome. Because these variables are independent of one another, each can be used to separately adjust the maternal age related risk, either up or down. The more variables are included in the screening protocol, the higher the sensitivity becomes for a fixed false positive rate. Worldwide, the protocols available through state funded care, or private care, are determined by resources, moral and ethical values.

A "combined" test describes a screening protocol where a number of ultrasound and biochemical variables are tested at approximately the same gestation, and their effects on the Down syndrome risk are superimposed. This term is used in the UK to describe the current NSC "gold standard" of Down syndrome screening which is an NT scan at 12 weeks gestation with first trimester PAPP-A and free β-hCG values between 10 and 13 weeks gestation. The performance of this test varies, but a recent position statement by the International Society for Prenatal Diagnosis quoted an 80 % sensitivity for a 3 % FPR. The FASP standard for the combined test is a sensitivity rate of 85 % for an FPR of between 1.8 and 2.5 %. Adding in examination for the nasal bone to the combined test increases the sensitivity to 91 %. Failure to achieve a technically satisfactory NT measurement remains a problem, especially in women with a raised BMI, and some women continue to book later than the NT window. Current UK recommendations are for these women to be offered the quadruple test as an alternative.

Integrated testing describes the biochemical testing of the pregnancy in both the first and second trimesters, with or without scan variables, and only giving a risk estimate after the second trimester component. Sensitivity rates comfortably exceed 90 % for a 3 % FPR; however, the risk estimate is provided relatively late in gestation and the protocols are resource heavy. *Contingency* screening is a compromise between combined and integrated testing. Following the first round of the screening protocol in the first trimester, only the women with borderline risk estimates go forward to the second stage. Women with a very high risk are offered invasive testing immediately and those with a very low risk are not offered the second round. Approximately 1 in 5 women will go forward to the second stage, and this significantly saves on resources without seriously compromising detection rates.

As testament to the efforts of research teams, and the Fetal Anomaly Screening Programme, detection rates for T21 have increased significantly, hand in hand with a reduction in the false positive rate. Fewer women are labelled "high risk" and have to face the dilemma of invasive testing, and yet the detection rate for T21 has continued to climb. However, the PPV of even the best screening protocols remains only 3–4 %, meaning that approximately 30 invasive tests are performed for every affected pregnancy detected. With a miscarriage risk of 0.5–1.0 % associated with amniocentesis and CVS, the potential for iatrogenic loss of an unaffected pregnancy remains evident.

Screening Using cfDNA

"Cell free" DNA (cfDNA) refers to fragments of DNA which circulate in plasma having been released from the nuclei of damaged or dying cells. They have a short life span but because they are continually escaping from cells there is a relatively steady state. The fragments are random in size and chromosomal origin but in totality cover the entire genome and give an indication of gene dosage, i.e., how many copies of a particular part of the genome exist in that individual. Tumour biologists recognised some time ago that cfDNA arising from tumour cells could provide non-invasive genetic information regarding a malignancy by the analysis of a simple blood test from an affected individual. Even though cfDNA from cancerous cells could not be physically isolated from the cfDNA of normal cells, somatic genetic mutations contributing to the malignant potential of a tumour could be identified by studying the cfDNA because their DNA sequences differed from those of the host DNA. In 1997, Lo [6] showed that a pregnancy also contributes to the pool of cfDNA circulating in a pregnant woman. As the "host" she would not be expected to have cfDNA derived from the Y chromosome in her circulation, and identification of such Y-chromosomal DNA fragments using sensitive PCR techniques applied to her plasma, from a simple blood draw, would indicate she was carrying a male fetus. This was the first application of this knowledge and technique to prenatal testing and was soon joined by the non-invasive testing of fetal Rhesus D blood group in pregnancies complicated by Rhesus D isoimmunisation. Rhesus D negativity is usually caused by a deletion of the entire RhD gene. A RhD negative woman with anti-D antibodies would not be expected therefore to have cfDNA fragments from the Rhesus D gene in her circulation if she was carrying a RhD negative fetus. A RhD positive fetus would contribute RhD DNA fragments to the total cfDNA pool, and these would then be detectable using PCR techniques. Prior to this non-invasive prenatal testing (NIPT), an amniocentesis would have been required to ascertain the RhD status where the father of the baby was RhD heterozygous. Both these applications are now common practice in clinical genetics and fetal medicine clinics, and there are a number of other single gene disorders that can be tested for non-invasively in this way. Until recently, however, the clinical applications in a prenatal setting have been limited to this relatively small group of specific indications. A shift in thinking and rapid progress in DNA sequencing technology have now moved NIPT into the realm of screening for the common trisomies and testing for some of the more common deletion syndromes.

These genetic disorders result in a quantitative change in DNA, rather than a qualitative change. Individuals with T21 do not have genetic mutations per se, they have an extra copy of the otherwise normal genes on chromosome 21. This initially excluded NIPT from this field of prenatal testing because the early techniques relied on a difference in sequence between the mother and her unborn baby. However, as our ability to sequence DNA fragments has improved exponentially, it is now possible to sequence literally millions of DNA fragments in a matter of hours. The chromosomal origin of these fragments can be identified because we have mapped the entire human genome. Although the feto-placental unit makes only a small contribution of its cfDNA to the total pool of cfDNA in the maternal circulation, this is sufficient to mean that if the fetus has an imbalance in its chromosomal make-up, this will be detectable in the maternal pool of cfDNA. So, a fetus with trisomy 21 will contribute more chromosome 21 fragments to the cfDNA pool, meaning that a greater proportion of the total pool of cfDNA fragments will come from chromosome 21, even though the fetal cfDNA cannot be identified separately from the maternal. The technology behind this is remarkable, and it is being improved and becoming cheaper all the time.

A number of different techniques have been developed, the details of which will not be described here. They each rely on meticulous laboratory standards and complex statistical algorithms to maximise the sensitivity and positive predictive value of the testing process.

The use of cfDNA in the testing of pregnancies for Down syndrome and other trisomies has been developed and promoted, until very recently, by the commercial sector, with biotechnology companies in North America and Hong Kong dominating the market. There are now a plethora of published studies attesting to the power of these new techniques (summarised in a meta-analysis by Taylor –Phillips [7]). However, the picture emerging is that NIPT *cannot* be considered a diagnostic test. The headlines quoting detection rates of 99 % and false positive rates of <0.1 % are eye-catching; however, the test may not perform quite as well when confined to the end of the first trimester, or when used in a general obstetric population, rather than the high risk groups common to many of these studies. A recent meta-analysis of 41 studies [7] also found publication bias, which will further overestimate test accuracy. The International Society for Prenatal Diagnosis [8] have recently calculated a positive predictive value of 56 % for cfDNA testing for Down syndrome, although the Taylor-Phillips meta-analysis put this at 91 %. The latter figure would mean that when a cfDNA test gave a high risk for Down syndrome, in 9 out of 10 cases a subsequent invasive test would confirm the diagnosis. All commercial providers firmly recommend invasive testing for women with a cfDNA test showing a "high likelihood of an affected pregnancy." Of course, when compared with the PPV of 3–4 % of current screening methods for Down syndrome, this is a major advance. Far fewer women are given a "high risk" result, and of those that are, nearly all will be carrying an affected pregnancy. Decision making will be easier, and the number of test-related miscarriages will fall dramatically if cfDNA is introduced widely.

The RAPID study [9] is the only one to date to use cfDNA testing for Down syndrome in a publicly funded "real life" healthcare system and, as such, gives the most valuable insight into how cfDNA testing would perform if it was introduced as part of a national screening programme. RAPID used cfDNA testing in a contingent manner, i.e., all women were offered the combined test or quadruple test as per current NSC guidelines. Those with a risk >1 in 1000 for Down syndrome were then offered NIPT. If this test indicated a high likelihood of Down syndrome, they were then offered invasive testing. In the final analysis, the RAPID team were able to set the threshold for the offer of NIPT at 1 in 150, 1 in 500 or 1 in 1000. At all thresholds, the overall detection for Down syndrome was increased above that of the current screening protocol, and there was a huge reduction in the number of invasive tests performed, and the number of test-related miscarriages. However, with current costs of cfDNA technology, only the use of a threshold of 1 in 150 kept costs for the screening programme neutral (in fact it had a small associated saving). As the costs of testing fall, the threshold of the primary screening test at which NIPT can be offered will also fall, with an associated increase in the proportion of Down syndrome pregnancies detected. This leads to the question as to whether cfDNA testing should be offered to all women, as the primary screening test. Costs are prohibitive currently for this option, and there are realistic concerns that test accuracy will fall, and the number of invasive tests performed will climb again, despite only a relatively small increase in the additional cases of Down syndrome detected. Concerns have been raised about losing the nuchal translucency scan, and the use of first trimester biochemical markers, because of the other pregnancy complications these test components can be a marker of.

The National Screening Committee in the UK has opened a consultation on the use of cfDNA as part of a contingency screening programme for Down syndrome, to be offered when the primary screening result is 1 in 150 or greater. If, and when, this becomes established practice, it remains to be seen how thresholds will change as the costs of testing come down.

Although there seems to be much to be gained, and little to lose, from the introduction of NIPT into national screening for T21, it is important to recognise that the test is unsuccessful in 1.9–6.4 % of cases. The original sample is usually run-again if the first run is inconclusive, and this can extend the time taken for a result to be issues well beyond a week. If the second run also fails, then the options are to proceed with invasive testing, or draw a second sample of blood (with no more than a 50 % chance that the test on this sample will be successful). The likelihood of success is closely related to the "fetal fraction," i.e., the proportion of total cell free DNA which is derived from the feto-placental unit. Laboratories usually require a minimum value of 4 % with maternal obesity recognised as a risk factor for lower levels. Trisomy 18 and 13 may also be associated with lower fetal fractions. Delay in obtaining a result will heighten anxiety levels, and the options for methods of termination of pregnancy may be limited at gestations beyond 12–13 weeks as gynaecologists become less comfortable with performing second trimester surgical abortions.

Screening for Trisomy 18 and 13

T13 and T18 are associated with a high risk of miscarriage and later *in utero* fetal death. Liveborns rarely survive more than a year, and most die within the first few days or weeks of life. Longer term survivors have major physical and learning disabilities. Although much less common than T21, the incidence of T18 and T13 has increased significantly with time, partly due to the increasing maternal age at conception, and partly due to the diagnosis of these trisomies in early pregnancies which would have previously gone unrecognised.

The number of diagnosed cases of T13 increased from 152 in 2004 to 213 in 2010 and for T18 from 369 to 514. Approximately 90 % of T13 cases are diagnosed in the antenatal period and 93 % of T18. Just over half are detected through first trimester screening for T21, a smaller proportion through second trimester screening and the remainder following investigations for structural anomalies or growth restriction identified on later scans. In the UK, until very recently, the only formal screening test for T13/T18 has been the second trimester anomaly scan. This occurs quite late in gestation, and does not detect all cases. Both first and second trimester screening tests for Down syndrome have resulted in the detection of T13/T18 as an unintentional "bi-product" of testing for T21. Because the nuchal translucency measurement tends to be raised in all three trisomies and the PAPP-A level at 9–14 weeks tends to be lower than normal, a raised risk for Down syndrome may also inadvertently be indicating a raised risk for T13/T18. Unlike T21, the β-HCG value in T13/T18 tends to be lower than in a normal pregnancy, rather than higher, as is the case with T21. The National Screening Committee has determined that during 2015, formal screening for T13/T18 should be introduced for all women in the first trimester, in isolation or addition to T21, depending on their preferences. The components of the screening test (NT and biochemical markers) are already in place. Using a risk threshold of ≥1 in 150 for T13/T18, followed by invasive testing, should result in first trimester detection rates of 80–90 %, with only a 0.2–0.5 % additional false positive rate above the 2–3 % FPR found with the use of the combined test for Down syndrome screening [1]. This will bring forward the point at which these trisomies are diagnosed, and ultimately result in a higher proportion of cases being detected prenatally. It remains to be determined if these women will be offered NIPT once this has become embedded in the NHS screening protocol for Down syndrome. The sensitivity of cfDNA screening for T13 and 18 (95–96 %) is slightly lower than that for T21 (99 %) and the positive predictive values calculated in the Warwick meta-analysis were 87 and 84 % respectively.

Screening in Multiple Pregnancies

Screening for Down syndrome in multiple pregnancies is even more complex. Deriving and interpreting the risk estimates is more complicated, and subsequent invasive testing and decision making in affected pregnancies is also significantly more difficult than in singletons. The population of women conceiving following assisted conception is older on average than those conceiving spontaneously, and therefore at greater risk of an aneuploid pregnancy (unless a donor oocyte is used). Data collected by the Human Fertilisation and Embryo Authority showed a UK multiple birth rate of 27 % of ongoing IVF/ICSI pregnancies in 2008 which fell dramatically to 16 % by 2014 due to the widespread adoption of single embryo transfer. However, it is clear that 1 in 6 couples conceiving through ART will still be faced by the complex issues of screening for Down syndrome in a multiple pregnancy. Monochorionic twins will always be monozygous and therefore genetically identical (except in a very small number of so-called heterokaryotypic monozgous twins). If one of the twin pair has Down syndrome, then they both will. Dichorionic twins may be dizygous or monozygous. Dizygous twins are genetically individual and each has its own independent risk of having a chromosomal disorder. It is very unlikely that both would be affected by the same condition. The likelihood of a dichorionic twin pair being monozygous will depend on the age of the woman, her ethnicity, whether she has had IVF and if so, how many embryos were transferred. In spontaneous dichorionic conceptions, approximately 90 % will be dizygous, with only a minority being monozygous. Dizygosity is more common in older women, and in Afro-Caribbeans. In a double embryo transfer IVF pregnancy, resulting dichorionic twins are more than likely to be dizygous (99 %). A dichorionic twin pair following single embryo transfer will almost certainly be monozygous (the exception being an additional spontaneous pregnancy in a frozen embryo natural cycle). Spontaneous dichorionic twins are assumed to be dizygous for screening purposes.

Age specific risks for Down syndrome are not available for twin pregnancies. The assumption is often made that the maternal age related risk for Down syndrome in a twin is the same as it would be for a singleton. This would be the risk that both twins would be affected if they are monochorionic, and the risk of at least one of a dichorionic (presumed dizygous) twin pair being affected would be twice this value. This assumption is incorrect. European registries have recently shown that the risk of Down syndrome per fetus/baby is lower in multiple pregnancies than it is in singletons [10, 11]. These data suggest that the risk of Down syndrome in monozygous twins is 0.34 times that of singleton pregnancies, and that the risk of at least one of a dizygous twin pair being affected by Down syndrome is 1.34 times that of singleton pregnancies (when the above assumption would predict a 2.0 fold greater risk). The intrauterine lethality of Down syndrome is thought to be greater in twin pregnancies, meaning fewer reach the screening gestation.

Even the first two steps in determining Down syndrome risk in twins are complicated. Firstly, there may be uncertainty regarding the zygosity of the twin pregnancy, and secondly there is a lack of robust age-related *a priori* risks to work from.

Nuchal translucency measurements can be taken for each fetus, allowing the *a priori* risk to be adjusted up or down. This assumes that the NT measurements are independent of one another, which unfortunately is probably not the case. The NT measurements can be particularly problematic in monochorionic twins where a large NT may also be the sign of impending twin to twin transfusion syndrome, cardiac or structural malformations. Furthermore, when the measurements are discordant, which they usually are, which should be used for the calculation? Evidence supports using the average of the two measurements, but the compromise remains clear. Using NT measurements in isolation for Down syndrome screening in twins limits the detection rate to 70 % at best, with a false positive rate of 5 %. However, serum biochemistry can also be performed [12]. Indeed, the combined test is now the FASP gold standard for screening for T21 in twin pregnancies, irrespective of chorionicity. In dichorionic twins, an individual risk for Down syndrome is given for each separate twin, whereas in a monochorionic twin pregnancy a single risk is given for both twins being affected. Appropriate correction factors need to be applied to the biochemistry to take account of the greater placental mass, and these vary depending on whether the pregnancy is monochorionic or dichorionic, particularly for PAPP-A where the MoM is 2.25 that of singleton pregnancies when the twins are dichorionic, and only 1.76 when they are monochorionic [13]. The actual shift in biochemistry values in twin pregnancies affected by Down syndrome is not known and assumptions have to be drawn from screening singleton pregnancies. Further adjustment should be made if the twins have been conceived through IVF/ICSI, as is the case with singletons (see below).

A recent meta-analysis of studies examining the performance of the combined test in twin pregnancies gave an overall detection rate of 89 %, although the false positive rate was 5.4 % [14]. It seems clear the detection rate is likely to be a little lower than that of the combined test in singletons pregnancies for the reasons cited above. This is intuitive for discordant dizygous twins, where the abnormal biochemistry of the affected twin is "masked" or "diluted" by the normal biochemistry of the euploid twin.

For women presenting too late for the combined test, or where NT measurements are not possible for both twins, the quadruple test is recommended and a single risk is given that at least one twin will be affected, irrespective of the chorionicity. FASP suggest that a detection rate of 40–50 % should be possible, with a false positive rate of approximately 3 %, but this clearly falls far below the standards of the other screening protocols.

In higher order pregnancies, nuchal translucency scanning alone is recommended, and an individual risk is derived for each fetus. The detection rate would be expected to be approximately 70 % for a false positive rate of 5 %.

Data on the use of NIPT are accumulating in twin pregnancies, and for twins concordant for aneuploidy it makes sense to believe that the sensitivity and specificity should be as high as that for singletons, perhaps even higher. A recent meta-analysis [7] has, however, reported an overall 9 % lower sensitivity of NIPT in all twin pregnancies. In a similar way to the first trimester biochemistry in discordant dizygous twins, the impact of the additional DNA fragments from the extra copy of chromosome 21 in the affected twin is lessened or masked by the normal contributions from the euploid twin.

Studies using early pregnancy scanning show that the incidence of twins at 11–14 weeks gestation is significantly less than the incidence earlier in the pregnancy. Between one and two fifths of all pregnancies showing two sacs or even two embryos, will undergo spontaneous embryo reduction by the end of the first trimester. This "vanishing twin" phenomenon has caused concerns regarding Down syndrome screening. Might the "non-viable" sac or embryo contribute to the levels of first trimester serum markers and falsely elevate the levels of PAPP-A and hCG? Although opinions vary, Spencer [15] has shown that free β-hCG MOMs are unchanged with a vanishing twin. PAPP-A levels increase if there is a measurable CRL in the non-viable twin, although not if there is just an empty sac. Current guidance recommends using only the nuchal translucency to give a Down syndrome risk if a second sac is visible and has a measurable embryo within it.

Invasive Testing in Multiples

We have seen that in monochorionic twin pregnancies the risk for T21 is the risk that both twins will be affected. In dichorionic twins, an individual risk for each fetus is generated and the assumption made that they are dizygous. In the event of a high risk screening results, it is usually considered essential in dichorionic twin pregnancies to sample the placenta or the amniotic fluid of each twin, and a variety of techniques can be employed. Chorionic villus sampling can be performed transabdominally or transcervically, and in twin pregnancies a combination of the two routes may be preferred. However the CVS is done, there must be certainty that both placentas are being sampled. If they are clearly separate, for example one on the anterior uterine wall, and one posterior, then this can be achieved without doubt. However, as the individual placental masses grow and their edges meet, the risk of sampling the same placenta twice is increased. Two needle insertions will be required if a transabdominal approach is taken, and sampling from widely separated placental areas is recommended, if possible. To avoid the risk of sampling error, amniocentesis may be preferred. Sampling amniotic fluid from either side of the inter-twin membrane is usually possible with two separate needle entries. Although the injection of indigo carmine into the first sampled sac can be employed to reassure the practitioner that the second sample is definitely from the second sac, this is usually unnecessary. A single needle insertion has also been employed when sampling dichorionic twins. The needle is advanced into the first sac and a sample taken. The needle is then moved into the second sac through the inter-twin membrane and a second sample taken.

Whichever technique is used, it is essential that the position of the fetuses and the placentas is mapped very carefully before the procedure, and that the samples are labelled very carefully. In dichorionic twin pregnancies, if one twin is affected, it is very unlikely that the co-twin will also be aneuploid. In the event of a request for selective termination it is vital that the obstetrician knows with certainty which is the affected fetus. In the absence of obvious structural anomalies, the fetal and placental map will be of crucial importance.

Monochorionic twins are monozygous and the fetuses should be genetically identical. A single sampling should, in theory, be sufficient therefore. However, there exists a very small risk of heterokaryotypia in monozygous twins, i.e., chromosomal discordance resulting from mitotic errors or postzygotic non-disjunction [16]. In this situation, single sampling would result in the erroneous belief that both twins were either aneuploid, or both euploid. Single sampling is considered acceptable if both twins of a monozygous pair look normal on careful scanning, but if there are any structural anomalies to find then both twins should be sampled, either by CVS, amniocentesis, or even a combination of the two.

FASP advise an added miscarriage risk, meaning loss of the entire pregnancy, of twin invasive testing of 2 %. A meta-analysis of cohort studies found a 3.84 % loss rate after twin CVS and 3.07 % risk following twin amniocentesis [17]. This includes the background risk of miscarriage (which is higher in twins than in singletons) and some have argued that the risk of procedure related miscarriage is not significantly higher in twins than it is in singletons.

When invasive testing confirms a chromosomal abnormality in a twin pregnancy, counselling from an experienced practitioner is required. An objective and non-directive discussion of the implications of the diagnosis and of the available management options is key. Written literature, suitable internet based resources and an opportunity to meet with a specialist paediatrician and parents of an affected child are examples of how information and experience can be shared. An affected monozygous twin pregnancy will pose a particular challenge to future parents because two children will be affected. An affected discordant dizygous twin pregnancy will pose a very difficult dilemma for the couple who would have chosen to terminate an affected singleton. Selective termination using intracardiac potassium chloride or lidocaine carries a 5–10 % risk of total pregnancy loss. It is clear that the offer of screening twin pregnancies for Down syndrome should be made by a knowledgeable clinician who is able to take the discussion through to invasive testing and subsequent options, in the event of an affected pregnancy. These decisions may be all the more difficult to make if the pregnancy has resulted from assisted reproductive technologies.

The Impact of Assisted Reproductive Technologies

There is no evidence that assisted reproduction *per se* increases the chances of conceiving a trisomic pregnancy when maternal age is controlled for. However, by virtue of the fact that women seeking out infertility treatment tend to be older than women conceiving spontaneously, the chances of a pregnancy being affected will be higher. For this group of women, subsequent screening and testing may prove to be even more challenging, and decision making even more difficult. A greater proportion of pregnancies resulting from assisted conception will be higher order (particularly twins) and this adds further to the complexity, as described before. By 2014, following the introduction of strategies to reduce multiple births such as single embryo transfer, the rate of multiple pregnancy following ART had fallen to 16 % [18]. This means that 1 in 6 couples still face the difficult decision of screening for fetal anomalies in a twin pregnancy. Evidence from Denmark and the Lebanon shows that fewer women conceiving through ART opt for Down syndrome screening or invasive testing. The reasons are complex, but it is reasonable to assume that anxiety over the loss of the pregnancy through procedure-related miscarriage contributes. Evidence suggests that couples pregnant following ART are just as concerned about the risk of fetal abnormality as those who have conceived naturally, but fears over the complications of testing would appear to prevent many pursuing prenatal screening and diagnosis [19, 20].

Numerous studies have demonstrated that ART is associated with changes in biochemical serum screening markers [21], and a few have even shown that NT measurements may be affected by the type of conception. However, the results of many of the studies are conflicting. Factors such as whether the embryo transfer was fresh or frozen, standard IVF or ICSI, and even how many oocytes were aspirated at the time of egg collection might all have an influence on subsequent levels of biochemical markers and have been suggested as reasons why these studies have failed to find a consistent effect. Most studies have shown no impact of ART on the NT measurement, but there is reasonable evidence to support the belief that PAPP-A levels are somewhat lower, and less suggesting that free hCG values are a little higher. Gjerris [22] found the PAPP-A multiple of the median to be 0.78 when compared with spontaneous conceptions, although this was confined to fresh embryo transfers. These changes would result in a higher risk for Down's syndrome being quoted, unless they were controlled for, so increasing the false positive rate in this group of women. The impact of using CRL for dating the pregnancy, rather than the date of oocyte retrieval, may be another factor of importance. Some laboratories will use adjustments in their Down syndrome calculation software, taking account of ART, although these are system specific. LifeCycle4, for example, does not correct PAPP-A levels following ART, but does assume a free β-hCG MoM of 1.12.

Translating this information into practical advice is very difficult. It is recommended that clinicians speak with their lead screening biochemists for local advice on which, if any, corrections are used and what false positive and detection rates should be quoted for women who have undergone ART.

Assisted reproduction may have involved the use of donor eggs. In calculating a risk for Down syndrome, and other trisomies, the age of the donor must be used for the *a priori* age related risk, not that of the woman undergoing the IVF.

Preimplantation genetic screening (PGS) is a technique employed by fertility specialists to maximise the chances of implantation and success in IVF cycles. Approximately half of all very early pregnancy losses occur because of aneuploidy, and this proportion rises with maternal age. If only euploid embryos are transferred at IVF, then the theory predicts that ongoing pregnancy rates would be much higher. One or two cells can be removed from the early embryo and tested using fluorescent in situ hybridisation or comparative genomic hybridisation to assess for major chromosomal anomalies, deletions and duplications. Only embryos with normal analyses are used in the transfer. This can seriously limit the number available and is one of the disadvantages of this technique. Furthermore, it is now understood that the early embryo is quite commonly "chaotic" from a chromosomal point of view. Not all cells in the early embryo have the same chromosomal makeup and so cells biopsied for PGS may not be representative of the cells destined to become the fetus. Potentially viable embryos might be discarded, and undue reassurance inferred about the embryos chosen for transfer. Large meta-analyses have reported no significant benefits on ongoing pregnancy rates following PGS, although there may yet be benefits in certain subgroups (e.g., older women). What advice should be given to a woman who has successfully conceived following PGS? There can be no guarantee that the fetus is euploid, because of the mosaicism commonly seen in early embryos. However, it is nonsensical to say that the risk has not been significantly reduced by the use of this technique. Many obstetricians will recommend Down syndrome screening anyway, but the counselling becomes very difficult when the combined risk is high, despite PGS. The use of cell-free DNA and NIPT, although expensive, is now a very sensible option for women in this position.

Screening for Structural Anomalies

Justifying and introducing a new screening test nationally requires a solid evidence base and convincing cost-effectiveness. Ultrasound screening for fetal abnormalities became an increasingly widespread practice throughout much of the world during the 1980s and 1990s as ultrasound machines became more powerful. The evidence underpinning this apparently welcome development was very poor. Across the UK, the provision, timing and standards of prenatal ultrasound scanning were highly variable. A survey in 1995 reported that only 82 % of UK maternity units were offering a mid-trimester anatomy scan. The value of a routine mid-trimester scan was still being debated at that time. A large RCT of routine second and third trimester scanning (RADIUS), published in 1993 [23], had failed to demonstrate any difference in perinatal mortality rates between routinely and selectively scanned groups. However, another trial from Helsinki [24, 25] showed that routine scanning did reduce perinatal mortality, and was cost-effective, mostly because of the better detection of major malformations followed by termination of pregnancy. A later systematic review further endorsed this view but pointed out that the benefits were only obvious if there was access to termination of pregnancy [26]. However, an HTA report by the same group emphasised the huge variability in detection rates for fetal abnormality across the studies included in their review, and called for national standards and training to be introduced across the UK. The overall detection of fetal anomalies across the four UK studies included in the analysis was 53 %, although this varied hugely between the individual studies and anomaly groups. "Reproductive choice" is a very important outcome from a fetal anomaly screening programme (i.e., whether to continue or discontinue a pregnancy), and it is widely believed that the knowledge of an anomaly prior to delivery can limit parental shock and distress at the time of birth (for example with facial clefting). New parents have time to assimilate information before their baby arrives, which would otherwise be given and received during the newborn period. There is accumulating evidence also that the outcome for babies with certain prenatally diagnosed anomalies is better. They can be delivered in tertiary paediatric units, with appropriately skilled teams present. Surgical and medical interventions can be initiated early, helping to limit deterioration in the newborn period. This is best evidenced in babies born with diaphragmatic hernia [27], or certain cardiac anomalies such as transposition without septal defect, and those with complex upper airway difficulties.

Although it is clear that the mid-trimester scan can cause significant anxiety amongst pregnant women and their partners, and that false positives are possible, it is nevertheless a very popular investigation with more than 95 % of women taking up the offer of a scan at this gestation. Furthermore, it provides a baseline for comparison of growth measurements later on in pregnancy, and an opportunity for future parents to begin to bond with their unborn child.

It was clear that ultrasound scanning for fetal abnormalities was here to stay. In 2004, the National Screening Committee tasked the Fetal Anomaly Screening Programme to develop a national, quality assured, obstetric ultrasound screening programme. They found still a huge variation in practice throughout the UK, and set about turning this into a well defined and standardised screening programme which would adhere to the principles of the other national screening programmes [28]. The International Society of Ultrasound in Obstetrics and Gynaecology (ISUOG) has also published practice guidelines for the performance of the routine mid-trimester fetal ultrasound scan [29]. All women should be offered a scan looking for structural abnormalities between 18 and 23 weeks gestation and the detection rates should be at least as high as the values given below for a number of key conditions:

- Anencephaly 98 %
- Open spina bifida 90 %
- Cleft lip 75 %
- Diaphragmatic hernia 60 %
- Gastroschisis 98 %
- Exomphalos 80 %
- Bilateral renal agenesis 84 %
- Lethal skeletal dysplasia 60 %
- Serious cardiac abnormalities (transposition of the great arteries, atrioventricular septal defect, Tetralogy of Fallot, hypolastic left heart syndrome) 50 %

ART and Structural Anomalies

There has been much understandable interest in whether ART is associated with an increased risk of structural congenital anomalies following early reports in the late 80s and early 90s suggesting that the incidence of neural tube defect and certain cardiac abnormalities was significantly increased. A number of case-controlled and population registry studies, of varying quality and methodology, have all pointed to a real increase of approximately 30–40 %, across all anomaly groups with particular focus on cardiac abnormalities, neural tube and limb reduction defects, and hypospadias [30]. A number of meta-analyses have produced relative risks of between 1.3 and 1.8, with ICSI contributing more to this increase than standard IVF in some of these [31–33]. Hypospadias has a particularly strong association with ICSI, and this is likely to be due to subtle Y chromosomal genetic defects, which are the cause of more minor anomalies of the male genitalia and azoo/oligospermia, being inherited by ICSI male offspring of infertile men.

It is interesting to speculate on the possible causes of this increased risk. Monozygous twinning is more common in ART pregnancies, and this has a well recognised association with greater congenital anomaly risk. However, the effect of ART persists when singleton pregnancies are examined in isolation from multiples, so this cannot account for more than a small contribution to the overall increase. It is possible that couples needing ART will be less likely to elect for termination in the event of discovery of a serious anomaly, but again this is an inadequate explanation on its own. There is a real possibility that the process of ovarian stimulation, egg collection, in vitro fertilisation and subsequent embryo transfer might bring about an increase in the risk of subsequent abnormality. Imprinting disorders such as Beckwith-Wiedemann (BWS) and Angelmann syndromes are more common in pregnancies following ART. The underlying aetiologies are very complex but a proportion of cases are caused by epigenetic mechanisms. These are non-sequence alterations to the DNA, such as a change in the methylation status of a gene. The techniques of IVF have been shown to alter methylation status and it is now widely accepted that the ART-associated increase in the risk of these rare imprinting disorders occurs through this mechanism [34].

A further possible explanation is that couples requiring ART have an intrinsically greater risk of having offspring with congenital anomalies that is somehow associated with their infertility. The link between hypospadias and male infants resulting from ICSI has already been discussed, and other similar mechanisms may exist. It is pertinent to note that couples who subsequently conceive spontaneously, following previous ART, have pregnancies at greater risk of congenital anomaly even in the absence of infertility treatments [35].

This academic discussion is fascinating, but in clinical practice the exact reasons why the anomaly risk is greater in pregnancies conceived through ART is less important than its potential consequences. Women and their partners who conceive with the help of ART are likely to be more anxious about the risk of fetal abnormality than those who conceive spontaneously. Many will also be aware that the risk of anomaly in their pregnancy is greater by virtue of the ART. How should the clinician respond? It is important to stress that the absolute increase in risk of anomaly is small and that the majority of babies born following ART will be normal. At the time of the scan, the couple can be reassured that the majority of major anomalies will be detected and that many can be corrected with a normal or near-normal long term outcome (e.g., cardiac defects). Some abnormalities will not be detectable by ultrasound scanning, e.g., hypospadias, but are readily correctable after birth. With the ever-increasing standards demanded by the Fetal Anomaly Screening Programme for the routine 18–20+6 week scan, it is unnecessary to recommend higher level "Fetal Medicine" scanning or fetal echocardiography by a paediatric cardiologist, unless concern is raised during the routine anatomy scan. However, if there is suspicion of a problem, the inherent greater risk is worth bearing in mind, and also the association between ART and imprinting disorders. An exomphalos, for example, is more likely to be a sign of BWS in a pregnancy following ART than it is in a spontaneously conceived pregnancy. The possibility of fetal abnormality is a situation which always necessitates great sensitivity. The added pre-existing anxieties of couples who have undergone ART also need to be accommodated and dealt with appropriately.

References

1. Fetal Anomaly Screening Programme Standards 2015–2016. https://www.gov.uk/government/publications/fetal-anomaly-screening-programme-standards. First trimester combined screening for trisomy 13 and trisomy 18. External review against programme appraisal criteria for the UK National Screening Committee (UK NSC), version 5. Bazian Ltd. October 2013. http://legacy.screening.nhs.uk/t18andt13.
2. Smith-Bindman R, Chu P, Goldberg JD. Second trimester prenatal ultrasound for the detection of pregnancies at increased risk of Down syndrome. Prenat Diagn. 2007;27:535–44.
3. Cuckle H, Maymon R. Role of second-trimester ultrasound in screening for Down syndrome. Ultrasound Obstet Gynecol. 2013;41:241–4.
4. Cuckle H, Benn P, Pergament E. Cell-free DNA screening for fetal aneuploidy as a clinical service. Circulating nucleic acids, a Clinical Biochemistry Special Issue. 2015;48(15): 932–41.
5. Agathokleous M, Chaveeva P, Poon LCY, Kosinski P, Nicolaides KH. Meta-analysis of second-trimester markers for trisomy 21. Ultrasound Obstet Gynecol. 2013;41:247–61.
6. Lo DYM, Corbetta N, Chamberlain P, Rai V, Sargent IL, Redman CWG, Wainscoat JS. Presence of fetal DNA in maternal plasma and serum. Lancet. 1997;350:485–7.
7. Taylor Phillips S, Freeman K, Geppert J, Madan J, Uthman O, Agbebiyi A, Clarke A, Quenby S. Systematic review and cost consequences assessment of cell-free DNA testing for T21, T18 and T13 in the UK – Final Report. 2015. In press and available through the FASP website.
8. Benn P, Borrell A, Chiu R, Cuckle H, Dugoff L, Brigitte F, Gross S, Johnson J, Maymon R, Norton M, Odibo A, Schielen P, Spencer K, Huang T, Wright D, Yaron Y. Position Statement from the Chromosome Abnormality Screening Committee on Behalf of the Board of the International Society for Prenatal Diagnosis. 2014; https://www.ispdhome.org/docs/ISPD/Society%20Statements/PositionStatement_Current_8Apr2015.pdf.
9. Chitty L, Cameron L, Daley R, Fisher J, Hill M, Jenkins L, Kroese M, McEwan A, McKay F, Morris S, Verhoef T, Wright D. RAPID non-invasive prenatal testing (NIPT) evaluation study: a report for the UK National Screening Committee (Executive Summary). 2015.
10. Jamar M, Lemarchal C, Lemaire V, Koulischer L, Bours V. A low rate of trisomy 21 in twin pregnancies: a cytogenetics retrospective study of 278 cases. Genet Couns. 2003;14: 395–400.
11. Boyle B, Morris J, McConkey R, Garne E, Loane M, Addor M, Gatt M, Haeusler M, Latos-Bielenska A, Lelong N, et al. Prevalence and risk of Down syndrome in monozygotic and dizygotic multiple pregnancies in Europe; implications for prenatal screening. BJOG. 2014;121:809–19.
12. Prats P, Rodriguez I, Comas C, Puerto B. First trimester risk assessment for trisomy 21 in twin pregnancies combining nuchal translucency and first trimester biochemical markers. Prenat Diagn. 2012;32:927–32.
13. Spencer K, Kagan K, Nicolaides K. Screening for trisomy 21 in twin pregnancies in the first trimester: an update of the impact of chorionicity on maternal serum markers. Prenat Diagn. 2008;28:49–52.
14. Prats P, Rodriguez I, Comas C, Puerto B. Systematic review of screening for T21 in twin pregnancies in 1st trimester combining NT and biochemical markers: a meta-analysis. Prenat Diagn. 2014;34:1077–83.
15. Spencer K, Staboulidou I, Nicolaides KH. First trimester aneuploidy screening in the presence of a vanishing twin: implications for maternal serum markers. Prenat Diagn. 2010;30: 235–40.
16. Lewi L, Blickstein I, Van Schoubroeck D, Gloning KP, Casteels M, Brandenburg H, Fryns JP, Deprest J. Diagnosis and management of heterokaryotypic monochorionic twins. Am J Med Genet. 2006;140:272–5.
17. Agarwal K, Alfirevic Z. Pregnancy loss after chorionic villus sampling and genetic amniocentesis in twin pregnancies. a systematic review. Ultrasound Obstet Gynecol. 2012;40:128–34.

18. Monni G, Iuculano A, Zoppi M. Screening and invasive testing in twins. J Clin Med. 2014;3:865–82.
19. Gjerris AC, Loft A, Pinborg A, Christiansen M, Tabor A. Prenatal testing amongst women pregnant after assisted reproductive techniques in Denmark 1995-2000: a national cohort study. Hum Reprod. 2008;23:1545–52.
20. Abu-Musa AA, Nassar AH, Usta IM. Attitude of women with IVF and spontaneous pregnancies towards prenatal screening. Hum Reprod. 2008;23:2438–43.
21. Tul N, Novak-Antolic Z. Serum PAPP-A levels at 10-14 weeks of gestation are altered in women after assisted conception. Prenat Diagn. 2006;26:1206–11.
22. Gjerris AC, Tabor A, Loft A, Christiansen M, Pinborg A. First trimester prenatal screening among women pregnant after IVF/ICSI. Hum Repro Update. 2012;18:350–9.
23. Ewigman BG, Crane JP, Frigoletto FD, LeFevre ML, Bain RP, McNellis D. Effect of prenatal ultrasound screening on perinatal outcome. RADIUS Study Group. N Engl J Med. 1993;329:821–7.
24. Saari Kemppainen A, Karjalainen O, Ylostalo P, Heinonen OP. Ultrasound screening and perinatal mortality: controlled trial of systematic one-stage screening in pregnancy. The Helsinki Ultrasound Trial. Lancet. 1990;336:387–91.
25. Leivo T, Tuominen R, Saari-Kemppainen A, Ylostalo P, Karjalainen O, Heinonen OP. Cost-effectiveness of one-stage ultrasound screening in pregnancy: a report from the Helsinki ultrasound trial. Ultrasound Obstet Gynecol. 1996;7:309–14.
26. Roberts T, Henderson J, Mugford M, Bricker L, Neilson J, Garcia J. Antenatal ultrasound screening for fetal abnormalities: a systematic review of studies of cost and cost effectiveness. BJOG. 2002;109:44–56.
27. Betremieux P, Gaillot T, de la Pintiere A, Beuchee A, Pasquier L, Habonimana E, Le Bouar G, Branger B, Milon J, Fremond B, Wodey E, Odent S, Poulain P, Pladys P. Congenital diaphragmatic hernia: prenatal diagnosis permits immediate intensive care with high survival rate in isolated cases. A population-based study. Prenat Diagn. 2004;24:487–93.
28. Kirwan D. NHS Fetal Anomaly Screening programme. 18+0 to 20+6 weeks fetal anomaly scan. National Standards and Guidance for England. 2010. http://www.bmfms.org.uk/UserFiles/documents/nhs_fasp_fa_standards_and_gudance_2010.pdf.
29. Salomon LJ, Alfirevic Z, Berghella C, Bilardo C, Hernandez-Andrade E, Johnsen SL, Kalache K, Leung KY, Malinger G, Munoz H, Prefumo F, Toi A. Practice guidelines for performance of the routine mid-trimester fetal ultrasound scan. Ultrasound Obstet Gynecol. 2011;37(1):116–26.
30. Williams C, Sutcliffe A, Sebire NJ. Congenital malformations after assisted reproduction: risks and implications for prenatal diagnosis and fetal medicine. Ultrasound Obstet Gynecol. 2010;35:255–9.
31. Rimm AA, Katayama AC, Diaz M, Katayama KP. A meta-analysis of controlled studies comparing major malformation rates in IVF and ICSI infants with naturally conceived children. J Assist Reprod Genet. 2004;21:437–43.
32. Hansen M, Bower C, Milne E, de Klerk N, Kurinczuk JJ. Assisted reproductive technologies and the risk of birth defects – a systematic review. Hum Reprod. 2005;20:328–38.
33. Pandey S, Shetty A, Hamilton M, Bhattacharya S, Maheshwari A. Obstetric and perinatal outcomes in singleton pregnancies resulting from IVF/ICSI: a systematic review and meta-analysis. Hum Repro Update. 2012;18:485–503.
34. Sutcliffe AG, Peters CJ, Bowdin S, Temple K, Reardon W, Wilson L, Calyton-Smith J, Brueton LA, Bannister W, Maher ER. Assisted reproductive therapies and imprinting disorders – a preliminary British survey. Hum Reprod. 2006;21:1009–11.
35. Zhu JL, Basso O, Obel C, Bille C, Olsen J. Infertility, infertility treatment, and congenital malformations: Danish national birth cohort. BMJ. 2006;333:679–81.

Chapter 8
Multiple Pregnancy Update: Issues Following Assisted Reproductive Techniques

Lisa J. Knight, Lisa A. Joels, and Myles J.O. Taylor

Introduction

It is estimated that infertility affects 1 in 7 couples of reproductive age in the United Kingdom [1]. Births following in vitro fertilisation (IVF) techniques are said to account for 2% of all births in the UK [2]. Approximately 13,000 IVF babies are born each year, with one in five IVF pregnancies resulting in multiple gestation compared with one in 80 from natural conceptions [2]. However, overall the trend is downwards, dropping from 26.6% in 2008 to 16.3% in 2014 [3] (Fig. 8.1). Multifetal conceptions are the single most important determinant of pregnancy and long-term outcomes for both the mother and baby and these risks increase exponentially with the number of fetuses. There is good evidence that IVF conceived pregnancies, even if a singleton pregnancy, are at increased risk of adverse outcomes for the majority of pregnancy complications and these risks increase further with multiple pregnancy [4]. Monozygosity (MZ) is associated with higher risks of adverse outcomes. While the majority of MZ twins are spontaneously conceived (22% compared with 2% of IVF twins), there are some technologies, which increase the risk of MZ twins with IVF [5]. Assisted conception technologies such as IVF increase the risk of these pregnancies by twofold, although overall incidence remains low [6].

L.J. Knight, BSc, BMBS, MRCOG, DipClinEd (✉)
Department of Obstetrics and Gynaecology, Royal Devon and Exeter Hospital, Exeter, UK
e-mail: lisaknight@doctors.org.uk

L.A. Joels, MB, ChB, MD, FRCOG, FHEA
Royal Devon and Exeter NHS Foundation Trust, Centre for Women's Health,
Wonford Hospital, Exeter, UK
e-mail: lisajoels@doctors.org.uk

M.J.O. Taylor, BA(Oxon), MRCGP, MRCOG, PhD
Royal Devon and Exeter NHS Foundation Trust, Centre for Women's Health, Exeter, UK
e-mail: mylesjotaylor@gmail.com

K. Jayaprakasan, L. Kean (eds.), *Clinical Management of Pregnancies following ART*, DOI 10.1007/978-3-319-42858-1_8

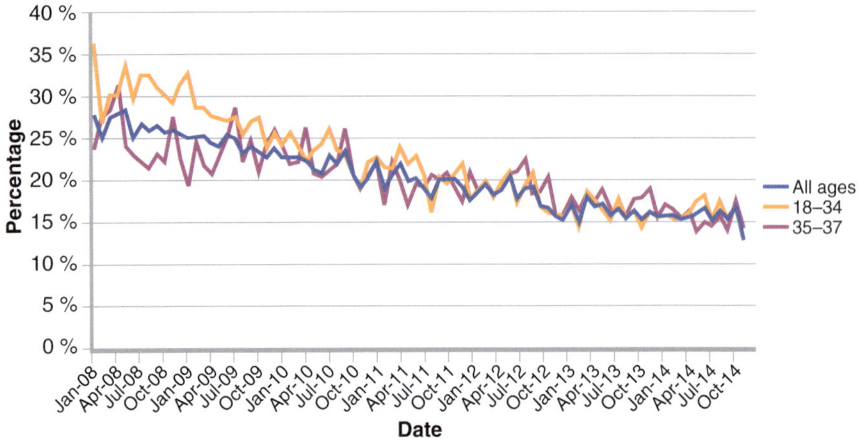

Fig. 8.1 Monthly multiple pregnancy rate (% of pregnancies) 2008–2014 (Source: Human Fertilisation and Embryology Authority (HFEA) [3])

What Are the Maternal, Fetal and Neonatal Risks Associated with Multiple Pregnancies?

Multiple pregnancy is considered to be the most common adverse outcome and largest health risk associated with assisted reproductive technologies (ARTs) [2]. Perinatal mortality rates are higher for multiple pregnancies. In 2009 the stillbirth rate was 12.3 per 1000 twin births and 31.1 per 1000 triplet and higher-order multiple births, compared with the singleton perinatal mortality rate, which is 5 per 1000 births [7, 8]. In multiple pregnancies 66 % of stillbirths are associated with growth restriction and birth weight less than 10th centile [7]. Approximately half of twin pregnancies will result in prematurity [2, 7]. Preterm birth is associated with an increased risk of long-term mental and physical handicap including cerebral palsy, mental disability, long-term learning difficulties and chronic lung disease [2]. The risks of producing a child with cerebral palsy are eight-times greater in twins and forty to fifty-times greater in triplets compared with singleton pregnancies [8]. Triplet pregnancies are associated with preterm birth before 37 weeks gestation in over 90 % of cases, leading to significant neonatal morbidity and mortality. Major congenital anomalies are 4.9 % more common in multiple pregnancies than in singletons [7].

These risks were highlighted in the 2006 Human Fertilisation and Embryology Authority (HFEA) report led by Professor Braude: "One Child at a Time" [9]. This investigation group was set up in response to growing concerns regarding the increasing rates of multiple pregnancies following ARTs as clinics often transferred more than one optimal embryo in order to increase pregnancy rates. As well as neonatal mortality, it also identified maternal risks, which include higher risks of miscarriage, gestational diabetes, pregnancy-induced hypertension, pre-eclampsia, impaired fetal growth and stillbirth, and problems during labour including

Table 8.1 Summary of the risks of multiple pregnancies to mother and baby

	Risk
Mother	Higher rates of **miscarriage**.
	Higher chance of **pregnancy induced hypertension**: 20 % in women pregnant with twins compared with 1–5 % in women pregnant with a singleton.
	Higher risk of **pre-eclampsia**: up to 30 % for twin pregnancies compared with 2–10 % in singleton pregnancies.
	Higher risk of **gestational diabetes**: up to 12 % in twin pregnancies compared with around 4 % for singleton pregnancies.
	Higher chance of **intervention in delivery**: elective and emergency caesarean section rates are higher for mothers of twins.
	Maternal mortality associated with multiple births is 2.5 times greater than with singletons.
Baby	**Premature Birth**. Preterm delivery rate is increased by 50 % compared with singleton pregnancies. 10 % twin births take place before 32/40 compared with 1.6 % singletons.
	Perinatal Mortality. Five times higher in twins in 2013 than singletons
	Neonatal Care/Admission to NICU. 40–60 % twins will be transferred to NICU when they are born, compared with 20 % IVF singletons
	Additional Health Complications:
	Respiratory distress
	Cerebral Palsy
	Delay in Language Development
	Disability
	Congenital malformations

Data from Braude [9]

intrapartum hypoxia, obstetric haemorrhage and increased need for elective and emergency caesarean section [6, 9] (Table 8.1).

The Barker Hypothesis predicts that adverse antenatal conditions can lead to long term consequences in the adult. Certainly the increased risks of multiple pregnancies with or without ARTs, such as hypertension and diabetes may lead to cardiac and metabolic disturbances in later life, which cannot be ignored. Epidemiological data are needed in IVF adolescents and adults [6].

Assisted Reproductive Technologies and Multiple Pregnancies: How Does It Happen?

Assisted reproduction technologies (ART) aim to approximate male and female gametes in order to create an embryo with the hope of subsequent embryo implantation leading to a clinical pregnancy. Techniques include intrauterine insemination (IUI) where motile sperm are placed in the uterine cavity close to the fundus in a woman with confirmed tubal patency or in-vitro fertilization (IVF) where embryos are created outside the body and subsequently replaced in the uterine cavity. Both

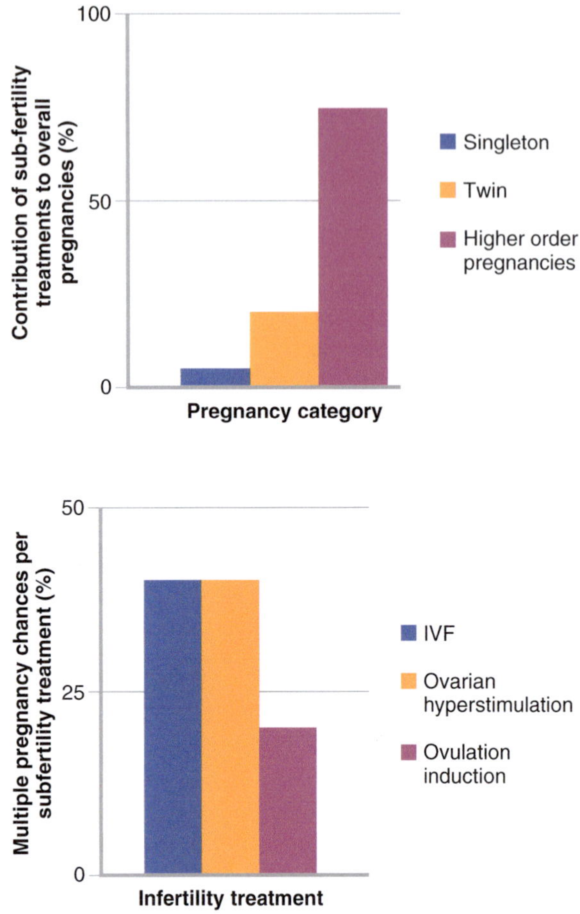

Fig. 8.2 Contribution of sub-fertility treatments to overall pregnancies (*upper graph*) and reported frequency of multiple pregnancies in relation to IVF, ovarian hyperstimulation and ovulation induction (*lower graph*) (Used with permission of Elsevier from Fauser et al. [11])

IUI and IVF treatments can be carried out in natural cycles but have disappointingly low results so that almost all treatments (97.6 % [3]) now include an element of ovulation induction to improve pregnancy rates. Gonadotrophins are the most common method of ovulation induction (OI) for ART inducing multi-follicular development. In IUI treatment, development of multiple follicles increases the risk of multiple pregnancy [10]. Methods to reduce the risk of multiple pregnancy with IUI include abandoning treatment, conversion to IVF, switching to oral estrogen antagonists and accepting lower success rates or considering fetal reduction in an established multi-fetal pregnancy. In IVF treatment the HFE Act permits the transfer of more than one embryo which also increases the risk of multiple pregnancy in selected groups. Strategies to reduce the risk include elective single embryo transfer (eSET) and blastocyst culture. Births resulting from infertility treatments account for around 1–3 % of all singleton births, 30–50 % of twin births and greater than 50 % of higher order multiples (Fig. 8.2) [11].

Ovulation Induction

The aim of OI is to use the lowest effective dose of fertility drug in order to achieve monofollicular ovulation for patients with anovulatory infertility [12]. This is then repeated monthly until pregnancy is achieved for up to six to nine cycles. The method of ovulation induction depends on the ovulatory disorder, classified by the World Health Organization [13]. The two groups that would benefit from ovulation induction are those with hypothalamic pituitary failure (Group I: hypothalamic amenorrhoea or hypogonadotrophic hypogonadism) and hypothalamic pituitary dysfunction (Group II: normogonadotrophic, predominantly polycystic ovary syndrome).

In WHO Group I, women may have low or normal serum FSH and LH, with low estradiol concentrations and normal or low testosterone. They do not have a withdrawal bleed with a progesterone challenge test [13]. Ovulation is induced either with pulsatile gonadotrophin-releasing hormone via a pump or with urinary (FSH and LH) or recombinant gonadotrophin (FSH) therapy. The aim is to support the growth of a single follicle until it reaches 16–18 mm size when hCG is administered to trigger ovulation. Usually a low-dose step up regime of gonadotrophins is used to minimise multifollicular development, reducing rates of multiple pregnancy and ovarian hyperstimulation [12]. If the trigger of hCG is administered in the presence of more than one large follicle the rates of multiple pregnancies exponentially increase, with reported rates of 50 % with greater than 3 large pre-ovulatory follicles [10]. It is therefore recommended to cancel the hCG trigger and to advise the couple to avoid unprotected sexual intercourse in that cycle if there are >3 pre-ovulatory follicles developed.

In WHO Group II disorders, clomifene citrate is used for stimulation of ovulation by blocking the estrogen receptors in the hypothalamus and blocking the negative feedback effect of estradiol [12], leading to increased endogenous FSH secretion and stimulating follicular development. Again the aim is to use the lowest necessary dose of clomifene in order to nurture one follicle. The risk of multiple pregnancy rises from the background rate of 1 in 80 to 1 in 10–20 with clomifene use, becoming more common with the use of higher doses of clomifene in those with PCOS [14]. Side effects of clomifene include Ovarian Hyperstimulation Syndrome (OHSS) (1–6 %) [12], visual disturbances, nausea, vomiting, dizziness and in some cases seizure activity.

In this same group of ovulation disorders, FSH can be used for women resistant to clomifene to achieve ovulation. As for the Group I disorders a low-dose step up regime is employed to reduce the risks of multiple pregnancy and OHSS. In some cases aromatase inhibitors such as letrozole have been used. They work by decreasing the aromatization of androgens to estrogens, decreasing the negative feedback cycle of estradiol and increasing follicular growth [12]. Pregnancy rates are promising with a lower incidence of multiple pregnancies, and a more favorable effect on the endometrium compared with clomifene [15].

Gonadotrophin Stimulation in Intrauterine Insemination (IUI)

IUI with controlled ovarian stimulation is widely used in cases of unexplained subfertility and mild male-factor infertility before resorting to more invasive options like IVF [16]. In contrast to older studies, more recent evidence has suggested that using IUI with gonadotrophin stimulation may correct subtle ovulation issues, leading to a greater number of oocytes and consequently a higher live pregnancy rate. The offset is of course multiple pregnancies, rates of which have been reported as high as 20–30 % in some centres regardless of the infertility cause [10, 11]. Reduction of the risk of a multiple pregnancy can be obtained by either avoiding any gonadotrophic stimulation (a 'natural cycle'), using strict cancellation regimes or using a low-dose step up regime similar to that described in the last section of this chapter. This can result in a reduction to 10 % multiple pregnancy rate without an overall impact on live birth rates [17]. Recent NICE guidelines [1] do not support using this method in those with unexplained infertility and instead suggest that it is restricted to those who are unable to have vaginal intercourse due to a disability or psychosexual problem, those in whom sperm washing is appropriate (such as HIV positive men) or those in same sex relationships. However, NICE are currently reviewing this recommendation which is therefore likely to change at the next update.

IVF/ICSI

In IVF procedures, controlled ovarian hyperstimulation can also be employed to generate the follicles for embryo creation *in vitro*. It is the *number* of embryos transferred which has a direct bearing on the chance of a multiple pregnancy. The risk of twins after double embryo transfer (DET) is 23.5 % for cleavage stage embryos (day 2–3 of development) and 36.4 % for blastocysts (day 5 of development). Elective single embryo transfer (eSET) in selected patient groups has shown promising success with clinical and live pregnancy rates, which are not dissimilar to those for double or higher order embryo transfers.

IVF itself appears to increase the risk of monozygotic twins by twofold compared with natural conception (0.8 % vs 0.4 %) although the overall incidence is low [6, 18]. The HFEA routinely collects outcome data from all IVF/ICSI treatment cycles across the UK and have reported that the incidence of twin pregnancy after eSET of a cleavage stage embryo is 0.6 %, identical to natural conception whereas eSET of a blastocyst embryo results in a more than doubling of the twin pregnancy rate to 1.9 % [3]. These are presumed to be monozygous pregnancies as the chance of simultaneous natural conception is thought to be very low.

Monozygosity itself is associated with higher adverse outcomes as two thirds of monozygous twins are monochorionic [7]. A twin pregnancy with a shared chorion is at increased risk of complications due to the vascular placental anastomoses that connect the umbilical circulations of both twins, leading to twin-to-twin transfusion syndrome (TTTS), which complicates 10–15 % of monochorionic pregnancies. This leads to haemodynamic and liquor discordance in the "donor" and "recipient" twin and in severe cases death of the recipient twin due to high output cardiac failure. In these cases death of the surviving twin can be as high as 12 % with the risk of neurological abnormalities in those that do survive being approximately 18 % [19]. Monochorionic pregnancies also have a higher chance of fetal loss greater than 24 weeks of gestation (3.3 % fetuses) compared with dichorionic pregnancies [19]. Overall these babies may also be more at risk of neurodevelopmental abnormalities.

IVF twins also seem to have a small but statistically significant increase in the risk of preterm labour, approximately by 23 % [6] compared with spontaneously conceived twins. Early fetal loss of one twin can lead to premature delivery of the remaining twin. Similarly IVF twins have shown an increased risk of low birth weight in IVF twins [6]. Rates of congenital anomalies are known to be 30–40 % higher in IVF pregnancies (septal heart defects, cleft lip, oesophageal atresia, anorectal atresia). The risk of anomalies after conventional ART is the same as natural conception but is higher after ICSI. This is much like a "chicken and egg" problem with ICSI. It is not completely clear if it is the process of ICSI (i.e., stripping cumulus cells and longer exposure to light and oxygen, which causes the anomalies) or if it is due to the underlying sperm dysfunction which provokes the need for ICSI in the first place. Most severe sperm dysfunction (<5 million sperm/ml) is probably genetic involving the Y chromosome, although there is no evidence to suggest that in multiple pregnancies this rate would be higher, especially for hypospadias [20, 21]. The risk of congenital heart disease in monochorionic twins has been shown to be higher [19, 22].

Overall, it should be acknowledged that factors that predispose to infertility are also linked with adverse perinatal outcomes. To determine whether a particular ART is leading to an adverse outcome or whether it is a consequence of other infertility causes and complex factors between the couple needs further investigation [6, 7].

The HFEA and Elective Single Embryo Transfers (eSET)

High multiple pregnancy rates are preventable. A recent publication from the HFEA examined the national picture of multiple pregnancies and births after fertility treatment [2]. In 2008 almost a quarter of births resulting from IVF treatment were multiple [2]. The HFEA mandated a target goal of reducing the multiple pregnancy rate to 10 % of all live births. Although the mandate was removed after a legal challenge, the HFEA continues to advise clinics to reduce multiple pregnancy rates. There has been a decrease in multiple pregnancy rates from 26.6 % in 2008 to 15.9 % in 2014 [3], which begs the question, why did this happen?

One of the goals set by Professor Braude's report, was for clinics to move from double embryo transfer (DET) to elective single embryo transfer (eSET) even if more than one embryo is available as a result of IVF preparation. This was quite a changing of the tide in reproductive medicine given the firmly held belief among professionals and the public that the number of embryos transferred positively equates to successful pregnancy outcomes. Couples who are in a desperate position to achieve a pregnancy balance the benefits of having two or more babies against the cost of repeating fertility treatment both financially and psychologically. The NHS funds approximately 40 % of IVF treatment cycles so the majority of the financial burden of treatment falls on the couples themselves. The HFEA publishes the results of the pregnancy rates for each fertility clinic in the UK, which becomes *de facto* a league table that produces a perverse incentive to maximise pregnancy rates by transfer of one or more embryo. In a competitive market the motivation of clinics to maximise pregnancy rates mirrors the desires of the couple and all of these motivations are not sufficiently offset by the known dangers of multiple pregnancy for the mother and her babies.

All the available evidence shows that increasing the number of embryos transferred increases pregnancy rates. Other countries in the world have less stringent laws on the number of embryos that may be transferred and consistently show higher pregnancy rates than the average in the UK [23]. The HFE Act restricts the number of embryos transferred to two in women under 40 years of age and three for older women. With restrictions on number of embryos to transfer, other strategies have been developed to maximise the chance of pregnancy. There is convincing evidence that for women aged less than 36 years with more than one optimal quality embryo, the chance of conception is almost the same with eSET as with DET of sub-optimal embryos. In women over 40 years of age there is reassuring evidence that eSET of an optimal embryo maintains pregnancy rates (21.7 %) similar to women having DET (21 %) where in most cases DET will have been chosen due not having an optimal embryo to transfer [3]. There is further evidence that blastocyst transfer increases pregnancy rates; however, this belies the fact that not all embryos have the potential to survive to day 5 in culture and therefore this option may not be suitable to all patients.

There has been encouraging data released by the HFEA in recent months. There has been a rise in eSET from 5 to 29 % overall, with a specific rise from 7 to 38 % in the 18–34 age range [2]. Despite the rise in eSET, pregnancy and birth rates have been maintained and have recently started to rise [2] (Fig. **8.3**). The average multiple birth rate in the fertility sector is now 15.9 % [3], closer to the 10 % target set by the HFEA than ever before. With eSET the risk of twins is only 1 in 50 pregnancies.

Fetal Reduction

The ethical rationale in relation to fetal reduction is that of a "consequentialist" approach, in which the parents and the clinician weigh the benefits and risks of the pregnancy continuing and make a "best interest" decision for the remaining fetus(es) and for the mother's health [24, 25].

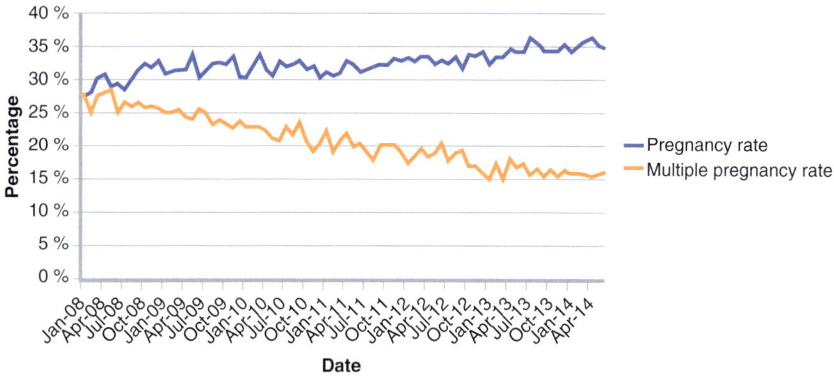

Fig. 8.3 Pregnancy rate (per embryo transfer) and multiple pregnancy rate (per pregnancy), fresh and frozen transfers: 2008 to mid-2014 (Source: Human Fertilisation and Embryology Authority (HFEA) [2])

Multifetal pregnancy reduction (MFPR) attempts to ameliorate the maternal and fetal risks of higher order pregnancies by reducing the number of fetuses to a more manageable number [8]. Epidemiological studies have shown that twin pregnancies produced a child with cerebral palsy 8 times more often than singletons and for triplet pregnancies this rate was 47 times higher [26]. For example, 8–12 % of triplet pregnancies will experience some kind of neurodevelopmental sequelae compared with twin pregnancies. This is likely to be even higher if the triplet pregnancy contains a monoamniotic pair [19]. Reducing the triplet pregnancy to twins significantly reduces the risk of preterm delivery without an increase in miscarriage rates [27]. Full fetal medicine assessment should be carried out before deciding on which fetus(es) to terminate. This is best carried out between 11 and 14 weeks gestation when the risk of spontaneous reduction has passed and in order to identify features of aneuploidy (i.e., nuchal translucency) [27]. Fetuses at lowest risk of aneuploidy, determined by nuchal translucency should be left intact as should those implanted closest to the cervix so as not to increase the risk of miscarriage of the entire pregnancy should the fetus closest to the cervix miscarry following MFPR. Studies to date do have major limitations, however, as many do not differentiate between trichorionic and non-trichorionic pregnancies, the latter in which a monochorionic pair exists, which of course will have a bearing on fetal outcomes (which will be discussed below). However, despite the controversies, reducing triplets to twins suggests that the chance of preterm labour before 32 weeks gestation drops by around 55 %, with very little increase in miscarriage [27], and the potential to take a live born baby home increases from 80 to 90 % [8]. However, it is clear that expectant management of a trichorionic triplet pregnancy does have a reasonable perinatal outcome.

MFPR does have a significant psychological impact on parents, most reporting acute stress, pain and fear [28]. The ethical dilemma of the parents must be taken into account, encompassing the emotional journey already experienced through the ART process balanced against their own ethical and religious beliefs.

Recommendations for Birth Choices and Intrapartum Care

When multiple pregnancy is diagnosed in a fertility unit, referral to specialist multidisciplinary team should be made, consisting of a specialist obstetrician, midwives and ultrasonographers, all of whom have experience of managing twin and triplet pregnancies. Within the clinic, the woman and her partner will receive specialist prenatal screening and diagnosis as well as initial counseling regarding selective fetal reduction if she has triplets or a higher order pregnancy [6]. She will also receive advice regarding nutrition, the antenatal course including frequency of scans and antenatal clinic appointments, information regarding the risks, signs and symptoms of preterm labour, advice regarding the likely timing and optional modes of delivery [7]. An enhanced support program should offer psychological, parenting and breastfeeding from those with the experience and knowledge relevant to twin and triplet pregnancies.

A study from Australia of IVF conceived twins compared perinatal adverse outcomes with spontaneously conceived (SC) twins and in particular dizygotic twins [5]. This showed clearly that IVF conceived twins have a greater risk of adverse events including preterm birth, low birth weight and death than SC twins. Obstetricians caring for women with IVF conceived twins should take this into consideration when developing management plans for these pregnancies.

Zygosity, Chorionicity, and Amnionicity

Risks to the fetuses in multiple pregnancies depend partly on amnionicity and chorionicity [7]. Zygosity refers to the genetic makeup of the twins. When a single zygote splits into two equal zygotes they share the same genetic material (monozygotic) and if two separate zygotes are simultaneously fertilized by two sperm they are genetically different (dizygotic). Chorionicity refers to the placentation and amnionicity refers to the relation of the amniotic membranes between the twins. Two amnions and two chorions lead to dichorionic, diamniotic pregnancies (DCDA). Dizygous twins are always DCDA. These are the most common types of twinning occurring in approximately two-thirds of multiple pregnancies and carry the lowest risks for the fetus and mother due to the complete separation of the placentas.

Monozygous twins can become DCDA twins if cleavage of the single zygote happens before day 3. This happens in 25–30 % of monozygous twinning. More commonly cleavage occurs after day 3 and before day 8 when the blastocyst has already formed, resulting in a monochorionic diamniotic (MCDA) pairing. Here each twin has its own amniotic sac but shares a placenta and occurs in 75 % cases. Much more rarely, cleavage of the blastocyst will occur after day 8 and before day 13. These twins will share both the placenta and amniotic sac in monochorionic

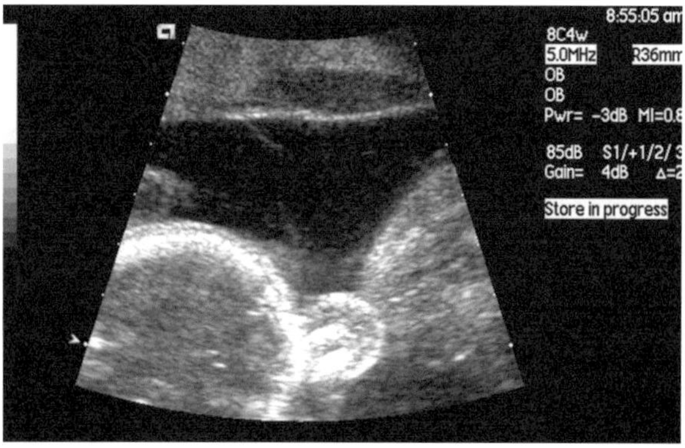

Fig. 8.4 "T sign" in Monochorionic Twins (Reproduced with permission of John Wiley and Sons from Taylor and Fisk [8])

monoamniotic pregnancy (MCMA). This type of twinning occurs in <2 % cases and is high risk for cord entanglement and stillbirth. Cleavage after day 13 results in conjoined twins. This is extremely rare and beyond the scope of this chapter. Around a third of twin pregnancies are monochorionic and can also occur in higher order multiples as well. Twin-twin transfusion syndrome (TTTS) is a condition associated with monochorionic twins and occurs in around 10–15 % of these pregnancies [19] and is associated with a 20 % risk of stillbirth [7]. This is discussed in more detail below.

Antenatal Care

First trimester screening in twin pregnancies allows accurate dating, screening for Downs Syndrome, determination of fetal number, amnionicity and chorionicity. The most accurate and reliable time is between 11^{+0} and 13^{+6} weeks gestation [7]. Ultrasound reveals either a "T sign" for monochorionic (Fig. 8.4) or a "lambda or twin peak" sign in dichorionic pregnancies (Fig. 8.5).

Twin-Twin Transfusion Syndrome

Determining chorionicity is the most important indicator of fetal outcome in twins and guides the antenatal management. A monochorionic placenta contains unique vascular architecture which include superficial arterio-arterial or veno-venous communications allowing bi-directional flow between the fetuses but also deep arterio-venous communications allowing only uni-directional flow. Thus intertwin transfusion is a normal event in MC twins – and is usually balanced. TTTS occurs

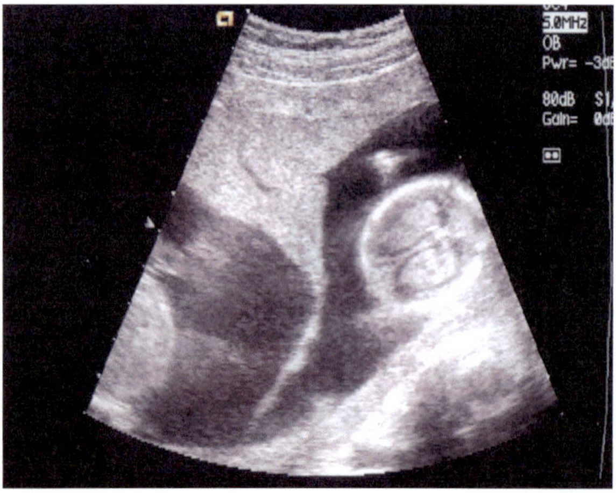

Fig. 8.5 "Twin peak" or "lambda" sign (Reproduced with permission of John Wiley and Sons from Taylor and Fisk [8])

when haemodynamic imbalance arises as a result of the particular arrangement of deep anastomoses, which overwhelms any compensation afforded by superficial anastomoses. Consequently the vascular abnormalities lead to hypovolaemia in one twin (the donor), which is thought to cause activation of the renin-angiotensin system leading to oligohydramnios and oliguria. Conversely in the recipient twin there may be increased secretion of atrial naturietic peptide leading to polyuria and polyhydramnios. Volume overload leads to cardiac hypertrophy, fetal hydrops, outflow tract obstruction and eventually death [8, 29]. TTTS occurs in 15 % of MCDA twins, affecting some 1600 pregnancies [30]. Scanning begins at 16 weeks and is carried out fortnightly until 24 weeks gestation, aiming to pick up the early signs of TTTS. Quintero staging [31] below (Table **8.2**) outlines the different stages of TTTS and what the defining ultrasound features are [29, 30].

In addition, screening for Downs Syndrome is an important point of discussion with parents, since there is a greater likelihood of Down's Syndrome with a twin or triplet pregnancy [7]. The likelihood of a false positive result is higher than in a singleton pregnancy, however, and as a consequence the offer of invasive testing is also increased. The risk is calculated based on nuchal translucency, beta-human chorionic gonadotrophin, pregnancy-associated plasma protein-A at 11^{+0} to 13^{+6} weeks gestation. A risk per baby is calculated in a dichorionic pregnancy compared with a risk for the pregnancy in monochorionic twins. Second trimester screening has limitations in dichorionic pregnancies as a risk per baby cannot be established accurately and therefore the rate of invasive testing is higher. Second trimester screening should not be used in triplet pregnancies [7]. Non-invasive prenatal testing (NIPT) of cell free fetal DNA can be used. However, any positive result will need confirming with invasive karyotyping, not least to determine with certainty, which, if any, is the affected fetus.

Table 8.2 Quintero staging for twin-twin transfusion syndrome

Stage	TOPS (O<2 cm, P>8 cm)	Absent bladder visualisation	Critical arterial Doppler (absent/reversed end diastolic flow)	Hydrops	Demise
I	+	–	–	–	–
II	+	+	–	–	–
III	+	+	+	–	–
IV	+	+	+	+	–
V	+	+	+	+	+

Data from Taylor and Fisk [29]
TOPS twin oligo-polyhydramnios (values refer to amniotic fluid pocket), *O* oligohydramnios, *P* polyhydramnios

With regard to IVF pregnancies and antenatal screening, it should be noted that PAPP-A levels are significantly lower in fresh transfer IVF pregnancies, hence potentially leading to a false positive result and increased risk of having CVS or amniocentesis [6].

Growth Restriction

The incidence of growth restriction in twin pregnancies has been reportedly as high as 29 % (4 % concordant and 25 % discordant) occurring in up to 42 % of monochorionic twins and 25 % of dichorionic twins [8]. Therefore standard antenatal care of twins employs regular growth scans in DCDA twins every 4 weeks and every 2–3 weeks in MCDA twins. Twenty-five percent growth discordancy or more between twins or triplets is considered to be a clinically significant measure of intrauterine growth restriction [7]. Management of discordant growth including timing of delivery is complex, and is a multi-disciplinary decision. Identification of IUGR at the extreme of prematurity, for example in DCDA twins, may warrant discussion with the parents to allow the pregnancy to continue in order to optimize the health of the larger twin, albeit potentially at the expense of the smaller twin [8].

In terms of screening for the maternal complications of multiple pregnancy, blood pressure and urine analysis is carried out at each antenatal visit to screen for the development of hypertension. Predicting preterm birth is less straightforward. Some studies have reported that cervical length measurements could be helpful. In twin pregnancies the mean cervical length at 24 weeks is similar to that of singletons, but one that is less than 25 mm (compared with 15 mm in singletons) may be predictive of preterm labour before 30 weeks gestation [8]. Progesterone supplementation has not been shown to be effective at preventing preterm labour in twin pregnancies [32]. Fetal fibronectin has also not been shown to be able to accurately provide a quantifiable risk of preterm labour as it has done in singletons and therefore is not recommended as a sole predictor of preterm labour [7].

Timing and Mode of Delivery

It is becoming common practice to consider an induction of labour at 40 weeks for those pregnancies resulting from assisted reproductive techniques, particularly IVF. However, these discussions are redundant with twins in light of the evidence stating the optimal safe timing of birth. Existing evidence has identified that in twin pregnancies that progressing beyond 38 weeks gestation leads to an increased rate of perinatal morbidity and mortality [33].

The Twins Timing of Birth Trial [34] randomised women with twin pregnancies to either elective birth at 37 weeks gestation or standard care/expectant management from 38 weeks gestation. An elective birth at 37 weeks was associated with a significant reduction in the serious adverse outcomes for the twins compared with expectant management allowing labour to progress beyond 38 weeks. Currently NICE recommendations [7] state that in DCDA twin pregnancies, labour should be induced between 37 and 38 weeks gestation and from 36 weeks gestation in MCDA twins, with steroid cover to aid lung maturity in preparation for delivery [7]. Most monochorionic monoamniotic twins (MCMA) have some degree of cord entanglement which can have significant implications for antenatal and intrapartum morbidity and mortality. Delivery is usually recommended by caesarean section from 32 weeks gestation [19]. In triplet and higher order pregnancies delivery decisions are taken on an individual basis and will be mostly driven by the growth and wellbeing of each of the fetuses. Triplet pregnancies containing a monochorionic pair have higher fetal loss rates than trichorionic triplets [19]. The general recommendation is that labour should not progress beyond 36 weeks in triplet pregnancies due to a higher risk of fetal death [7]. Elective birth is usually offered from 35 weeks gestation following a course of antenatal steroids.

Mode of delivery in twin pregnancies is based on the principles of the presentation of the first twin (cephalic being preferred), fetal growth and wellbeing [8]. The Twin Birth Study Collaborative Group [35] randomized uncomplicated twin pregnancies between 32^{+0} and 38^{+6} weeks gestation to a trial of planned caesarean section or vaginal delivery between 37^{+5} and 38^{+6} weeks delivery and compared the maternal and fetal outcomes. Findings concluded that an elective caesarean birth does not significantly increase or decrease perinatal complications and mortality compared with vaginal birth. However, it is worth noting that there was a high intrapartum caesarean section rate in the vaginal delivery group of around 39.6 % for both twins and 4.2 % for combined vaginal-caesarean delivery [35]. The twin birth study did, however, exclude pregnancies with a significant size discrepancy between twins. A consensus hasn't been reached regarding the timing of delivery in these twins. In general the current authors would consider a growth discrepancy of around 20 % to indicate that growth restriction is evident, which is echoed in the current literature, though NICE guidance recommends 25 % discordance as the best indicator of selective growth restriction [36]. In a recent multi-centre, prospective trial of 1000 women in Ireland, the Evaluation of Sonographic Predictors of Restricted Growth in Twins (ESPRiT) trial revealed that a difference of 18 % or more in twin birth weights is associated with an increased risk of fetal or neonatal death, bowel complications, breathing difficulties, infection and admission to the neonatal intensive care unit [37]. Taking into account additional measures of fetal wellbeing (e.g., gestation, middle cerebral arterial doppler and ductus venosus Doppler measurements of each twin, liquor volumes and presentation of twin 1, the presence of any obstetric complications and whether steroids have been administered), a discussion can take place between the obstetrician and the mother regarding the appropriate mode of delivery.

It is appropriate to aim for a vaginal birth in uncomplicated monochorionic twin pregnancies providing there is no clinical indication for Caesarean section such as twin one presenting breech or a previous caesarean section [19]. Evidence of acute transfusion in labour is reported in the literature, and has been described as high as 10 % therefore continuous monitoring of the fetuses should be employed in labour [19]. In higher order pregnancies caesarean section is usually recommended to avoid the challenges of intrapartum monitoring and potential birth trauma from internal podalic versions and breech extraction procedures that may be required [19].

Strategies to Promote Single Embryo Transfer

Now the focus of research is on selecting the best quality embryo for transfer using techniques such as time-lapse imaging of embryo growth, extended culture to blastocyst, metabolomics or controversial pre-implantation screening.

The challenge for IVF clinics is to move away from the focus on their position in the HFEA leagues tables in terms of pregnancy rates and to move towards a holistic approach to creating a family that isn't burdened by bereavement or long-term health problems of their ART-conceived children. In order to do this, strategies could include increasing conception rates with eSET or changing funding arrangements.

Research into increasing pregnancy rates with eSET has focused on better selection of embryos and methods of improving the chance of implantation of the embryo. Using the technique of blastocyst culture has continually shown potential in research studies to improve clinical pregnancy rates [38, 39]. Blastocyst culture involves extended culture of the embryos from the traditional day 2 cleavage stage to day 5 (blastocyst stage) [38]. Cochrane reviews have shown that the live birth rate is as much as 40 % higher in favour of the blastocyst stage culture [39]. However, blastocyst eSET doubles the risk of monozygotic twins compared to cleavage stage embryos and the risk of congenital malformations and preterm birth are significantly higher [6]. There is a lack of long-term safety data and of the long term health effects of prolonged embryo culture. Blastocyst culture reduces the number of additional embryos available for freezing meaning that women face a further episode of ovarian stimulation. Given the concerns about an increased risk of borderline ovarian tumours with repeated cycles of OI [40], the long term consequences of a wholesale move to blastocyst transfer are unknown.

In vivo maturation involves the maturation of immature oocytes from antral follicles with minimal or no gonadotrophin stimulation followed by maturation and fertilization in the laboratory [41]. Avoiding gonadotrophins has the additional benefit of reducing the risk of ovarian hyperstimulation mentioned earlier in this chapter and therefore reducing the multiple pregnancy rate. Its use would be particularly beneficial for those at risk of hyperstimulation and hence multiple conceptions, such as polycystic ovarian syndrome patients and those with a high antral follicle count. The advantages aside from multiple pregnancy reduction are that it is less costly, safe and convenient. The main disadvantage is that, at present, the live birth rate is lower [41]. However, it may be that this could be improved in the future with optimized protocols and laboratory training. Follow-up developmental studies in children have thus far been promising [41, 42].

Time lapse photography without removing the embryos from the incubator has been proposed as a better method of assessing normal development of embryos than the traditional approach of intermittent microscopy when embryos are removed from the incubator and assessed by an embryologist [43]. It is suggested that closer analysis of stages of cleavage will result in better embryo selection and increase pregnancy rates but the evidence to support this is yet to be sufficiently convincing to justify the additional costs in changing laboratory equipment given those costs will drive up costs to the patients even further. Since most IVF cycles in the UK are funded by the couple, an unintended consequence of time lapse photography may be to push up DET rates.

It has been suggested that investigating the metabolomics of the embryos will improve embryo selection. This involves analyzing metabolites in the culture medium in which the embryos have developed with the suggestion that this will identify the optimum embryo for eSET but results to date have been disappointing [44].

It is recognized that embryo implantation is an immunological process involving cross-talk between the secretory phase endometrium and the hatching day six embryo. Focusing on improving implantation rates after transfer of a single optimal embryo has centred on these immunological processes but use of steroids has not resulted in significant improvements in pregnancy rates apart from in women with antiphospholipid syndrome [45]. An alternative approach has been to cause damage to the endometrium to provoke a healing response with a migration of natural killer cells, which alters the immune environment in the uterine cavity. There is some evidence of increased pregnancy rates for women with recurrent implantation failure (more than two failed IVF treatments after transfer of optimal embryos) but this has not provided a solution to improving pregnancy rates after eSET for all other patients.

The alternative approach adopted by Sweden, Finland and Belgium is to increase state funding of IVF eSET cycles. In Belgium couples can now have up to 6 eSET cycles funded by the health service [5]. A liberal approach to funded IVF combined with eSET in Sweden and Finland has resulted in a reduction for IVF twins to 6 % of cycles [6]. The increased costs of providing more IVF treatment has been offset by a significant reduction in the obstetric, neonatal, pediatric and long-term costs of dealing with the consequences of complications linked with multiple pregnancy.

Conclusion

In 1984, Baroness Warnock produced a report assessing the Human Fertilisation and Embryology Association following the birth of Louise Brown, the first IVF baby in 1978 [46]. In her report she discussed the ethical, social and spiritual aspects of assisted reproductive techniques. She concluded that "childlessness is a source of stress to even those who have chosen it… it can disrupt the picture of the whole future of their lives… unable to fulfill their own and other people's expectations." She explained that infertility is a condition meriting treatment and that it should not be limited to the private sector and should be offered within the NHS. Achieving a family is incredibly important to many people and should be supported in as safe a way as possible. The long term outcomes for the majority of children born from IVF are reassuring once prematurity and multiple gestations are taken out of the equation.

From this chapter it would be safe to conclude that the burden on society, the parents and the children themselves from iatrogenic, avoidable multiple pregnancies is too high [38]. Financial pressures for the NHS are worsening and the costs of neonatal and postnatal resources are high for those children born prematurely or with neurodevelopmental morbidities. Measures need to be continued in reproductive medicine clinics to drive the multiple pregnancy rates down, such as elective single embryo transfers. We now have the evidence to demonstrate that live pregnancy rates are not reduced by eSET in the under 36 year old age group. It remains to be seen from audit figures whether those in the advanced maternal age category would also benefit from this approach with a similar reassuring improvement in live birth rates. Promotion of singleton birth as the 'norm' in IVF clinics is already in progress and we hope will continue.

References

1. NICE Guidelines CG156: fertility: assessment and treatment for people with fertility problems. 2013.
2. Human Fertilisation and Embryology Authority (HFEA). Improving outcomes for fertility patients: multiple births. London: HFEA; 2015. http://www.hfea.gov.uk/docs/Multiple_Births_Report_2015.pdf.
3. Human Fertilisation and Embryology Authority (HFEA). Fertility treatment 2014: trends and figures. London: HREA; 2016. http://www.hfea.gov.uk/docs/HFEA_Fertility_treatment_Trends_and_figures_2014.pdf.
4. Pandey S, Shetty A, Hamilton M, Bhattacharya S, Maheshwari A. Obstetric and perinatal outcomes in singleton pregnancies resulting from IVF/ICSI: a systematic review and meta-analysis. Hum Reprod Update. 2012;18(5):485–503.
5. Hansen M, Colvin L, Petterson B, Kurinczuk JJ, deKlerk N, Bower C. Twins born following assisted reproductive technology: perinatal outcome and admission to hospital. Hum Reprod. 2009;24(9):2321–31.
6. RCOG Press and British Fertility Society (BFS). In vitro fertilisation: perinatal risks and early childhood outcomes. Scientific Impact Paper No. 8. May 2012.

7. NICE Guidelines CG129: multiple pregnancy: the management of twin and triplet pregnancies in the antenatal period. 2011.
8. Taylor M, Fisk N. Multiple pregnancy. Obstet Gynaecol. 2000;2:2–10.
9. Braude P. One child at a time. Reducing multiple births after IVF. Report of the Expert Group on Multiple Births after IVF. London: HFEA; 2006. http://www.oneatatime.org.uk/images/MBSET_report_Final_Dec_06.pdf.
10. Homberg R. Ovulation induction and controlled ovarian stimulation. Switzerland: Springer International Publishing; 2014.
11. Fauser BC, Devroey P, Macklon NS. Multiple birth resulting from ovarian stimulation for subfertility treatment. Lancet. 2005;365:1807–16.
12. Gorthi S, Balen AH, Tang T. Current issues in ovulation induction. Obstet Gynaecol. 2012;14:188–96.
13. Rowe PJ, Comhaire FH, Hargreave TB, Mellows HJ. WHO manual for the standardized investigation and diagnosis of the infertile couple. Cambridge: Cambridge University Press; 1997.
14. Baden AH, Jacobs HS. Infertility in practice. New York: Churchill Livingstone; 1997.
15. Casper RF, Mitwally MF. Review: aromatase inhibitors for ovulation induction. J Clin Endocrinol Metabol. 2006;91:760–71.
16. Nandi A, Homburg R. Unexplained subfertility: diagnosis and management. Obstet Gynaecol. 2016. doi:10.1111/tog.12253.
17. Ragni G, Caliari I, Nicolosi AE, Arnoldi M, Somigliana E, Crosignani PG. Preventing high-order multiple pregnancies during controlled ovarian hyperstimulation and intrauterine insemination: 3 years' experience using low-dose recombinant follicle-stimulating hormone and gonadotropin releasing hormone antagonists. Fertil Steril. 2006;85:619–24.
18. Vitthala S, Gelbaya TA, Brison DR, Fitzgerald CT, Nardo LG. The risk of monozygotic twins after assisted reproductive technology: a systematic review and metanalysis. Hum Reprod Update. 2009;15(1):45–55.
19. RCOG. Green Top Guideline No. 51. Management of monochorionic twin pregnancy. London: RCOG Press; 2008.
20. Seoud MA, Toner JP, Kruithoff C, Muasher SJ. Outcome of twin, triplet, and quadruplet in vitro fertilization pregnancies: the Norfolk experience. Fertil Steril. 1992;57(4):825–34.
21. Ericson A, Källén B. Congenital malformations in infants born after IVF: a population-based study. Hum Reprod. 2001;16(3):504–9.
22. Best KE, Rankin J. Increased risk of congenital heart disease in twins in the North of England between 1998 and 2010. Heart. 2015;101(22):1807–12.
23. Fertility Success Rates: United States. 2014. http://fertilitysuccessrates.com/report/United-States/women-35-37/data.html.
24. Brinsden PR. Textbook of in vitro fertilization and assisted reproduction. Oxon: Taylor & Francis Group; 2005.
25. Hope T. Medical ethics. A very short introduction. Oxford: Oxford University Press; 2004.
26. Petterson B, Nelson KB, Watson L, Stanley F. Twins, triplets, and cerebral palsy in births in Western Australia in the 1980s. BMJ. 1993;307(6914):1239–43.
27. Wimalasundera RC. Selective reduction and termination of multiple pregnancies. Semin Fetal Neonatal Med. 2010;15(6):327–35.
28. Bergh C, Moller A, Nilsson L, Wikland M. Obstetric Outcome and psychological follow-up of pregnancies after embryo reduction. Hum Reprod. 1999;14(8):2170–5.
29. Taylor MJO, Fisk N. Management of twin-twin transfusion syndrome. In: High risk pregnancy. Blickenstein; 2005.
30. Smith RP, Denbow ML. Review: twin to twin transfusion syndrome. Obstet Gynaecol. 2006;8:1–6.
31. Quintero RA, Morales WJ, Allen MH, Bornick PW, Johnson PK, Kruger M. Staging of twin-twin transfusion syndrome. J Perinatol. 1999;19:550–5.
32. Normal JE, Mackenzie F, Owen P, Mactier H, Hanretty K, Cooper S, et al. Progesterone for the prevention of preterm birth in twin pregnancy (STOPPIT): a randomised, double-blind, placebo-controlled study and meta-analysis. Lancet. 2009;373(9680):2034–40.

33. Hartley RS, Emanuel I, Hitti J. Perinatal mortality and neonatal morbidity rates among twin pairs at different gestational ages: optimal delivery timing at 37 to 38 weeks' gestation. Am J Obstet Gynaecol. 2001;184(3):451–8.
34. Dodd J, Crowther C, Haslam R, Robinson J. Elective birth at 37 weeks of gestation versus standard care for women with an uncomplicated twin pregnancy at term: the Twins Timing of Birth Randomised Trial. BJOG. 2012;119:964–74.
35. Barrett JFR, Hannah ME, Hutton EF, Willan AR, Allen AC, Armson BA, Gafni A, Joseph KS, Mason D, Ohlsson A, Ross S, Sanchez JJ, Asztalos EV. A randomized trial of planned caesarean or vaginal delivery for twin pregnancy. N Engl J Med. 2013;369:1295–305.
36. Breathnach FM, McAuliffe FM, Geary M, Daly S, Higgins JR, Dornan J, Morrison JJ, Burke G, Higgins S, Dicker P, Manning F. Optimum timing for planned delivery of uncomplicated monochorionic and dichorionic twin pregnancies. Obstet Gynecol. 2012;119(1):50–9.
37. Kent EM, Breathnach FM, Gillan JE, McAuliffe FM, Geary MP, Daly S, Higgins JR, Hunter A, Morrison JJ, Burke G, Higgins S. Placental pathology, birthweight discordance, and growth restriction in twin pregnancy: results of the ESPRiT Study. Am J Obstet Gynecol. 2012;207(3):220–e1.
38. Scientific Impact Paper. Multiple pregnancy following assisted reproduction. RCOG Press; 2011.
39. Blake DA, Farquhar CM, Johnson N, Proctor M. Cleavage stage versus blastocyst stage embryo transfer in assisted conception. Cochrane Database System Rev. 2007;(4):CD002118.
40. Klip H, Burger CW, Kenemans P, van Leeuwen FE. Cancer risk associated with subfertility and ovulation induction: a review. Cancer Causes Control. 2000;11:319–44.
41. Vitek W, Robins JC. In vitro maturation. Obstet Gynaecol. 2013;15:215–9.
42. Söderström-Anttila V, Salokorpi T, Pihlaja M, Serenius-Sirve S, Suikkari AM. Obstetric and perinatal outcome and preliminary results of development of children born after in vitro maturation of oocytes. Hum Reprod. 2006;21:1508–13.
43. Campbell A, Fishel S, Bowman N, Duffy S, Pedler S, Fonte Lidemann Hickme C. Modeling a risk classification of aneuploidy in human embryos using non-invasive morphokinetics. Reprod BioMed Online. 2013;26(5):477–85.
44. Vergow CG, Heymans MW, Hardson T, Sfontouris IA, Economou KA, Ahlstrom A, Rogberg L, Lainas TG, Sakkas D, Kieslinger DC, Kostelijk EH, Hompes PGA, Schats R, Lambalk CB. No evidence that embryo selection by near-infrared spectroscopy in addition to morphology is able to improve live birth rates: results from an individual patient data meta-analysis. Hum Reprod. 2014;29(3):455–61.
45. Nardo LG, El-Toukhy T, Stewart J, Balen AH, Potdar N. British Fertility Society Policy and Practice Committee: adjuvants in IVF: evidence for good clinical practice. Hum Fertil. 2015;18(1):2–15.
46. Dame Mary Warnock DBE. Department of Health and Social Security: report of the committee of inquire into human fertilisation and embryology. London: Her Majesty's Stationary Office; 1984.

Chapter 9
Maternal Medical Complications in Pregnancy Following Assisted Reproductive Technology

Margaret Ramsay and Shobhana Parameshwaran

Introduction

There has been an increase in the demand for assisted reproductive technology (ART) in the last 30 years. Assisted reproductive techniques have proved effective in achieving successful conception as well as outstanding live birth rates of 51–72 % after up to 6 treatment cycles; for women younger than 35 years the live birth rates are even better at 65–86 % [1]. Assisted reproductive technology refers not only to In Vitro Fertilization (IVF) but also to several other procedures related to the reason for subfertility, including intrauterine insemination. These procedures are usually paired with drugs to enhance ovulation. Women undergoing ART need it for various reasons: chronic anovulation due to polycystic ovarian syndrome (PCOS), diminishing ovarian function due to advanced age, tubal disease and male factor subfertility. However, these women may also have other significant problems which affect not only their fertility but also their risk for problems occurring should they achieve pregnancy, e.g., raised body mass index (BMI), pre-existing medical conditions including hypertension, diabetes or endocrine problems.

The use of ART has been linked with adverse pregnancy outcomes, including gestational hypertension, pre-eclampsia and gestational diabetes. Maternal medical complications, especially pre-eclampsia, are known to be exaggerated in those who conceive a twin or higher-order multiple pregnancy following ART. [2] In a large prospective study of singleton pregnancies, the pregnancy outcomes for 34,286

M. Ramsay, MA, MB, BChir, MD, MRCP, FRCOG (✉)
Department of Fetomaternal Medicine and Obstetrics, Nottingham University Hospitals, Queen's Medical Centre Campus, Nottingham, UK
e-mail: mmramsay@doctors.org.uk

S. Parameshwaran, MBBS, MS, MRCOG
Department of Obstetrics and Gynaecology, Sheffield Teaching Hospitals, Sheffield, UK
e-mail: pshobhana@hotmail.com

K. Jayaprakasan, L. Kean (eds.), *Clinical Management of Pregnancies following ART*, DOI 10.1007/978-3-319-42858-1_9

women who spontaneously conceived were compared with 1222 women who had been given ovulation induction therapy and 554 who had undergone IVF treatment [3]. An increased incidence of gestational hypertension and pre-eclampsia was found in the IVF group as compared to the spontaneous conception group; the adjusted odds ratio for pre-eclampsia was 2.7 (with 95 % confidence interval 1.7–4.4), which reached a high degree of statistical significance ($p<0.01$). Ovulation induction was found to be associated with increased risk for gestational diabetes (adjusted odds ratio 1.5 with 95 % confidence interval 1.1–2.2). The question raised was whether these pregnancy complications were due to the ART techniques themselves, or to the innate characteristics of the patients undergoing a particular treatment modality [4].

A systematic review concentrating on 15 cohort studies (11 of which were matched) of singleton pregnancies conceived following IVF as compared to spontaneous conceptions concluded that the relative risk for hypertensive complications was 1.49 (95 % confidence interval 1.39–1.59) [5]. This review estimated that the absolute increase in risk for hypertensive complications was about 2 %. The same review reported the findings of 6 cohort studies (4 of which were matched) regarding risks for gestational diabetes. The findings were of a relative risk for gestational diabetes of 1.48 (95 % confidence interval 1.33–1.66) in the IVF group compared to spontaneous conceptions; this was an absolute increase in risk of approximately 1 % [5].

Others studies have disagreed and did not find an association between use of ART and higher incidence of gestational hypertension or diabetes [6, 7]. One of these studies was a cohort of 242,715 women in Japan, where 3 study groups divided by the type of ART procedure (ovulation induction alone, intrauterine insemination and IVF) were compared with matched controls to adjust for maternal characteristics including age, parity, BMI, smoking and alcohol consumption and pre-existing medical complications [7]. This study found no differences in hypertensive complications between the groups but did find overall that the ART pregnancies had more adverse outcomes including preterm delivery and low birthweight infants; the incidence of gestational diabetes was not reported. The study concluded that maternal factors associated with infertility contribute to adverse pregnancy outcomes and it is not anything to do with the ART procedures themselves.

Other authors have used Propensity Scoring (a statistical tool to minimise selection bias and confounding factors in observational studies) in their analysis of prospectively recruited subjects, who conceived with or without IVF techniques. They found the association between IVF and pre-eclampsia to be much weaker than previously described [8].

There are, however, some circumstances when maternal medical complications may be anticipated following ART.

Problems Arising due to Advanced Maternal Age

Childbearing at advanced maternal age is becoming increasingly common, especially in affluent countries. Assisted reproductive techniques, including IVF and egg donation, contribute to an increasing incidence of pregnancies in women outside of the normal reproductive age. In England and Wales the average age at childbearing has increased progressively since the mid-1970s from 26.4 to 29.5 years in 2010, with 48 % of all babies born to mothers aged more than 30 years [9].

Advanced maternal age (more than 35 years) is associated with subfertility, chromosomal abnormalities, miscarriage, multiple gestation, low birth weight, placenta praevia and caesarean delivery [10, 11]. In addition, advanced maternal age is associated with an increased risk of pregnancy complications including gestational diabetes, pregnancy-induced hypertension and pre-eclampsia [10–12]. A national prospective cohort of more than 1.5 million maternities in Sweden found the odds ratios for maternal death in women aged 40–44 years (as compared to the age group 20–29 year) to be 16.2 (with 95 % confidence intervals 6.38–41.2); in the age group >45 years, the odds ratio was even higher (121, with 95 % confidence intervals 27–542) [10]. There are also adverse perinatal outcomes including antepartum stillbirth, intrapartum-related perinatal death, early neonatal death and neonatal unit admission [10, 11]. However, in all these studies it is acknowledged that there are many confounding factors. In a prospective cohort of singleton pregnancies, there were no difference in the incidence of gestational hypertension or pre-eclampsia once race, body mass index, parity, smoking, other medical disorders, previous adverse outcomes and use of ART had been controlled for; only gestational diabetes became more common with advancing maternal age (adjusted odds ratio of 2.4 in women over 40 years, compared to those less than 35 years) [11].

A retrospective cohort study looked at the interaction between maternal age, use of ART and maternal pregnancy complications [13]. There were 330 women aged 40 years or more, of whom 242 had conceived spontaneously (SC) and 88 had conceived with IVF (all with autologous embryos); these were compared with 450 women aged 30–34 years (of whom 422 had conceived spontaneously and 28 following IVF). The respective incidence in these groups of pregnancy induced hypertension was 7.9 % (SC), 20.5 % (IVF) in the older mothers; 2.6 % (SC) and 14.3 % IVF in the younger mothers. Pregnancy induced hypertension was more common in all women who had conceived following IVF, compared to those who had conceived spontaneously; however, it was overall more common in the older mothers, regardless of mode of conception.

Risk Assessment, Identification, and Management of Specific Pregnancy Complications

Hypertensive Complications of Pregnancy

Women should have risk assessment at booking (Table 9.1) and those at high risk of developing pregnancy induced hypertension or pre-eclampsia should be offered low dose aspirin (75 mg daily) [14]. These women should also have a plan

Table 9.1 Pre-eclampsia risk assessment and prevention

Assessment should be made in early pregnancy, to allow for initiation of prophylactic low-dose aspirin treatment from 12 weeks gestation and appropriate surveillance of blood pressure and urinanalysis throughout pregnancy [14].
High Risk
Women with the following conditions are high risk for developing pre-eclampsia. These women should also be started on aspirin 75 mg from 12 weeks until delivery, unless there are contraindications to its use.
Hypertensive disorders during a previous pregnancy
Chronic kidney disease
Autoimmune disease such as Systemic Lupus Erythematosis or Antiphospholipid syndrome
Type 1 or type 2 Diabetes
Chronic Hypertension
Moderate Risks
If a woman has *two* or more of the following risk factors she should be started on aspirin 75 mg from 12 weeks until delivery, unless there are contraindications to its use.
First pregnancy
Age 40 years or older
Pregnancy interval of more than 10 years
Body mass index of 35 kg/m^2 or more at first visit
Family history of pre -eclampsia
Multiple pregnancy

for closer maternal and fetal surveillance especially in the third trimester (Table 9.2) [15].

Gestational Diabetes

Women who are at high risk of developing gestational diabetes (GDM) on the basis of their age, having BMI ≥30 kg/m^2, South Asian ethnicity, previous macrosomic baby of 4.5 kg or more, personal prior history or close family history of diabetes should be screened at 26–28 weeks with a glucose tolerance test (GTT) [16]. If the GTT is abnormal, referral should be made to the multidisciplinary obstetric-diabetic clinic. Dietary assessment and modification, use of oral hypoglycaemic agents (Metformin) and/or insulin may be necessary to ensure normo glycaemia.

Thromboembolism

Women should have a risk assessment early in pregnancy based on their age, parity, family and personal history of thromboembolism, medical history and current health to assess their risk of thrombosis during pregnancy (Table 9.3) [17]. A decision about whether thromboprophylaxis should be offered during or after pregnancy

Table 9.2 Recommended frequency of maternal surveillance for those deemed at high risk of developing pre-eclampsia

24–32 weeks gestation	32 weeks gestation until delivery
No more than 3 week interval between assessments	No more than 2 week interval between assessments
Women to be included in this schedule are those who have one or more of the following factors:	
First pregnancy	
Previous pregnancy complicated by pre-eclampsia	
Interval of ≥10 years since last pregnancy	
Age ≥ 40 years	
BMI ≥ 35 kg/m^2	
Family history of pre-eclampsia (in mother or sister)	
Diastolic blood pressure at booking ≥80 mmHg	
Proteinuria at booking visit	
Multiple pregnancy	
Medical conditions (pre-existing hypertension, renal disease, diabetes, antiphospholipid syndrome)	

can be made on this assessment. Factors occurring during pregnancy may also influence decisions about the need for short-term thromboprophylaxis, e.g., if ovarian hyperstimulation has been triggered, or the woman is hospitalised, immobile or unwell with a pyrexia.

Multiple Gestation

Women with twin pregnancies have at least double the incidence of gestational hypertension and pre-eclampsia as those with singleton pregnancies [18]. In a cohort study of multiple pregnancies conceived either spontaneously or after ART (either ovulation induction alone or IVF), those women who received ART were twice as likely to develop preeclampsia, after adjustment for age and parity [19].

Risk Assessment, Identification, and Management of Specific Pregnancy Complications

Hypertensive Complications of Pregnancy

Consideration should be given to the use of prophylactic aspirin 75 mg daily (Table 9.1) and enhanced blood pressure surveillance throughout pregnancy (Table 9.2). Serial ultrasound examinations are required to document fetal growth and umbilical artery Doppler velocimetry.

Table 9.3 Assessment of risk factors for venous thromboembolism at booking

Pre existing factors
Previous VTE
Family history of VTE
Thrombophilia
Inherited
Antithrombin deficiency
Protein C or S deficiency
Factor V Leiden
Prothrombin gene variant
Acquired (Antiphospholipid syndrome)
Persistent lupus anticoagulant
Persistent moderate/high titre anticardiolipin or beta-2 glycoprotein 1 antibodies
Age over 35 years
Obesity (BMI >30 kg/m^2 or weight >90 kg at booking)
Parity ≥ 3
Smoking
Medical morbidities, e.g.,
Heart or Lung disease
SLE
Cancer
Inflammatory bowel disease
Inflammatory polyarthropathy
Nephrotic syndrome
Sickle cell disease
Intravenous drug user
Gross varicose veins
Paraplegia

Pregnancy following ART is itself considered a risk factor for VTE, as is a multiple pregnancy (e.g., twins). Each of the above factors should also be considered in order to determine whether the woman's individual risks for VTE justify antenatal thromboprophylaxis with low molecular weight heparin. There are also temporary factors (e.g., surgery, dehydration, hyperemesis, ovarian hyperstimulation, systemic infection, immobility, long distance travel) which would heighten VTE risk and could be managed with short-term thromboprophylaxis (until the risk period is passed). It is advised that VTE risk is reassessed upon admission to hospital and after delivery [17]

Thromboembolism

Having conceived as a result of ART and having a multiple gestation are both risk factors for venous thromboembolism. These should be considered along with other factors to help decide if specific thromboprophylactic measures (including daily administration of low molecular weight heparin) are indicated during or after pregnancy (Table 9.3).

Pre-existing Hypertension

Hypertensive disorders occur in about 10 % of pregnancies and are responsible for a third of severe maternal morbidity, as well as many maternal deaths [14]. Chronic hypertension is present in about 1–2 % of pregnant women with rates increasing as maternal age increases [10, 11]. Chronic hypertension may be primary (essential) in approximately 90 % of cases with the remaining 10 % secondary to one or more underlying diseases such as renal disease, collagen vascular disease, endocrine disorders, or coarctation of the aorta. Pre-existing hypertension is a well-recognised risk factor for pre-eclampsia and all its associated sequaelae [14]. There are no specific studies comparing the incidence of hypertensive complications in women with and without pre -existing hypertension who have conceived following ART.

Pregnancy Care for Women with Underlying Hypertension

Women with pre-existing hypertension on Angiotensin Converting Enzyme (ACE) inhibitors, Angiotensin Receptor Blockers (ARB) or Chlorthiazide should be informed about the increased risk of congenital abnormalities and later pregnancy complications if these are taken during pregnancy. Antihypertensive medication should be changed to labetolol, methyl dopa, or other drugs that are known to be safe to use in pregnancy, ideally prior to commencement of ART schedules [14]. Low dose Aspirin (75 mg daily) should be prescribed in this group of women (Table 9.1). There is no evidence of benefit in starting low dose aspirin periconceptually [20].

Polycystic Ovarian Syndrome

Women with polycystic ovarian syndrome (PCOS) more often need ART to achieve pregnancy than women without this diagnosis; 13.7 % in a large Swedish study of 3787 births to women with PCOS, compared to a background rate of 1.5 % in more than one million women without PCOS [21]. The study also found these women were almost twice as likely to be obese. There were strong associations between PCOS and pre-eclampsia (adjusted odds ratio 1.45, with 95 % confidence interval 1.24–1.69) and between PCOS and gestational diabetes (adjusted odds ratio 2.32, with 95 % confidence interval 1.88–2.88) [21]. Adjustments in the odds ratios quoted here had been made for maternal age, parity, BMI, ART, smoking, year of delivery and years of education.

Another study looked at the adverse pregnancy outcomes in obese and non-obese women with PCOS who underwent ART, compared to obese and non-obese controls, who had ART for tubal factor infertility [22]. As this was an Asian population, obesity was defined as BMI more than 25 kg/m^2. No differences in the incidence of pregnancy-induced hypertension were found between the 4 groups; however, it was the obese women from PCOS and control groups who had the highest incidence of gestational diabetes (10.5 % and 8.6 %, respectively) [22].

Pregnancy Care for Women with PCOS

A risk assessment should be performed early in pregnancy to assess individualised risks for pre-eclampsia, gestational diabetes and venous thromboembolism (Tables 9.1 and 9.3). Most of these women will qualify for low dose aspirin and enhanced fetal and maternal surveillance (Table 9.2). Although in the United Kingdom, PCOS is not identified as a screening criterion for gestational diabetes (16), many women will qualify for screening on the basis of weight, racial origin or family history and thought should be given to offering women a glucose tolerance test (GTT) at 26–28 weeks. If the woman has a BMI more than 40 kg/m^2, then consideration should be given to performing an additional, earlier GTT at 16–18 weeks.

Thyroid Dysfunction

It is important to check thyroid function and correct clinical hypothyroidism or hyperthyroidism prior to ART. Derangement of thyroid function is likely to be a major contributor to subfertility. However, it is also apparent that subclinical hypothyroidism (i.e., elevated thyroid stimulating hormone levels in the presence of normal circulating free thyroxine and tri-iodothyronine levels) and the presence of thyroid antibodies are associated with adverse pregnancy outcomes. In a meta-analysis of women with subclinical hypothyroidism compared to those with normal thyroid function higher risks for pre-eclampsia (Odds Ratio 1.7, with 95 % confidence intervals 1.1–2.6) and perinatal mortality (Odds Ratio 2.7, with 95 % confidence intervals 1.6–4.7) were found [23]. Thyroid antibodies were associated with higher risks for miscarriage, recurrent miscarriage, preterm birth and maternal thyroiditis in the postpartum period [23].

Another systematic review looked at randomised controlled trials of levothyroxine versus placebo treatment for women with subclinical hypothyroidism or thyroid autoimmunity who were undergoing ART [24]. The conclusions (from 3 trials totalling 220 patients) were that levothyroxine treatment lowers miscarriage rate, increases live delivery rate, but no changes could be demonstrated in the incidence of pre-eclampsia [24].

Pregnancy Care for Women with Thyroid Dysfunction

Clinical or Subclinical Hypothyroidism, Thyroid Autoimmunity

Adequate maternal thyroid hormone production is especially important in the first trimester, when fetal brain developments start and the fetus does not produce its own thyroid hormones. Pre-conceptually and throughout pregnancy, the aim should be to keep thyroid stimulating hormone (TSH) in the range 2–2.5 iu/l. This usually necessitates an increase in daily dose of levothyroxine of the order of 25–50 mcg. The TSH levels should be checked each trimester.

Clinical Hyperthyroidism

During pregnancy, mild hyperthyroidism, in which TSH is low but free thyroxine (T4) and tri-iodothyronine (T3) are normal, does not require treatment. More severe hyperthyroidism is treated with medication to suppress thyroid hormone production. While both Propylthiouracil and Carbamizole can be used, propylthiouracil is the preferred antithyroid agent in pregnancy. Antithyroid medication crosses the placenta in small amounts and can decrease fetal thyroid hormone production, so the lowest possible dose should be used to avoid hypothyroidism in the baby. During pregnancy, TSH, free T3 and T4 should be monitored, with medication adjusted to maintain FT4 levels at the upper limit of the normal range.

Other Intercurrent Medical Conditions

Any woman with a chronic medical condition who is aiming to conceive with ART should be counselled about the likely effects of their condition on pregnancy outcome, the effects of pregnancy on their medical condition and they should have their drug medication reviewed for safety. A multidisciplinary approach may be required, as there can be a conflict of interest with respect to what may be best for the mother and what for the fetus. In these circumstances, skilled counselling about the safest and most sensible course is needed. For some conditions, multidisciplinary review may conclude that pregnancy is very hazardous; in which case, proceeding with ART would be unethical.

An example of inadequate pre-conceptual preparation was reported by the French Study Group for Oocyte Donation, who looked at the maternal and fetal outcomes of pregnancies achieved by oocyte donation in women with Turner's Syndrome [25]. There were 93 patients in this study, of whom only 35 had undergone echocardiography or cardiac magnetic resonance imaging in preparation for ART and only 6 had documented aortic root diameters. Of the 82 women whose pregnancies continued beyond 20 weeks, 31 had hypertensive complications, including 4 cases of eclampsia. Two mothers died from aortic rupture, with evidence of aortic root dilatation. Almost a third of the babies were growth-restricted and there was one fetal death attributed to maternal eclampsia. Only 40 % of the reported pregnancies resulted in normal fetal and maternal outcomes.

Pregnancy Care for Women with Underlying Medical Conditions

For most *chronic inflammatory conditions* (e.g., autoimmune arthritis, inflammatory bowel disease), keeping the disease processes quiescent during pregnancy is critical for a favourable pregnancy outcome. Anti-inflammatory and disease-modifying drugs can be adjusted to those with the best safety record for use in pregnancy. It is not generally advisable to withdraw drugs that are keeping inflammation under control, since managing a serious disease flare during pregnancy could involve use of much larger doses of drugs, with greater fetal exposure to them overall with the additional risks to the pregnancy of inflammation which is associated with preterm labour.

Meticulous glycaemic control periconceptually and in early pregnancy is vital for good outcomes in women with *diabetes mellitus*. High dose folic acid supplements (5 mg daily) are recommended [16].

For women with *epilepsy*, periconceptual review of anticonvulsant drug treatment and use of high dose folic acid supplements are important [26].

Women with *renal disease* need careful assessment prior to ART as they may be on medication (e.g., ACE inhibitors) that should be changed prior to conception. Baseline blood pressure and proteinuria should be established. Meticulous blood pressure control during pregnancy is essential, as are serial tests of renal function, including quantitative proteinuria. Women with renal disease are at increased risk for pre-eclampsia during pregnancy, so should be given aspirin prophylaxis and have enhanced maternal surveillance (Tables 9.1 and 9.2).

Women with *bleeding or clotting problems* need careful planning for their initial ART procedures, as well as for the risks they may encounter during pregnancy; those with thrombophilia or a prior history of thromboembolism may require thromboprophylaxis to cover ovarian stimulation schedules.

Multidisciplinary care for these and other less common conditions needs to continue during pregnancy to ensure the best maternal and fetal outcomes.

Maternal Obesity

Obesity has become an increasing problem over the last 30 years, including in pregnant women. Maternal obesity has significant health implications during pregnancy, contributing to increased morbidity and mortality for both mother and baby

Table 9.4 Pregnancy risks associated with increased maternal BMI

	Overweight (BMI 25–30)	Obese class 1 (BMI 30–35)	Obese class 2 (BMI 35–40)	Obese class 3 (BMI>40)
Hypertension	1.9	3.5	5.0	6.6
Gestational diabetes	1.7	3.7	6.0	8.5
Labour induction	1.2	1.3	1.4	1.6
Caesarean Section	1.4	1.8	2.5	2.8
Postpartum haemorrhage	1.4	1.8	2.4	2.7
Macrosomia >4 kg	1.5	1.9	2.1	3.2

Odds ratios for pregnancy outcomes in the BMI groups, compared with women of normal weight (BMI 20–25 kg/m^2) from a retrospective study of 30,298 women over 8 years [27]

[27–29]. As BMI increases, so do the risks for gestational diabetes, thromboembolism, gestational hypertension, including pre-eclampsia (Table 9.4) [27]. Obese women are less likely to go into labour spontaneously, more likely to have a prolonged pregnancy and have labour induced, less likely to achieve a normal delivery and more likely to deliver by caesarean section [27, 30]. Intrapartum and postpartum complications are more common in obese mothers, such as uterine rupture associated with a previous uterine scar, primary postpartum haemorrhage, and postpartum infection [27, 28, 31]. Obesity is also associated with a higher risk of adverse neonatal outcomes, including congenital anomalies, macrosomia, shoulder dystocia, neonatal intensive care admission, and perinatal death [27, 28, 30, 31].

Obesity also affects the responses to ART. The higher a woman's BMI, the more days of gonadotrophin stimulation she is likely to need and the greater the chance of cancellation of an IVF treatment cycle [32, 33]. An interesting observation from a report of 152,500 ART cycle starts in the years 2007–8, for women of known BMI, was that the failure to achieve a clinical intrauterine pregnancy, which became more common as BMI increased, was more marked in fresh cycles using autologous, as opposed to donor eggs [34]. The incidence of fetal death and stillbirth also increased as maternal BMI increased. It is evident that obesity creates an adverse environment for the oocyte, embryo and fetus through many endocrine and inflammatory mechanisms [34, 35]. A meta-analysis of studies of IVF outcomes after fresh donor oocytes in recipients of known BMI (totalling 4758 women) confirmed that there were no worse outcomes for miscarriage and live births in women with BMI ≥30 kg/m^2 [36]. These results were interpreted to show that oocyte quality is more important in terms of getting a good outcome from IVF in obese women than endometrial receptivity. These studies did not, however, look at maternal complications during pregnancy.

There has been much discussion about the ethics and economic aspects of offering IVF to those of high BMI. The risks of failure to achieve an intrauterine pregnancy and miscarriage rise with maternal BMI, but are significantly worse even in the "overweight" women whose BMI is 25–29.9 kg/m^2, as compared to those whose BMI is less than 25 kg/m^2 [37]. Recommendations for the BMI cut-off for being offered IVF varies between countries and Societies: less than 30 kg/m^2 in the United

Kingdom for National Health Service-funded cycles [38], and less than 32 kg/m^2 in New Zealand [39]. However, some have argued that restriction of access to ART on the basis of BMI is unjust and that it is worse to defer pregnancy until suitable weight loss has occurred, since advancing maternal age brings even more problems [39].

Pregnancy Care for Obese Women

It is recommended that increased folic acid doses of 5 mg daily are given periconceptually to obese women, as neural tube defects are twice as likely to occur in this group, compared to normal-weight women [40]. Individualised risk assessment for thromboembolism, gestational hypertension and gestational diabetes at the start of pregnancy will lead to decisions about the need for thromboprophylaxis, low dose aspirin and screening for gestational diabetes in the second trimester (Tables 9.1 and 9.3). Dietary and healthy lifestyle advice and support is also important, to try and reduce gestational weight gain to 5–10 kg [28]. Vitamin D supplements of 10 mcg daily are also recommended, due to a higher incidence of vitamin D deficiency in obese women.

Pregnancy Post-bariatric Surgery

Women with high BMI who have failed to lose weight with dietary modification and exercise alone, may consider the option of undergoing bariatric surgery which may lead to rapid weight loss, return of periods and ovulation [28, 41]. If these women do not spontaneously conceive, they are more likely to be at an optimal BMI for ART. Pregnancy will then be safer for them, than if they were still morbidly obese. Bariatric surgery involves either restrictive procedures such as gastric banding or sleeve gastrotomy alone or restrictive plus malabsorptive procedures, such as Roux-en Y bypass. Women are advised not to conceive during the period of rapid weight loss following surgery and should ideally wait 12–18 months before trying to conceive.

There is a potential for nutritional deficiencies of protein, iron, calcium, folate, vitamin B12 and vitamin D, particularly after malabsorptive bariatric surgical procedures. An assessment of serum levels of these factors should be done at the start of pregnancy and repeat assessments in each trimester. Adequate nutritional replacements should be provided, based on these results [28, 41].

For women who have had gastric banding procedures, surgical complications can happen during pregnancy, including band slippage and migration, which causes severe vomiting. There are also reports of intestinal herniation, obstruction and perforation following bariatric surgery. These complications may be difficult to diagnose during pregnancy, so symptoms of epigastric pain or vomiting should not be ignored [41].

Pregnancies Following Gamete Donation

Pregnancies that are created from oocyte, sperm or embryo donation have for a long time been suspected of having a high incidence of gestational hypertension and pre-eclampsia. A retrospective cohort of 72 women who had conceived with sperm, ooctye or embryo donation were compared with age and parity-matched women who conceived either spontaneously or with intrauterine insemination with their partner's sperm. [42] The incidence of gestational hypertension and pre-eclampsia in the gamete donation group overall was 12.5 % and 18.1 %, respectively; compared with 2.8 % and 1.4 % in the control group. Other, larger studies reporting pregnancy complications after intrauterine insemination (IUI) with either partner or donor sperm confirmed higher incidence of pre-eclampsia after donor insemination (3.7 % difference, with 95 % confidence interval −0.8 to +7.8 %) [43]. Logistic regression analysis found that the highest incidence of pre-eclampsia was in women who conceived with donor sperm after only a few cycles of IUI.

A single-centre study of 71 donor oocyte recipients and 108 women (aged over 38 years) who conceived with IVF using autologous oocytes addressed maternal and fetal pregnancy complications [44]. Multivariate analysis found that, after controlling for multiple gestation, the use of donor oocytes was not a major risk factor for adverse obstetric outcomes (adjusted odds ratio for pre-eclampsia 1.25, with 95 % confidence intervals 0.53–2.93). However, the two groups were not well matched for age and there were far more multiple pregnancies in the donor oocyte group; these factors may have confounded the findings. It was observed that in women over the age of 38 years, twin or higher-order multiple pregnancies were more likely following the use of donor oocytes, even if fewer embryos were transferred in the IVF process. The increased risk of pre-eclampsia that multiple pregnancy brings is well recognised [2].

The largest cohort study to address the impact of oocyte donation followed 205 women who conceived with donor oocytes and compared them with 205 women who had undergone IVF, specifically intracytoplasmic sperm injection (ICSI) with autologous oocytes; thus all the pregnancies had arisen from the same ART technique [45]. Cases were individually matched for age, ethnicity, parity and number of fetuses. All the cycles were with fresh oocytes. This study confirmed that oocyte donation was associated with a significantly increased risk for gestational hypertension (incidence 19.1 % in donor oocyte pregnancies versus 8.3 % in autologous oocyte pregnancies). When singleton and twin pregnancies were separated, the most marked difference in incidence of gestational hypertension was in the twin pregnancies (24.6 % in donor oocyte group versus 7 % in autologous oocyte group). There was a higher, but statistically non-significant, incidence of pre-eclampsia in donor oocyte pregnancies, but no differences in the incidence of gestational diabetes. There were no differences between the groups for overall perinatal outcomes.

Pregnancy Care for Women Following Gamete Donation

Use of prophylactic low-dose aspirin should be considered in this group, due to the higher risks of gestational hypertension, especially in multiple pregnancies (Table 9.1), with enhanced blood pressure surveillance (Table 9.2).

Conclusion

Pregnancies resulting from ART may have increased risks for maternal medical complications, especially gestational hypertension, pre-eclampsia, thromboembolism and gestational diabetes. These risks largely arise due to the characteristics of the women who undergo ART and are most marked in older women, those with high body mass index or polycystic ovary syndrome and in multiple pregnancies; but risks especially for pre-eclampsia are high when donor gametes have been used.

The important principle for good pregnancy care is that of thorough risk assessment for each of these complications in early pregnancy, in order to plan surveillance *including* additional blood pressure surveillance and glucose tolerance tests or to institute prophylactic treatment such as low dose aspirin, low molecular weight heparin, high dose folic acid and others as appropriate.

Women with significant underlying medical conditions need careful assessment prior to commencement of ART protocols to consider maternal and fetal risks in pregnancy, plan appropriate health surveillance during pregnancy and consider adjustment of medication.

Finally, the clear information about adverse pregnancy outcomes for those with high BMI and in those with twin or higher order multiple pregnancies should guide appropriate ART practices including single embryo transfers, mild stimulation protocols and weight reduction prior to ART.

References

1. Mallizia BA, Hacker MR. Cummulative live birth rates after in vitro fertilization. N Engl J Med. 2009;360:236–43.
2. Pinborg A, Loft A, Schmidt L, Langhoff-Roos J, Andersen AN. Maternal risks and perinatal outcome in a Danish national cohort of 1005 twin pregnancies: the role of in vitro fertilization. Act Obstet Gynecol Scand. 2004;83:75–84.
3. Shevell T, Malone FD, Vidaver J, Porter TF, Luthy DA, Comstock CH, et al. Assisted reproductive technology and pregnancy outcome. Obstet Gynecol. 2005;106:1039–45.
4. Thomopoulos C, Tsioufis C, Michalopoulou H, Makris T, Papademetriou V, Stefanadis C. Assisted reproductive technology and pregnancy-related hypertensive complications: a systematic review. J Hum Hypertens. 2013;27:148–57.
5. Pandey S, Shetty A, Hamilton M, Bhattacharya S, Maheshwari A. Obstetric and perinatal outcomes in singleton pregnancies resulting from IVF/ICSI: a systematic review and meta-analysis. Hum Reprod Update. 2012;18:485–503.

6. Farhi A, Reichman B, Boyko V, Hourvitz A, Ron-El R, Lerner-Geva L. Maternal and neonatal health outcomes following assisted reproduction. Reprod Biomed Online. 2013;26:454–61.
7. Hayashi M, Nakai A, Satoh S, Matsuda Y. Adverse obstetric and perinatal outcomes of singleton pregnancies may be related to maternal factors associated with infertility rather than the type of assisted reproductive technology procedure used. Fertil Steril. 2012;98:922–8.
8. Watanabe N, Fujiwara T, Suzuki T, Jwa SC, Taniguchi K, Yamanobe Y, et al. Is in vitro fertilization associated with preeclampsia? A propensity score matched study. BMC Pregnancy Childbirth. 2014;14:69.
9. Office for National Statistics. Live births by characteristics of mother. England and Wales, 2010.
10. Jacobsson B, Ladfors L, Milsom I. Advanced maternal age and adverse perinatal outcome. Obstet Gynecol. 2004;104:727–33.
11. Cleary-Goldman J, Malone FD, Vidaver J, Ball RH, Nyberg DA, Comstock CH, et al. Impact of maternal age on obstetric outcome. Obstet Gynecol. 2005;105:983–90.
12. Lao T, Ho L-F, Chan BCP, Leung W-C. Maternal age and prevalence of gestational diabetes mellitus. Diabetes Care. 2006;29:948.
13. Toshimitsu M, Nagamatsu T, Nagasaka T, Iwasa-Kawai Y, Komatsu A, Yamashita T, et al. Increased risk of pregnancy-induced hypertension and operative delivery after conception induced by in vitro fertilization/intracytoplasmic sperm injection in women aged 40 years and older. Fertil Steril. 2014;102:1065–70.
14. NICE guideline CG 107: Hypertension in pregnancy. 2011. https://www.nice.org.uk/guidance/cg107/evidence.
15. PRECOG: The pre-eclampsia community guideline. http://action-on-pre-eclampsia.org.uk/wp-content/uploads/2012/07/PRECOG-Community-Guideline.pdf.
16. NICE guideline NG 3: Diabetes in pregnancy. 2015. https://www.nice.org.uk/guidance/ng3/evidence.
17. RCOG. Thrombosis and embolism during pregnancy and the puerperium, reducing the risk (Green-top Guideline No. 37a). 2009. https://www.rcog.org.uk/globalassets/documents/guidelines/gtg37areducingriskthrombosis.pdf.
18. Sibai BM, Hauth J, Caritis S, Lindheimer MD, MacPherson C, Klebanoff M, et al. Hypertensive disorders in twin versus singleton gestations. Am J Obstet Gynecol. 2000;182:938–42.
19. Lynch A, McDuffie R, Murphy J, Faber K, Orleans M. Preeclampsia in multiple gestation: the role of assisted reproductive technologies. Obstet Gynecol. 2002;99:445–51.
20. Groeneveld E, Lambers MJ, Lambalk CB, Broeze KA, Hapsamo M, de Sutter P, et al. Preconceptional low-dose aspirin for the prevention of hypertensive pregnancy complications and preterm delivery after IVF: a meta-analysis with patient data. Hum Reprod. 2013;28:1480–8.
21. Roos N, Kieleer H, Sahlin L, Ekman-Ordeberg G, Falconer H, Stephansson O. Risk of adverse pregnancy outcomes in women with polycystic ovary syndrome: population based cohort study. BMJ. 2011;343:d6309. doi:10.1136/bmj.d6309.
22. Han AR, Kim HO, Cha SW, Park CW, Kim JY, Yang KM, et al. Adverse pregnancy outcomes with assisted reproductive technology in non-obese women with polycystic ovary syndrome: a case-control study. Clin Exp Reprod Med. 2011;38:103–8.
23. Van den Boogaard E, Vissenberg R, Land JA, van Wely M, van der Post JAM, Goddijn M, Bisschop PH. Significant of (sub)clinical thyroid dysfunction and thyroid autoimmunity before conception and in early pregnancy: a systematic review. Hum Reprod Update. 2011;17:605–19.
24. Velkeniers B, Van Meerhaeghe A, Poppe K, Unuane D, Tournaye H, Haentjens P. Levothyroxine treatment and pregnancy outcomes in women with subclinical hypothyroidism undergoing assisted reproduction technologies: systematic review and meta-analysis of RCTs. Hum Reprod Update. 2013;19:251–8.
25. Chevalier N, Letur H, Lelannou D, Ohl J, Cornet D, Chalas-Boissonnas C, et al. Materno-fetal cardiovascular complications in Turner syndrome after oocyte donation: insufficient prepregnancy screening and pregnancy follow-up are associated with poor outcome. J Clin Endocrinol Metab. 2011;96:E260–7.

26. Abe K, Hamada H, Yamad T, Obata-Yasuoka M, Minakami H, Yoshikawa H. Impact of planning a pregnancy in women with epilepsy on seizure control during pregnancy and on maternal and fetal outcomes. Seizure. 2014;23:112–6.
27. Scott-Pillai R, Spence D, Cardwell CR, Hunter A, Holmes VA. The impact of body mass index on maternal and neonatal outcomes: a retrospective study in a UK obstetric population, 2004-2011. BJOG. 2013;120:932–9.
28. Fitzsimons KJ, Modder J, Greer IA. Obesity in pregnancy: risks and management. Obstet Med. 2009;2:52–62.
29. Centre for Maternal and Child Enquiries (CMACE). Saving mothers' lives: reviewing maternal deaths to make motherhood safer: 2006–2008. The Eighth Report on Confidential Enquiries into Maternal Deaths in the United Kingdom. BJOG. 2011;118(Suppl 1):1–203.
30. Cedegren MI. Maternal morbid obesity and the risk of adverse pregnancy outcome. Obstet Gynecol. 2004;103:219–24.
31. Hibbard JU, Gilbert S, Landon MB, Hauth JC, Leveno KJ, Spong CY, et al. Trial of labor or repeat caesarean delivery in women with morbid obesity and previous caesarean delivery. Obstet Gynecol. 2006;108:125–33.
32. Maheshwari A, Stofberg L, Bhattacharya S. Effect of overweight and obesity on assisted reproductive technology – a systematic review. Hum Reprod Update. 2007;13:433–44.
33. Dokras A, Baredziak L, Blaine J, Syrop C, VanVoorhis BJ, Sparks A. Obstetric outcomes after in vitro fertilization in obese and morbidly obese women. Obstet Gynecol. 2006;108:61–9.
34. Luke B, Brown MB, Missmer SA, Bukulmez O, Leach R, Stern JE. The effect of increasing obesity on the response to and outcome of assisted reproductive technology: a national study. Fertil Steril. 2011;96:820–5.
35. Brewer CJ, Balen AH. The adverse effects of obesity on conception and implantation. Reproduction. 2010;140:347–64.
36. Jungheim ES, Schon SB, Schulte MB, DeUgarte DA, Fowler SA, Tuuli MG. IVF outcomes in obese donor oocyte recipients: a systematic review and meta-analysis. Hum Reprod. 2013;28:2720–7.
37. Rittenberg V, Seshadri S, Sunkara SK, Sobaleva S, Oteng-Ntim E, El-Toukhy T. Effect of body mass index on IVF treatment outcome: an updated systematic review and meta-analysis. Reprod Biomed Online. 2011;23:421–39.
38. NICE guideline CG 156: Fertility: assessment and treatment for people with fertility problems. 2013. https://www.nice.org.uk/guidance/cg156/evidence.
39. Pandey S, Maheshwari A, Bhattacharya S. Should access to fertility treatment be determined by female body mass index? Hum Reprod. 2010;25:815–20.
40. Anderson JL, Waller DK, Canfield MA, Shaw GM, Watkins ML, Werler MM. Maternal obesity, gestational diabetes, and central nervous system birth defects. Epidemiology. 2005;16:87–92.
41. Khan R, Dawatly B, Chappatte O. Pregnancy outcome following bariatric surgery. Obstet Gynaecol. 2013;15:37–43.
42. Salha O, Sharma V, Dada T, Nugent D, Rutherford AJ, Tomlinson AJ, et al. The influence of donated gametes on the incidence of hypertensive disorders of pregnancy. Hum Reprod. 1999;14:2268–73.
43. Kyrou D, Kolibianakis EM, Devroey P, Fatemi HM. Is the use of donor sperm associated with a higher incidence of pre- eclampsia in women who achieve pregnancy after intrauterine insemination? Fertil Steril. 2010;93:1124–7.
44. Krieg SA, Henne MB, Westphal LM. Obstetric outcomes in donor oocyte pregnancies compared with advanced maternal age in vitro fertilization pregnancies. Fertil Steril. 2008;90:65–70.
45. Stoop D, Baumgarten M, Haentjens P, Polyzos NP, De Vos M, Verheyen G, et al. Obstetric outcome in donor oocyte pregnancies: a matched pair analysis. Reprod Biol Endocrinol. 2012;10:42.

Chapter 10
Fetal Complications During Pregnancy

Catherine E.M. Aiken and Jeremy Brockelsby

Introduction

Since the introduction of artificial reproductive technology (ART) into clinical practice in 1978 [1] there has been considerable concern regarding effects on the resulting fetus, and the long-term outcomes for the offspring. In particular, concerns were widely voiced that the 'by-passing' of normal gamete selection processes during conception would result in a much greater chance of children being born with genetic or structural anomalies. However, as more pregnancies following ART have been conceived and their outcomes reported, many of the initial fears have subsided. There have now been over five million births worldwide following the use of ART and the rates of assisted conceptions continue to rise [2]. In 2011, approximately 1.5 % of all pregnancies in the US were conceived using ART [3], hence any increase in adverse fetal outcomes resulting from the use of this technology would constitute a significant public health issue. While some perinatal complications are more common in fetuses resulting from ART, difficulties arise in many studies with defining the risk of complications that is attributable to the process of ART itself. There are a number of important confounding factors that may well contribute to adverse fetal outcomes in pregnancies conceived using ART, including the high incidence of:

- Multiple pregnancies
- Underlying subfertility

C.E.M. Aiken, PhD, MRCP, MRCOG
Department of Fetal and Maternal Medicine, Addenbrooke's Hospital, Cambridge, UK
e-mail: Cema2@cam.ac.uk

J. Brockelsby, MBBS, PhD, MRCOG (✉)
Department of Obstetrics and Gynaecology,
Cambridge University Hospitals NHS Trust, Cambridge, UK
e-mail: Jeremy.brockelsby@addenbrookes.nhs.uk

K. Jayaprakasan, L. Kean (eds.), *Clinical Management of Pregnancies following ART*, DOI 10.1007/978-3-319-42858-1_10

- Poor gamete quality
- Advanced maternal age

All of these factors contribute to increased risk for adverse fetal outcomes independent of the actual processes of assisted conception. Nonetheless pregnancies conceived using ART do have a higher risk of fetal complications, regardless of whether these have a causal association with the use of ART or are merely associated through other indirect factors such as maternal age. Perhaps most concerning for clinicians caring for couples who have undergone assisted conception are data from meta-analyses that show an increase in perinatal mortality following ART by up to 2.4-fold (OR 2.4; CI 1.59–3.63), even in singleton pregnancies [4, 5].

This chapter aims to examine the magnitude and the nature of increased fetal complications during pregnancies conceived using ART, and where possible to disentangle the mechanisms leading to an association between mode of conception and fetal complications. Early pregnancy loss prior to fetal development and later childhood outcomes are not considered in detail here as they are discussed elsewhere.

Factors Contributing to Fetal Complications in Pregnancies Conceived with ART

One of the most important factors giving rise to fetal complications from pregnancies conceived using ART is the effect of maternal age. Higher maternal age is a risk factor for adverse fetal outcomes, regardless of mode of conception. Increased complications include a higher risk of chromosomal anomalies, intrauterine growth restriction and both iatrogenic and spontaneous preterm births [6]. Maternal age is readily ascertainable in most cohorts and is relatively easily controlled for. However, there are numerous other risk factors that are more common in older mothers that need to be accounted for in determining relative risk and these are often not adjusted for, particularly in retrospective cohorts. Pre-existing maternal medication conditions, for example hypertension and type 2 diabetes, are more common in older mothers [7]. These conditions may have an important influence on fetal complications during pregnancy, but are commonly missing data in less well-characterised cohorts.

Increased use of ART with donor oocytes has allowed pregnancy to become more common at the extremes of reproductive age, where the risks of hypertensive disease and operative delivery are much increased [8]. The effects of these adverse maternal outcomes on the fetus may be difficult to disentangle from other background risks.

Aside from maternal age, socioeconomic factors may be significantly different between populations of parents who conceive spontaneously and using ART, with one study observing more than twice the number of pregnancies conceived by ART in the highest versus the lowest socioeconomic status groups [9]. These factors are often not controlled for when making comparisons between groups. Particularly, information regarding the father (age, smoking status, and socioeconomic factors such as occupation) is often not accounted for in retrospective cohorts, although his input both biologically and socially may be germane to successful fetal outcomes.

The extent to which adverse maternal and fetal complications of any pregnancy can be separated is limited due to the nature of the intrinsic interplay of the materno-placento-fetal axis in maintaining a successful pregnancy. It is therefore necessary to consider the incidence of adverse fetal outcomes arising indirectly through maternal complications of pregnancies conceived using ART. The rate of maternal gestational diabetes for example is increased in pregnancies conceived using ART [9–11], and may lead to important fetal complications such as macrosomia and birth trauma. Similarly, high rates of maternal complications such as pregnancy-induced hypertension, antepartum haemorrhage and pre-eclampsia [11–13] may lead to an increase in iatrogenic preterm birth, even in the absence of any direct fetal complications. The maternal consequences of ART are dealt with in detail elsewhere, but must be born in mind as they are not independent of many of the fetal complications of pregnancy.

More complicated is the role of the underlying aetiology for the parental subfertility. In many studies this is not well recorded or controlled for. Even when the categorisation of subfertility is reliably ascertained many broad categories of infertility classification, such as 'unexplained' will contain a multitude of different pathologies, many of which might impact on the fetal course during pregnancy. There is evidence that both maternal complications of pregnancy and immediate neonatal outcomes (as assessed by Apgar scores) are influenced by the nature of the subfertility diagnosis [14, 15].

A further difficulty in interpreting and comparing studies is that not all ART techniques necessarily carry similar risks [16] and, particularly in small studies, there is a tendency to conflate groups that are not necessarily comparable. In addition, different techniques are more suitable for particular patient groups, and there may be systematic biases between the women who underwent each treatment [16]. The use of frozen embryo transfer, for example, is often associated with a non-hormonally stimulated endometrial environment (potentially influencing implantation and placental development) and may be more likely to contain women with some selection advantage, as this group by definition has produced a surplus of good-quality embryos during a previous cycle. Hence the outcomes from frozen cycles might be expected to be marginally better than from fresh cycles [12, 17]. Concerns have been raised regarding higher rates of genetic and chromosomal abnormalities in pregnancies conceived using ICSI, particularly where testicular biopsy is used to retrieve sperm [18]; however, there is little objective evidence as yet that this is the case [19]. Studies that do not take adequate account of technique and population-related factors risk over-estimating the adverse effects of ART on fetal outcome.

Fetal Complications During Pregnancy

Fetal Genetic and Chromosomal Disorders

A considerable number of infertility treatments are undertaken in order to perform preimplantation genetic diagnosis and hence reduce the risk of passing on genetic diseases that are known to be present in the parents. However, the risk of an unrecognized chromosomal anomaly being present in the parents is higher in the population requiring fertility treatment than in the general population. Azoospermic or oligozoospermic men requiring fertility treatment have a risk of autosomal translocations or inversions of 4.6–13.7 % [20]. Female partners of males requiring infertility treatments also have a higher risk than the general population of chromosomal anomalies for reasons that are not well understood. One series has suggested a sevenfold increase in reciprocal balanced translocations in the female partners in couples undergoing assisted conception [21]. In addition to heritable autosomal rearrangements, micro-deletions of the Y chromosome are a common finding in males with oligo- or azoospermia, occurring in up to 5–15 % of cases [22, 23]. If intracytoplasmic sperm injection (ICSI) is performed (overcoming the effects of a very low sperm count), then these Y deletions can be passed on to male offspring. It has further been suggested that other deletions may occur *de novo* in assisted conceptions, and there is some preliminary clinical evidence that expansion of existing Y chromosomal problems may occur hence creating a more severe phenotype in the subsequent generation [24].

Fetal Imprinting Disorders

Epigenetic imprinting is responsible for stable regulation of the possible expression patterns of an individual's genome. The most common modes of imprinting genes are via methylation, histone modification or DNA-binding proteins. Early in development, two distinct waves of imprinting (in the unfertilized egg and in the preimplantation embryo) wipe and then re-establish the correct epigenetic patterns for normally regulated development. Concern has arisen regarding the potential for disruption to the highly complex process of imprinting by ART techniques, particularly the techniques of superovulation and culture of the early embryo *in vitro*. Reports have suggested an excess incidence of the imprinted hypomethylation disorders Angelman and Beckwith-Weidermann syndrome following ART [25–27]. Whilst such disorders are very rare (with an estimated risk of Beckwith-Weidermann syndrome in pregnancies conceived using ART of <1 % [28]) and clearly do not affect the majority of fetuses arising from assisted conceptions, the concern regarding subtle epigenetic changes in the cultured embryo persists [29, 30]. Embryos cultured *in vitro* are exposed to a wide variety of stimuli that they do not encounter in unassisted conceptions including artificial culture media, temperature fluctuations and light exposure. All of these exposures have been suggested as potential stimuli to subtly disrupt the normal patterns of methylation and other epigenetic patterns established during early development. Differences in DNA methylation patterns at various loci have been demonstrated in children conceived using ART [31], although this finding is inconsistent across studies [32]. In particular, the functional significance of variations in methylation patterns remains uncertain [33]. The developmental programming hypothesis postulates that a suboptimal early environment (for example culture *in vitro*) may have subtle but profound effects on long-term offspring health, and that these adverse effects could be mediated via epigenetic modulation [34, 35]. Furthermore, developmental programming effects can persist across generations [36], thus impacting not only on the later health of the current offspring, but also health outcomes in future generations. As the first children born using ART are currently in their mid-thirties and few have yet reproduced, there is no available evidence that could refute or support these concerns regarding health in later adulthood in human populations.

Clinical Practice Points

Where structural problems are seen the clinician should consider whether there might be subtle chromosome rearrangements as a contributory factor. Genetic advice may be taken and consideration given to micro-array testing if karyotyping is undertaken

Fetal Structural Anomalies

Collecting data to determine whether the rate of fetal structural anomalies is increased following ART is subject to a number of methodological complexities. The first is that the rate of spontaneous miscarriage may be higher in pregnancies conceived using ART, and hence the number of structural anomalies observed at term may be reduced. Conversely, couples that have conceived using ART may be less likely to undergo invasive testing (carrying a risk of miscarriage) or to terminate pregnancies where a structural anomaly is identified, hence inflating the rate of congenital structural anomalies observed at birth. This creates difficulty in designing an ideal study to determine the risk of structural anomalies. Collecting data at the time of birth risks missing a substantial proportion of anomalies in pregnancies that ended prior to birth, whereas collecting data at the time of detailed anomaly scans will not account for anomalies that are not detectable or were not detected on scan but were present at birth. The ideal study would therefore prospectively recruit pregnancies at the time of booking, collect detailed information on subfertility risks in the parents and include all structural anomalies observed both during fetal surveillance and at the time of delivery, regardless of ultimate pregnancy outcome. In the absence of such cohorts, retrospective analyses of anomalies that were present at delivery in neonates can still give important information.

Concerns regarding higher levels of fetal structural anomalies in pregnancies resulting from ART have most often been raised in the context of more invasive technologies, for example ICSI or blastomere sampling for pre-implantation genetic diagnosis. These techniques raised concerns that structural or biochemical damage to the ovum or early embryo would result in higher rates of congenital anomalies. The higher-than-expected incidence of monozygotic twin pregnancies arising from ART [37] suggests that there is some influence of *in vitro* micromanipulation on the structure of the early embryo. The true magnitude of the embryo-splitting effect in ART is masked by the number of dichorionic diamniotic twin pregnancies that are presumed to be dizygous following multiple embryo transfer; there is evidence, however, to suggest that a significant proportion of such pregnancies actually arise from a single conceptus [38, 39].

Numerous cohort studies have been performed to determine whether the incidence of fetal structural anomalies is higher in children following the use of ART (reviewed in [19]), including some more recent prospective cohorts [40]. Many of these studies have found a significantly increased rate of various structural problems [41–43], but the type and frequency found is not consistent across studies [44, 45]. Specific congenital malformations that have been found with a higher incidence in children conceived using ART include anorectal malformations [46], congenital cardiac lesions [40, 47, 48], nervous system [40, 49] and genital structural anomalies [40, 50]. One study has found subtle effects of conception via ART on cardiac morphology (including thickened ventricular walls and mild atrial dilatation) in the neonate that persist until at least 6 months of age, but the study was prevented from drawing robust conclusions by small sample size and inability to control for several potentially important confounding factors such as fetal growth restriction [48]. It has also been suggested that the rate of congenital abnormality is dependent on the technology utilized; some studies have found higher rates of structural abnormalities in children conceived following ICSI than after IVF [43, 51], although this is not consistently observed [52]. Several major meta-analyses have been performed to determine the rates across various populations, and conclude that the odds ratio of congenital structural anomalies is higher in any type of assisted conception than in spontaneously conceived pregnancy [52–54] with odds ratios ranging from 1.37 (95 % CI 1.26–1.48) to 2.01 (95 % CI 1.49–2.69). However, more recent work suggests that much of the excess risk of congenital abnormalities in pregnancies conceived using ART may be due to underlying infertility issues [50] rather than exposure to ART per se. A reworking of one of the largest meta-analyses thus far performed to assess congenital malformations in ART cohorts suggested that there was no statistically significantly increased risk of congenital anomalies after conception via ART when subfertility was adequately controlled for with an odds ratio of 1.01 (95 % CI 0.82–1.23) [55]. After adequate controlling for infertility and other parental factors, other studies have also concurred that there may be no increased risk of fetal structural anomalies with the use of IVF [56] and that the increased risk in such pregnancies may be attributable to underlying parental factors rather than the actual process of assisted conception. The chance of birth defects in spontaneously conceived pregnancies in women with a history of prior assisted-conception is higher than for those who have never previously required fertility treatment; OR 1.24, CI 1.01–1.56 [56].

Clinical Practice Points

All women in the UK are offered screening for structural anomalies at 18–20+6 weeks. No additional surveillance for structural problems is recommended

Fetal Growth

There is some evidence from cohort studies and meta-analyses that fetal growth may be reduced in pregnancies conceived using ART [3, 5, 9, 11, 57–60]. Most studies use low birth weight as evidence of intrauterine fetal growth restriction rather than serial scan measurements during gestation, although differences in fetal growth trajectory have been reported between different ART protocols [61]. Despite the high number of cohorts that have reported low birth weight associated with the use of ART, the relative contribution of underlying subfertility may account for more of the variation in birth-weight than the technique used for conception [49, 62]. Importantly, a study that directly compared children conceived via ART with their spontaneously conceived siblings found no evidence of decreased birth weight in the ART group [63], hence many of the differences found on a whole population level may be attributable to intrinsic parental factors. Moreover, fetal growth restriction leading to low birth weight is more common in women diagnosed with subfertility regardless of mode of conception [64]. An increase in hypertensive diseases of pregnancy has also been observed in mothers who conceived after ART [60], which suggests a higher rate of placentation anomalies potentially leading indirectly to higher rates of fetal growth restriction.

Interestingly, several well-powered studies have observed a higher average birth-weight in children conceived using ART who were the result of frozen embryo transfer rather than fresh [12, 17, 51, 65]. This finding is difficult to explain, but may relate to the baseline characteristics of parents who had surplus embryos to freeze after initial treatment, or to the fact that the intrauterine environment is less likely to be acutely influenced by hormonal stimuli [66]. The mechanisms by which mode of conception is linked to differences in fetal growth velocity remain to be fully established, but the increased birth-weights of children conceived after cryopreservation could point to a key role for the endometrial environment around implantation leading to better establishment of placentation.

It has been suggested that early *in vitro* culture of human embryos during ART can directly influence birth weight, regardless of other maternal and placental factors. One such study quasi-randomized embryos during the IVF process to culture in one of two commercially available media, and showed a difference in birth weight between the two groups [67]. While the imprinting of key growth genes such as IGF2 was not affected by method of conception, there were differences in other genes, including the regulator of pre-RNA processing small nuclear ribonucleoprotein peptide N (SNRPN) which may contribute to dysregulation of fetal growth [68]. Similar effects are noted in animal model of *in vitro* culture [69], where epigenetic differences in growth-related genes including IGF2 have been noted [70].

Clinical Practice Points

The RCOG guideline "Investigation and Management of the Small-for-gestational-age Fetus" (Green-top Guideline No. 31, revised January 2014) considers use of IVF as a minor risk factor for fetal growth restriction. Increased surveillance of fetal growth in the absence of other risk factors is not currently recommended.

Preterm Delivery

Many large and well-controlled cohorts have demonstrated an increase in the incidence of preterm delivery in pregnancies conceived using ART and this has been confirmed in several meta-analyses [4, 5, 9–11, 57, 60, 66, 71]. Some studies have estimated that the risk of any preterm birth is at least doubled in pregnancies conceived via ART compared to the spontaneously conceived population, with even higher odds of an early preterm birth [72]. This increase in the magnitude of risk is approximately the same in a mother with a history of prior preterm birth, making ART potentially a major risk factor for prematurity [72, 73]. Distinguishing retrospectively between spontaneous and iatrogenic preterm delivery is complex, but extremely important in determining the precise mechanism that could link mode of conception to gestation at delivery. Unfortunately there are few cohorts in which information specifically regarding the aetiology of the prematurity is available. There is evidence of both increased rates of preterm rupture of membranes and antepartum haemorrhage in pregnancies conceived using ART, either of which could potentially make substantial contributions to the rate of spontaneous preterm birth [60]. However, there is also evidence of increased incidence of maternal disease in pregnancies conceived using ART, particularly hypertensive disease, which could substantially increase the rate of iatrogenic preterm birth [11]. Iatrogenic preterm delivery rates may also be increased due to the increased propensity to placental abruption observed in association with conception using ART in several cohorts [13, 74]. However, no excess risk of preterm birth was found between sibling pairs conceived spontaneously and via ART, suggesting that in common with fetal growth, the propensity to preterm labour may be more associated with maternal factors than with exposure to ART per se [63]. In particular, a history of maternal subfertility, as assessed by time to conception, is independently associated with the risk of preterm birth [75].

In common with fetal growth restriction, the incidence of preterm birth among ART conceptions appears to be lower where embryo cryopreservation was used than in fresh cycles [17]. The decreased incidence of preterm birth may be linked to lower rates of antepartum haemorrhage in the cryopreservation group [66]. Furthermore, it may be the case that blastocyst rather than cleavage stage embryo replacement further increases the risk of a preterm or very preterm delivery [76]; however, more work is needed to disentangle the causative effect from potential confounding factors.

Clinical Practice Points

There is no current evidence to suggest that additional surveillance or testing would be of benefit in reducing the rates of preterm birth in pregnancies conceived using ART.

Stillbirth

Several large cohorts and meta-analyses demonstrate increased risks of perinatal death in pregnancies conceived using ART [4, 5, 11, 73]; however, the meta-analysis results are heavily influenced by a single case-control study from the US that showed a very high rate of perinatal death in the ART group [77]. When spontaneously and ART-conceived siblings pairs were studied the rates of perinatal death were comparable, and may have been reduced in the ART group. The issue of excess perinatal mortality rates in ART-conceived pregnancies is further complicated by the high rates of ART use in mothers who had previously experienced a perinatal death [63]. Perinatal deaths appear to be increased in women with a history of subfertility regardless of whether ART is utilized [78], making interpretation of the attributable risk of ART to perinatal death extremely complex. While perinatal death as whole may be increased by the use of ART, few studies are powered to look at normally formed singleton stillbirths. While there is some evidence that the stillbirth rate overall is increased in IVF pregnancies (OR 1.49 for IVF versus spontaneous conceptions) [9], the causal link is yet to be established.

Clinical Practice Points

Detection of fetal growth restriction can reduce stillbirth rates, therefore surveillance for growth restriction is recommended for pregnancies conceived using ART in the presence of additional risk factors.

Multiple Pregnancies

Much of the excess incidence of adverse perinatal outcome associated with ART has been attributed to the vast increase in multiple pregnancies associated with these techniques. In the US, the incidence of twin pregnancies increased by 100-fold since the widespread introduction of ART in the 1980s [79]. A considerable percentage of all multiple pregnancies in the US are the result of use of ART, despite international attempts to move towards more single embryo transfers [3]. Multiple pregnancy can be considered the most likely fetal complication of conception using ART.

Twin Pregnancies

While twin pregnancies in general are much more vulnerable to fetal complications than singleton pregnancies, conflicting data exist on whether the use of ART increases the risk of adverse outcomes above spontaneously conceived multiple pregnancies [80]. Some studies have found higher rates of adverse fetal outcomes after the use of ART, including risks of fetal structural anomalies [81], growth restriction [82], preterm birth [83, 84] and perinatal mortality [85]. However, in other studies, twin pregnancies conceived using ART have a comparable rate of major perinatal complications to those conceived spontaneously [86–88], and in some studies are even estimated to have a lower perinatal mortality rate [73]. The association between growth restriction and ART seen in singleton pregnancies does not appear to hold true in multiple pregnancies [58].

Chorionicity is a major factor in determining outcome in twin pregnancy, and while most twins resulting from ART are the result of double embryo transfer (and hence dichorionic and diamniotic), there is also a higher rate of monozygous twin pregnancy with ART compared to spontaneous conception, which cannot be circumvented using single embryo transfer [37]. Various explanations for this phenomenon have been suggested, including a direct effect of *in vitro* culture, higher likelihood of embryo manipulations, e.g., blastomere sampling for preimplantation genetic diagnosis [89]. It is well established that monozygotic twins are at higher risk of adverse perinatal outcomes (regardless of mode of conception) including prematurity, low birth weight, congenital anomalies [90] and perinatal death [90], compared to dizygous twins. In particular twins that are monoamniotic have additional risks, including cord entanglement [91]. There are case reports of conjoined twin pregnancies occurring after the use of ART, but there are insufficient data to judge whether the risk of this extremely rare outcome is substantially elevated [92]. Congenital anomalies in general do not appear to be more common in twins conceived using ART than in spontaneous conceptions [50], with the possible exceptions of neural tube defects [93] and anencephaly [81].

Higher-Order Multiples

The number of triplet pregnancies born to older mothers has increase fourfold in recent decades, primarily due to increased use of ART [94]. In 2007, 1.2 % of all deliveries following ART were of triplets. Such pregnancies may have significant adverse effects on maternal and neonatal outcomes [95, 96]. The relative rarity of spontaneous higher-order multiple pregnancies and the frequency of adverse outcomes [97–99] regardless of mode of conception limits the strength of the conclusions that can be drawn about the contribution of the ART process to fetal complications. The ability to draw conclusions regarding pregnancy outcomes is further complicated by the number of higher-order multiple pregnancies that subsequently undergo selective fetal reduction [100, 101]. There is limited evidence from studies of multiple pregnancies including both twins and triplets to suggest that outcomes following ART conception are not worse than spontaneous conception [102, 103]. A recent study suggests that fetal outcomes of triplets conceived using ART may be improved by selective fetal reduction, particularly in terms of increasing birth weight and decreasing prematurity for no extra increase in pregnancy loss [98].

Clinical Practice Points

In the UK the National Institute for Health and Clinical Excellence (NICE) has produced guidelines for the management of multiple pregnancies. Management of ART assisted multiple pregnancies should be in line with the guidance.

Placental Complications

The increase in fetal complications from pregnancies resulting from ART may be in part attributable to increased placental complications, particularly fetal growth restriction, stillbirth and iatrogenic preterm delivery.

Vasa Praevia

Vasa praevia may be rapidly fatal to the fetus if bleeding occurs from the unprotected vessels traversing the membranes either with premature rupture of the membranes or during delivery. Over 50 % of neonates born following pregnancy complicated by vasa praevia require transfusion after delivery, and the perinatal death rate remains high [104]. Examination of placentas from both twin and singleton pregnancies conceived using ART has demonstrated a higher incidence of cord-insertion variants [105, 106], including vasa praevia [107, 108], and has estimated that the frequency of velamentous cord insertion in twins conceived via IVF may be as high as 10 % [109]. The reason for the increased incidence of vasa praevia in pregnancies conceived using ART remains uncertain, but it has been suggested that the normal process of blastocyst orientation at the time of implantation may be impaired by mechanical replacement of the embryo in the uterine cavity [109]. It has been further postulated that the increase in incidence of fetal growth restriction observed in pregnancies conceived using ART may be causally linked with abnormal cord insertion, although this hypothesis requires further verification [106]. The increased incidence of vasa praevia in IVF pregnancies, and its association with severe fetal complications has lead to the suggestion that specific screening of IVF pregnancies using transvaginal colour Doppler to detect vasa praevia should be undertaken [108]. Despite the low incidence of vasa praevia and the increasingly high proportion of pregnancies conceived using ART, transvaginal screening in IVF pregnancies may represent a cost-effective pregnancy intervention to prevent severe fetal morbidity [110].

Placenta Praevia/Accreta

Placenta praevia increases the risk of fetal complications during pregnancy, particularly with regard to antepartum haemorrhage, stillbirth and iatrogenic preterm delivery [111]. The overall incidence of clinically significant placenta praevia persisting until term is higher in ART-associated pregnancies than in those conceived spontaneously, with some studies suggesting an increase in risk as high as sixfold [9–11, 26, 59, 71, 112]. Some evidence exists that blastocyst transfer may be associated with higher rates of placenta praevia than cleavage-stage transfer [59]. When ART and spontaneously conceived pregnancies of the same mother were compared, the risk of placenta praevia still remained threefold higher in the ART group, implying that the increased risk is a direct effect of the ART process rather than a result of an underlying maternal structural complication such as Asherman's syndrome [113]. However, the increased risk is unlikely to result simply from low placement of the transferred blastocyst within the cavity, as the rates of placenta praevia are also elevated in pregnancies conceived using gamete intra-fallopian transfer (GIFT), where replacement occurs much higher in the maternal reproductive tract [13]. The incidence of both placenta praevia and associated antepartum haemorrhage may be reduced in pregnancies where cryopreservation rather than fresh transfer was used [112], which may relate to the fact that the endometrium is much less likely to have undergone stimulation prior to transfer in frozen cycles ("natural" cycles). More direct evidence that the unstimulated endometrium is less associated with placenta praevia comes from a large retrospective cohort Australian cohort, where the risk of placenta praevia was elevated fourfold in fresh cycles compared to "natural" unstimulated frozen cycles [114]. Importantly, this study was also able to include a group of women who had stimulated frozen cycles for comparison and in this group the incidence of placenta praevia was comparable to fresh cycles [114]. These findings strongly suggest that the stimulated endometrium may be the key risk factor for developing placenta praevia in this context, rather than the conceptus or underlying maternal factors. This finding correlates well with the risk of postpartum haemorrhage in pregnancies conceived using frozen cycle ART, which is lower in natural cycles than those using endometrial stimulation [13].

Placenta accreta has been observed at higher rates in pregnancies conceived using ART than in spontaneous pregnancies [115, 116], although this finding is not consistent across all cohorts [112]. The rarity of placenta accreta means that many studies are not sufficiently powered to assess invasive placentation as a separate outcome. It is remains uncertain whether the observed increase in placenta accreta in several studies may be due to intrinsic implantation dysregulation attributable to the ART process. Other possible explanations for the increased risk are maternal factors either linked to the requirement for ART (such as advanced maternal age) or linked to the underlying subfertility (such as previous endometrial resection [115]). In contrast with other fetal complications, the incidence of placenta accreta has recently been observed in a large Japanese cohort to be higher in ART cycles where cryopreservation was used than in fresh cycles [12].

Placental Insufficiency

The commonly observed phenotype of low birth weight in neonates born following the use of ART [3, 9, 12, 58, 59] has led to speculation regarding placental insufficiency in these pregnancies as a possible aetiological factor. Moreover, it has been observed that several key growth-related genes are up regulated in placental tissue from pregnancies conceived using IVF/ICSI techniques. These genes include H19 and PHLDA2, which are important mediators of intrauterine growth [61]. It is important to note, however, that no definite causal link to adverse fetal outcomes has been established.

Some studies have also suggested that the risk of early onset pre-eclampsia is higher in ART-conceived pregnancies [117], a relationship that persisted even after correction for possible aetiological factors including maternal age and pre-existing conditions [117]. This implies increased likelihood of a phenotype of insufficient trophoblast invasion; however, results from other studies are equivocal about the relationship between use of ART and development of early onset pre-eclampsia [59, 112].

Clinical Practice Points

In view of the increased risk of vasa praevia in ART-conceived pregnancies, if a low-lying placenta is seen at the time of routine fetal anomaly scanning, a transvaginal scan to look for vasa praevia should be undertaken.

Conclusions

There is evidence of an increased incidence of several important fetal complications in pregnancy following the use of ART [118]; however, it is important to note that the process of ART may not be the direct proximal cause of the observed adverse outcomes. Two potentially key aetiological factors are emerging from the developing body of literature on outcomes of pregnancies conceived using ART. Firstly, an increase in adverse outcomes is also seen in spontaneously conceived pregnancies of couples with subfertility [63] implying that the major under-lying factor behind the increase in fetal complications in pregnancies conceived using ART may be the underlying parental subfertility rather than an effect of the process of ART itself [71]. The second factor that may be an important determinant of pregnancy complications is stimulation of the endometrium. In particular, placenta-related complications are reduced in 'natural' cycles, where frozen embryos are replaced into an unstimulated uterine environment [13, 114]. The identification of endometrial stimulation as a factor increasing the risk of adverse fetal outcomes is especially important for the management of pregnancies conceived using ART as it is a modifiable risk factor and can be taken into account when designing optimal treatment protocols. Regardless of the aetiology of the increased rates of fetal complications, the demonstrable increase in complication rates for these pregnancies naturally leads to the question of whether any routinely increased surveillance of these pregnancies is indicated and whether it could be of benefit in improving outcomes. The most beneficial intervention remains the avoidance of multiple pregnancy through the use of single embryo transfer where appropriate [80]. There is further evidence that routine transvaginal screening for vasa praevia may be cost-effective [110]. In view of the increase in perinatal mortality seen in the neonates of subfertile couples and the established links between subfertility, placental dysfunction and intrauterine growth restriction, serious consideration should be given to introducing routine third trimester monitoring of fetal growth via ultrasound for singleton pregnancies conceived using ART. For twin pregnancies, where increased surveillance is already in place during gestation, the increased risks of subfertility and ART are probably too subtle to justify any additional antenatal care needs [80]. Women who have conceived using ART should be made aware of a higher risk of induction of labour or Caesarean section [118], particularly with advancing maternal age.

Later-life outcomes for the children resulting from pregnancies conceived using ART are a matter of important debate, but are outside the scope of this chapter. Recent expert opinion based on systematic review implies that regardless of immediate fetal complication, there may be no long-term cognitive or developmental disadvantage to ART for the offspring [19]. This is highly reassuring, even in light of the evidence that suggests there may be an increase in fetal complications. However, we are still a long way from fully understanding these effects and from creating studies free of confounding to improve our understanding. Much more evidence is needed from well-designed prospective studies to disentangle causal effects contributing to fetal complications seen in association with conception using ART. Beyond this lies the requirement for more evidence regarding the mechanisms by which fetal complications might arise from the use of ART. Better understanding of the underlying mechanisms is vital in developing interventions to ameliorate these adverse effects.

References

1. Steptoe PC, Edwards RG. Birth after the reimplantation of a human embryo. Lancet. 1978;2(8085):366.
2. Ferraretti AP, Goossens V, de Mouzon J, Bhattacharya S, Castilla JA, Korsak V, et al. Assisted reproductive technology in Europe, 2008: results generated from European registers by ESHRE. Hum Reprod. 2012;27(9):2571–84.
3. Sunderam S, Kissin DM, Crawford SB, Folger SG, Jamieson DJ, Barfield WD, et al. Assisted reproductive technology surveillance--United States, 2011. MMWR Surveill Summ. 2014;63(10):1–28.
4. McDonald SD, Murphy K, Beyene J, Ohlsson A. Perinatal outcomes of singleton pregnancies achieved by in vitro fertilization: a systematic review and meta-analysis. J Obstet Gynaecol Can. 2005;27(5):449–59.
5. Jackson RA, Gibson KA, Wu YW, Croughan MS. Perinatal outcomes in singletons following in vitro fertilization: a meta-analysis. Obstet Gynecol. 2004;103(3):551–63.

6. Johnson JA, Tough S, Society of O, Gynaecologists of C. Delayed child-bearing. J Obstet Gynaecol Can. 2012;34(1):80–93.
7. Segev Y, Riskin-Mashiah S, Lavie O, Auslender R. Assisted reproductive technologies: medical safety issues in the older woman. J Womens Health (Larchmt). 2011;20(6):853–61.
8. Kort DH, Gosselin J, Choi JM, Thornton MH, Cleary-Goldman J, Sauer MV. Pregnancy after age 50: defining risks for mother and child. Am J Perinatol. 2012;29(4):245–50.
9. Raisanen S, Randell K, Nielsen HS, Gissler M, Kramer MR, Klemetti R, et al. Socioeconomic status affects the prevalence, but not the perinatal outcomes, of in vitro fertilization pregnancies. Hum Reprod. 2013;28(11):3118–25.
10. Grady R, Alavi N, Vale R, Khandwala M, McDonald SD. Elective single embryo transfer and perinatal outcomes: a systematic review and meta-analysis. Fertil Steril. 2012;97(2):324–31.
11. Yang X, Li Y, Li C, Zhang W. Current overview of pregnancy complications and live-birth outcome of assisted reproductive technology in mainland China. Fertil Steril. 2014;101(2):385–91.
12. Ishihara O, Araki R, Kuwahara A, Itakura A, Saito H, Adamson GD. Impact of frozen-thawed single-blastocyst transfer on maternal and neonatal outcome: an analysis of 277,042 single-embryo transfer cycles from 2008 to 2010 in Japan. Fertil Steril. 2014;101(1):128–33.
13. Healy DL, Breheny S, Halliday J, Jaques A, Rushford D, Garrett C, et al. Prevalence and risk factors for obstetric haemorrhage in 6730 singleton births after assisted reproductive technology in Victoria Australia. Hum Reprod. 2010;25(1):265–74.
14. Grigorescu V, Zhang Y, Kissin DM, Sauber-Schatz E, Sunderam M, Kirby RS, et al. Maternal characteristics and pregnancy outcomes after assisted reproductive technology by infertility diagnosis: ovulatory dysfunction versus tubal obstruction. Fertil Steril. 2014;101(4):1019–25.
15. Kjerulff LE, Sanchez-Ramos L, Duffy D. Pregnancy outcomes in women with polycystic ovary syndrome: a metaanalysis. Am J Obstet Gynecol. 2011;204(6):558 e1–6.
16. Kallen B, Finnstrom O, Nygren KG, Olausson PO. In vitro fertilization (IVF) in Sweden: infant outcome after different IVF fertilization methods. Fertil Steril. 2005;84(3):611–7.
17. Pinborg A, Loft A, Aaris Henningsen AK, Rasmussen S, Andersen AN. Infant outcome of 957 singletons born after frozen embryo replacement: the Danish National Cohort Study 1995-2006. Fertil Steril. 2010;94(4):1320–7.
18. Devroey P, Liu J, Nagy Z, Goossens A, Tournaye H, Camus M, et al. Pregnancies after testicular sperm extraction and intracytoplasmic sperm injection in non-obstructive azoospermia. Hum Reprod. 1995;10(6):1457–60.
19. Fauser BC, Devroey P, Diedrich K, Balaban B, Bonduelle M, Delemarre-van de Waal HA, et al. Health outcomes of children born after IVF/ICSI: a review of current expert opinion and literature. Reprod Biomed Online. 2014;28(2):162–82.
20. Van Assche E, Bonduelle M, Tournaye H, Joris H, Verheyen G, Devroey P, et al. Cytogenetics of infertile men. Hum Reprod. 1996;11 Suppl 4:1–24; discussion 5–6.
21. Schreurs A, Legius E, Meuleman C, Fryns JP, D'Hooghe TM. Increased frequency of chromosomal abnormalities in female partners of couples undergoing in vitro fertilization or intracytoplasmic sperm injection. Fertil Steril. 2000;74(1):94–6.
22. Silber SJ, Alagappan R, Brown LG, Page DC. Y chromosome deletions in azoospermic and severely oligozoospermic men undergoing intracytoplasmic sperm injection after testicular sperm extraction. Hum Reprod. 1998;13(12):3332–7.
23. Kurinczuk JJ, Bhattacharya S. Rare chromosomal, genetic, and epigenetic-related risks associated with infertility treatment. Semin Fetal Neonatal Med. 2014;19(4):250–3.
24. Lee SH, Ahn SY, Lee KW, Kwack K, Jun HS, Cha KY. Intracytoplasmic sperm injection may lead to vertical transmission, expansion, and de novo occurrence of Y-chromosome microdeletions in male fetuses. Fertil Steril. 2006;85(5):1512–5.
25. Cox GF, Burger J, Lip V, Mau UA, Sperling K, Wu BL, et al. Intracytoplasmic sperm injection may increase the risk of imprinting defects. Am J Hum Genet. 2002;71(1):162–4.
26. Halliday J, Oke K, Breheny S, Algar E, Amour DJ. Beckwith-Wiedemann syndrome and IVF: a case-control study. Am J Hum Genet. 2004;75(3):526–8.

27. Manipalviratn S, DeCherney A, Segars J. Imprinting disorders and assisted reproductive technology. Fertil Steril. 2009;91(2):305–15.
28. Bowdin S, Allen C, Kirby G, Brueton L, Afnan M, Barratt C, et al. A survey of assisted reproductive technology births and imprinting disorders. Hum Reprod. 2007;22(12):3237–40.
29. El Hajj N, Haaf T. Epigenetic disturbances in in vitro cultured gametes and embryos: implications for human assisted reproduction. Fertil Steril. 2013;99(3):632–41.
30. Fauque P. Ovulation induction and epigenetic anomalies. Fertil Steril. 2013;99(3):616–23.
31. Turan N, Katari S, Gerson LF, Chalian R, Foster MW, Gaughan JP, et al. Inter- and intra-individual variation in allele-specific DNA methylation and gene expression in children conceived using assisted reproductive technology. PLoS Genet. 2010;6(7), e1001033.
32. Oliver VF, Miles HL, Cutfield WS, Hofman PL, Ludgate JL, Morison IM. Defects in imprinting and genome-wide DNA methylation are not common in the in vitro fertilization population. Fertil Steril. 2012;97(1):147–53 e7.
33. Gomes MV, Huber J, Ferriani RA, Amaral Neto AM, Ramos ES. Abnormal methylation at the KvDMR1 imprinting control region in clinically normal children conceived by assisted reproductive technologies. Mol Hum Reprod. 2009;15(8):471–7.
34. Fernandez-Twinn DS, Ozanne SE. Early life nutrition and metabolic programming. Ann N Y Acad Sci. 2010;1212:78–96.
35. Gluckman PD, Hanson MA, Cooper C, Thornburg KL. Effect of in utero and early-life conditions on adult health and disease. N Engl J Med. 2008;359(1):61–73.
36. Aiken CE, Ozanne SE. Transgenerational developmental programming. Hum Reprod Update. 2014;20(1):63–75.
37. Aston KI, Peterson CM, Carrell DT. Monozygotic twinning associated with assisted reproductive technologies: a review. Reproduction. 2008;136(4):377–86.
38. Knopman JM, Krey LC, Oh C, Lee J, McCaffrey C, Noyes N. What makes them split? Identifying risk factors that lead to monozygotic twins after in vitro fertilization. Fertil Steril. 2014;102(1):82–9.
39. van Jaarsveld CH, Llewellyn CH, Fildes A, Fisher A, Wardle J. Are my twins identical: parents may be misinformed by prenatal scan observations. BJOG. 2012;119(5):517–8.
40. Farhi A, Reichman B, Boyko V, Mashiach S, Hourvitz A, Margalioth EJ, et al. Congenital malformations in infants conceived following assisted reproductive technology in comparison with spontaneously conceived infants. J Matern Fetal Neonatal Med. 2013;26(12):1171–9.
41. Sagot P, Bechoua S, Ferdynus C, Facy A, Flamm X, Gouyon JB, et al. Similarly increased congenital anomaly rates after intrauterine insemination and IVF technologies: a retrospective cohort study. Hum Reprod. 2012;27(3):902–9.
42. Olson CK, Keppler-Noreuil KM, Romitti PA, Budelier WT, Ryan G, Sparks AE, et al. In vitro fertilization is associated with an increase in major birth defects. Fertil Steril. 2005;84(5):1308–15.
43. Bonduelle M, Wennerholm UB, Loft A, Tarlatzis BC, Peters C, Henriet S, et al. A multi-centre cohort study of the physical health of 5-year-old children conceived after intracytoplasmic sperm injection, in vitro fertilization and natural conception. Hum Reprod. 2005;20(2):413–9.
44. Yan J, Huang G, Sun Y, Zhao X, Chen S, Zou S, et al. Birth defects after assisted reproductive technologies in China: analysis of 15,405 offspring in seven centers (2004 to 2008). Fertil Steril. 2011;95(1):458–60.
45. Picaud JC, Chalies S, Combes C, Mercier G, Dechaud H, Cambonie G. Neonatal mortality and morbidity in preterm infants born from assisted reproductive technologies. Acta Paediatr. 2012;101(8):846–51.
46. Zwink N, Jenetzky E, Schmiedeke E, Schmidt D, Marzheuser S, Grasshoff-Derr S, et al. Assisted reproductive techniques and the risk of anorectal malformations: a German case-control study. Orphanet J Rare Dis. 2012;7:65.

47. Tararbit K, Lelong N, Thieulin AC, Houyel L, Bonnet D, Goffinet F, et al. The risk for four specific congenital heart defects associated with assisted reproductive techniques: a population-based evaluation. Hum Reprod. 2013;28(2):367–74.
48. Valenzuela-Alcaraz B, Crispi F, Bijnens B, Cruz-Lemini M, Creus M, Sitges M, et al. Assisted reproductive technologies are associated with cardiovascular remodeling in utero that persists postnatally. Circulation. 2013;128(13):1442–50.
49. Bergh T, Ericson A, Hillensjo T, Nygren KG, Wennerholm UB. Deliveries and children born after in-vitro fertilisation in Sweden 1982-95: a retrospective cohort study. Lancet. 1999;354(9190):1579–85.
50. Zhu JL, Basso O, Obel C, Bille C, Olsen J. Infertility, infertility treatment, and congenital malformations: Danish national birth cohort. BMJ. 2006;333(7570):679.
51. Belva F, Henriet S, Van den Abbeel E, Camus M, Devroey P, Van der Elst J, et al. Neonatal outcome of 937 children born after transfer of cryopreserved embryos obtained by ICSI and IVF and comparison with outcome data of fresh ICSI and IVF cycles. Hum Reprod. 2008;23(10):2227–38.
52. Wen J, Jiang J, Ding C, Dai J, Liu Y, Xia Y, et al. Birth defects in children conceived by in vitro fertilization and intracytoplasmic sperm injection: a meta-analysis. Fertil Steril. 2012;97(6):1331–7 e1–4.
53. Hansen M, Bower C, Milne E, de Klerk N, Kurinczuk JJ. Assisted reproductive technologies and the risk of birth defects – a systematic review. Hum Reprod. 2005;20(2):328–38.
54. Rimm AA, Katayama AC, Diaz M, Katayama KP. A meta-analysis of controlled studies comparing major malformation rates in IVF and ICSI infants with naturally conceived children. J Assist Reprod Genet. 2004;21(12):437–43.
55. Rimm AA, Katayama AC, Katayama KP. A meta-analysis of the impact of IVF and ICSI on major malformations after adjusting for the effect of subfertility. J Assist Reprod Genet. 2011;28(8):699 705.
56. Davies MJ, Moore VM, Willson KJ, Van Essen P, Priest K, Scott H, et al. Reproductive technologies and the risk of birth defects. N Engl J Med. 2012;366(19):1803–13.
57. Ishihara O, Adamson GD, Dyer S, de Mouzon J, Nygren KG, Sullivan EA, et al. International committee for monitoring assisted reproductive technologies: world report on assisted reproductive technologies, 2007. Fertil Steril. 2015;103(2):402–13 e11.
58. Schieve LA, Meikle SF, Ferre C, Peterson HB, Jeng G, Wilcox LS. Low and very low birth weight in infants conceived with use of assisted reproductive technology. N Engl J Med. 2002;346(10):731–7.
59. Sazonova A, Kallen K, Thurin-Kjellberg A, Wennerholm UB, Bergh C. Obstetric outcome in singletons after in vitro fertilization with cryopreserved/thawed embryos. Hum Reprod. 2012;27(5):1343–50.
60. Pandey S, Shetty A, Hamilton M, Bhattacharya S, Maheshwari A. Obstetric and perinatal outcomes in singleton pregnancies resulting from IVF/ICSI: a systematic review and meta-analysis. Hum Reprod Update. 2012;18(5):485–503.
61. Nelissen EC, Dumoulin JC, Busato F, Ponger L, Eijssen LM, Evers JL, et al. Altered gene expression in human placentas after IVF/ICSI. Hum Reprod. 2014;29(12):2821–31.
62. Cooper AR, O'Neill KE, Allsworth JE, Jungheim ES, Odibo AO, Gray DL, et al. Smaller fetal size in singletons after infertility therapies: the influence of technology and the underlying infertility. Fertil Steril. 2011;96(5):1100–6.
63. Romundstad LB, Romundstad PR, Sunde A, von During V, Skjaerven R, Gunnell D, et al. Effects of technology or maternal factors on perinatal outcome after assisted fertilisation: a population-based cohort study. Lancet. 2008;372(9640):737–43.
64. De Geyter C, De Geyter M, Steimann S, Zhang H, Holzgreve W. Comparative birth weights of singletons born after assisted reproduction and natural conception in previously infertile women. Hum Reprod. 2006;21(3):705–12.

65. Nakashima A, Araki R, Tani H, Ishihara O, Kuwahara A, Irahara M, et al. Implications of assisted reproductive technologies on term singleton birth weight: an analysis of 25,777 children in the national assisted reproduction registry of Japan. Fertil Steril. 2013;99(2):450–5.
66. Maheshwari A, Pandey S, Shetty A, Hamilton M, Bhattacharya S. Obstetric and perinatal outcomes in singleton pregnancies resulting from the transfer of frozen thawed versus fresh embryos generated through in vitro fertilization treatment: a systematic review and meta-analysis. Fertil Steril. 2012;98(2):368–77 e1–9.
67. Dumoulin JC, Land JA, Van Montfoort AP, Nelissen EC, Coonen E, Derhaag JG, et al. Effect of in vitro culture of human embryos on birthweight of newborns. Hum Reprod. 2010;25(3):605–12.
68. Whitelaw N, Bhattacharya S, Hoad G, Horgan GW, Hamilton M, Haggarty P. Epigenetic status in the offspring of spontaneous and assisted conception. Hum Reprod. 2014;29(7):1452–8.
69. McEvoy TG, Robinson JJ, Sinclair KD. Developmental consequences of embryo and cell manipulation in mice and farm animals. Reproduction. 2001;122(4):507–18.
70. Young LE, Fernandes K, McEvoy TG, Butterwith SC, Gutierrez CG, Carolan C, et al. Epigenetic change in IGF2R is associated with fetal overgrowth after sheep embryo culture. Nat Genet. 2001;27(2):153–4.
71. Hayashi M, Nakai A, Satoh S, Matsuda Y. Adverse obstetric and perinatal outcomes of singleton pregnancies may be related to maternal factors associated with infertility rather than the type of assisted reproductive technology procedure used. Fertil Steril. 2012;98(4):922–8.
72. McGovern PG, Llorens AJ, Skurnick JH, Weiss G, Goldsmith LT. Increased risk of preterm birth in singleton pregnancies resulting from in vitro fertilization-embryo transfer or gamete intrafallopian transfer: a meta-analysis. Fertil Steril. 2004;82(6):1514–20.
73. Helmerhorst FM, Perquin DA, Donker D, Keirse MJ. Perinatal outcome of singletons and twins after assisted conception: a systematic review of controlled studies. BMJ. 2004;328(7434):261.
74. Caserta D, Bordi G, Stegagno M, Filippini F, Podagrosi M, Roselli D, et al. Maternal and perinatal outcomes in spontaneous versus assisted conception twin pregnancies. Eur J Obstet Gynecol Reprod Biol. 2014;174:64–9.
75. Henriksen TB, Baird DD, Olsen J, Hedegaard M, Secher NJ, Wilcox AJ. Time to pregnancy and preterm delivery. Obstet Gynecol. 1997;89(4):594–9.
76. Maheshwari A, Kalampokas T, Davidson J, Bhattacharya S. Obstetric and perinatal outcomes in singleton pregnancies resulting from the transfer of blastocyst-stage versus cleavage-stage embryos generated through in vitro fertilization treatment: a systematic review and meta-analysis. Fertil Steril. 2013;100(6):1615–21 e1–10.
77. Dhont M, De Sutter P, Ruyssinck G, Martens G, Bekaert A. Perinatal outcome of pregnancies after assisted reproduction: a case-control study. Am J Obstet Gynecol. 1999;181(3):688–95.
78. Draper ES, Kurinczuk JJ, Abrams KR, Clarke M. Assessment of separate contributions to perinatal mortality of infertility history and treatment: a case-control analysis. Lancet. 1999;353(9166):1746–9.
79. Chauhan SP, Scardo JA, Hayes E, Abuhamad AZ, Berghella V. Twins: prevalence, problems, and preterm births. Am J Obstet Gynecol. 2010;203(4):305–15.
80. Jauniaux E, Ben-Ami I, Maymon R. Do assisted-reproduction twin pregnancies require additional antenatal care? Reprod Biomed Online. 2013;26(2):107–19.
81. Ben-Ami I, Edel Y, Barel O, Vaknin Z, Herman A, Maymon R. Do assisted conception twins have an increased risk for anencephaly? Hum Reprod. 2011;26(12):3466–71.
82. Hansen M, Colvin L, Petterson B, Kurinczuk JJ, de Klerk N, Bower C. Twins born following assisted reproductive technology: perinatal outcome and admission to hospital. Hum Reprod. 2009;24(9):2321–31.
83. Adler-Levy Y, Lunenfeld E, Levy A. Obstetric outcome of twin pregnancies conceived by in vitro fertilization and ovulation induction compared with those conceived spontaneously. Eur J Obstet Gynecol Reprod Biol. 2007;133(2):173–8.

84. McDonald SD, Han Z, Mulla S, Ohlsson A, Beyene J, Murphy KE, et al. Preterm birth and low birth weight among in vitro fertilization twins: a systematic review and meta-analyses. Eur J Obstet Gynecol Reprod Biol. 2010;148(2):105–13.
85. Chaveeva P, Carbone IF, Syngelaki A, Akolekar R, Nicolaides KH. Contribution of method of conception on pregnancy outcome after the 11-13 weeks scan. Fetal Diagn Ther. 2011;30(1):9–22.
86. Moise J, Laor A, Armon Y, Gur I, Gale R. The outcome of twin pregnancies after IVF. Hum Reprod. 1998;13(6):1702–5.
87. Olivennes F, Kadhel P, Rufat P, Fanchin R, Fernandez H, Frydman R. Perinatal outcome of twin pregnancies obtained after in vitro fertilization: comparison with twin pregnancies obtained spontaneously or after ovarian stimulation. Fertil Steril. 1996;66(1):105–9.
88. Vasario E, Borgarello V, Bossotti C, Libanori E, Biolcati M, Arduino S, et al. IVF twins have similar obstetric and neonatal outcome as spontaneously conceived twins: a prospective follow-up study. Reprod Biomed Online. 2010;21(3):422–8.
89. Sills ES, Moomjy M, Zaninovic N, Veeck LL, McGee M, Palermo GD, et al. Human zona pellucida micromanipulation and monozygotic twinning frequency after IVF. Hum Reprod. 2000;15(4):890–5.
90. Hack KE, Derks JB, Elias SG, Franx A, Roos EJ, Voerman SK, et al. Increased perinatal mortality and morbidity in monochorionic versus dichorionic twin pregnancies: clinical implications of a large Dutch cohort study. BJOG. 2008;115(1):58–67.
91. Desai N, Lewis D, Sunday S, Rochelson B. Current antenatal management of monoamniotic twins: a survey of maternal-fetal medicine specialists. J Matern Fetal Neonatal Med. 2012;25(10):1913–6.
92. Mercan R, Oktem O, Salar Z, Nuhoglu A, Balaban B, Urman B. Conjoined twins after intracytoplasmic sperm injection and transfer of day-3 embryos. Fertil Steril. 2011;96(2):e111–4.
93. Pinborg A. IVF/ICSI twin pregnancies: risks and prevention. Hum Reprod Update. 2005;11(6):575–93.
94. Oleszczuk JJ, Keith LG, Oleszczuk AK. The paradox of old maternal age in multiple pregnancies. Obstet Gynecol Clin North Am. 2005;32(1):69–80, ix.
95. Badgery-Parker T, Shand AW, Ford JB, Jenkins MG, Morris JM, Roberts CL. Multifetal pregnancies: preterm admissions and outcomes. Aust Health Rev. 2012;36(4):437–42.
96. Strauss A, Winkler D, Middendorf K, Kumper C, Herber-Jonat S, Schulze A. Higher order multiples – socioeconomic impact on family life. Eur J Med Res. 2008;13(4):147–53.
97. Chibber R, Fouda M, Shishtawy W, Al-Dossary M, Al-Hijji J, Amen A, et al. Maternal and neonatal outcome in triplet, quadruplet and quintuplet gestations following ART: a 11-year study. Arch Gynecol Obstet. 2013;288(4):759–67.
98. Shiva M, Mohammadi Yeganeh L, Mirzaagha E, Chehrazi M, Bagheri Lankarani N. Comparison of the outcomes between reduced and nonreduced triplet pregnancies achieved by Assisted Reproductive Technology. Aust N Z J Obstet Gynaecol. 2014;54(5):424–7.
99. Kaufman GE, Malone FD, Harvey-Wilkes KB, Chelmow D, Penzias AS, D'Alton ME. Neonatal morbidity and mortality associated with triplet pregnancy. Obstet Gynecol. 1998;91(3):342–8.
100. Boulot P, Vignal J, Vergnes C, Dechaud H, Faure JM, Hedon B. Multifetal reduction of triplets to twins: a prospective comparison of pregnancy outcome. Hum Reprod. 2000;15(7):1619–23.
101. American College of O, Gynecologists. ACOG Committee opinion no. 553: multifetal pregnancy reduction. Obstet Gynecol. 2013;121(2 Pt 1):405–10.
102. Shah V, Alwassia H, Shah K, Yoon W, Shah P. Neonatal outcomes among multiple births </= 32 weeks gestational age: does mode of conception have an impact? A cohort study. BMC Pediatr. 2011;11:54.

103. Fitzsimmons BP, Bebbington MW, Fluker MR. Perinatal and neonatal outcomes in multiple gestations: assisted reproduction versus spontaneous conception. Am J Obstet Gynecol. 1998;179(5):1162–7.
104. Oyelese Y, Catanzarite V, Prefumo F, Lashley S, Schachter M, Tovbin Y, et al. Vasa previa: the impact of prenatal diagnosis on outcomes. Obstet Gynecol. 2004;103(5 Pt 1):937–42.
105. Salafia CM, Yampolsky M, Shlakhter A, Mandel DH, Schwartz N. Variety in placental shape: when does it originate? Placenta. 2012;33(3):164–70.
106. Cai LY, Izumi S, Koido S, Uchida N, Suzuki T, Matsubayashi H, et al. Abnormal placental cord insertion may induce intrauterine growth restriction in IVF-twin pregnancies. Hum Reprod. 2006;21(5):1285–90.
107. Gavriil P, Jauniaux E, Leroy F. Pathologic examination of placentas from singleton and twin pregnancies obtained after in vitro fertilization and embryo transfer. Pediatr Pathol. 1993;13(4):453–62.
108. Baulies S, Maiz N, Munoz A, Torrents M, Echevarria M, Serra B. Prenatal ultrasound diagnosis of vasa praevia and analysis of risk factors. Prenat Diagn. 2007;27(7):595–9.
109. Jauniaux E, Englert Y, Vanesse M, Hiden M, Wilkin P. Pathologic features of placentas from singleton pregnancies obtained by in vitro fertilization and embryo transfer. Obstet Gynecol. 1990;76(1):61–4.
110. Cipriano LE, Barth Jr WH, Zaric GS. The cost-effectiveness of targeted or universal screening for vasa praevia at 18-20 weeks of gestation in Ontario. BJOG. 2010;117(9):1108–18.
111. Norgaard LN, Pinborg A, Lidegaard O, Bergholt T. A Danish national cohort study on neonatal outcome in singleton pregnancies with placenta previa. Acta Obstet Gynecol Scand. 2012;91(5):546–51.
112. Korosec S, Ban Frangez H, Verdenik I, Kladnik U, Kotar V, Virant-Klun I, et al. Singleton pregnancy outcomes after in vitro fertilization with fresh or frozen-thawed embryo transfer and incidence of placenta praevia. Biomed Res Int. 2014;2014:431797.
113. Romundstad LB, Romundstad PR, Sunde A, von During V, Skjaerven R, Vatten LJ. Increased risk of placenta previa in pregnancies following IVF/ICSI; a comparison of ART and non-ART pregnancies in the same mother. Hum Reprod. 2006;21(9):2353–8.
114. Rombauts L, Motteram C, Berkowitz E, Fernando S. Risk of placenta praevia is linked to endometrial thickness in a retrospective cohort study of 4537 singleton assisted reproduction technology births. Hum Reprod. 2014;29(12):2787–93.
115. Esh-Broder E, Ariel I, Abas-Bashir N, Bdolah Y, Celnikier DH. Placenta accreta is associated with IVF pregnancies: a retrospective chart review. BJOG. 2011;118(9):1084–9.
116. Farhi J, Ben-Haroush A, Andrawus N, Pinkas H, Sapir O, Fisch B, et al. High serum oestradiol concentrations in IVF cycles increase the risk of pregnancy complications related to abnormal placentation. Reprod Biomed Online. 2010;21(3):331–7.
117. Carbone IF, Cruz JJ, Sarquis R, Akolekar R, Nicolaides KH. Assisted conception and placental perfusion assessed by uterine artery Doppler at 11-13 weeks' gestation. Hum Reprod. 2011;26(7):1659–64.
118. Allen VM, Wilson RD, Cheung A, Genetics Committee of the Society of O, Gynaecologists of C, Reproductive Endocrinology Infertility Committee of the Society of O. Pregnancy outcomes after assisted reproductive technology. J Obstet Gynaecol Can. 2006;28(3):220–50.

Chapter 11
The Intrapartum and Postpartum Care of Women Following Assisted Reproduction Techniques (ART)

Sonia Asif and Srini Vindla

Introduction

Birth planning for women after assisted reproduction is an important facet of care. Understanding the complex literature to identify which aspects are pertinent to women who may have complex pregnancies not as a result of ART but because of their individual characteristics is challenging. In this chapter we aim to create an understanding of what the evidence presents about birth and outcomes for babies after ART.

Planning for birth must include an understanding of the psychological issues, the various pre-pregnancy risk factors, the progress of the pregnancy, and the expectations and needs of the parents.

Recognition of the Psychological Effects of ART

The need to understand the psychology of couples who have been through ART, and the impact that this has on both them and their maternity team is vital. Undergoing fertility treatment is physically, psychologically and financially demanding and not

S. Asif, MBChB, MRCOG (✉)
Division of Obstetrics, Gynaecology, and Child Health,
Queens Medical Centre, Nottingham, UK
e-mail: mda99sa@yahoo.co.uk

S. Vindla, MB, BS, BSc, FRCOG, DM
Department of Obstetrics and Gynaecology,
Sherwood Forest Hospitals NHS Foundation Trust,
Sutton-In-Ashfield, UK
e-mail: srini.vindla@sfh-tr.nhs.uk

K. Jayaprakasan, L. Kean (eds.), *Clinical Management of Pregnancies following ART*, DOI 10.1007/978-3-319-42858-1_11

unlike being on an "emotional rollercoaster" [1]. Recognition of the potential for significantly increased psychological and emotional needs of couples is helpful to those involved in care [2, 3]. Women with IVF pregnancies have been shown to be more anxious throughout pregnancy [4]. Patients who have conceived through IVF present with antenatal complaints earlier and more frequently, increasing personal and medical anxiety [5]. This has also been shown to have a "knock-on" effect on medical intervention [6, 7]. They are more likely to be admitted when presenting with problems and may need more reassurance that normal symptoms of pregnancy, such as backache, are not something more serious [8].

There is evidence that obstetricians and midwives view patients who conceive through ART differently with regard to how they manage birth. Elective caesarean section (CS) rates for maternal request are higher in most countries in pregnancy after ART, with rates of 50 % or more being seen in some countries.

This protective attitude is especially evident in older women who may have had multiple attempts to conceive and in whom achieving another pregnancy may prove challenging. Concern about minimising adverse fetal outcomes and fear of litigation lead to a lower threshold for intervention, induction of labour, or operative delivery.

The mental well-being and psychological coping strategies of women who conceive with ART are also different from spontaneously conceived pregnancies. Some studies [9] cite that the emotionally demanding aspects of fertility treatment positively prepares some women to deal with the unexpected complications of childbirth whereas other authors state that these same factors can lead to anxiety about delivery [10]. Interestingly parents of both IVF and naturally conceived pregnancies find parenthood similarly stressful [11].

Birth Outcomes After ART?: How Do They Differ?

In the UK national guidance on antenatal care advises that women conceiving with ART do not have to be booked under an obstetrician unless there are additional risk factors [12]. However, before deciding on whether consultant led care is required, it is important that a full assessment of the obstetric risks associated with non-spontaneous conception is undertaken. Antenatal assessment of risk factors is discussed in other chapters.

The clinician managing labour may not have been involved in the delivery of antenatal care and so a thorough understanding of those risks that will be pertinent to labour is important.

Data from two large robust systematic reviews [13, 14] concluded that singleton IVF pregnancies compared to naturally conceived pregnancies, were more likely to have preterm (<37 weeks), very preterm (<32 weeks), low birth weight (<2500 g), very low birth weight (<1500 g) and small for gestational age babies. Recent data from Australia suggest that the larger part of this risk appears to be related to the infertility itself rather than the assisted conception, as risks were actually highest in pregnancies conceived spontaneously after a period of prolonged infertility [15]. Few studies have examined actual outcomes in labour for women after assisted conception compared to control groups. On large study from the Netherlands where pregnancies were very carefully matched at booking showed that the outcomes for labour were not significantly different except that delivery occurred approximately 3 days earlier on average in the IVF group amongst women who spontaneously laboured. There were more elective CS in the IVF group and slightly more assisted vaginal deliveries in the control group. Induction rates were no different. Birthweight centiles were slightly lower for babies born after IVF but neonatal outcomes for term babies were similar [16].

Approach for Birth Planning

Pre-birth planning should be undertaken with every woman, regardless of method of conception. The appropriate professional to undertake this may be the midwife in the UK, if the pregnancy has progressed normally and there are no additional fetal or maternal risks identified. Conversely the obstetric team may have to fulfil this role, where midwives are not available or where complications or risks have been identified or where a couple wish to discuss alternative birth options to those offered by the midwife. Many women who have conceived after ART but are otherwise well are keen to avoid medicalisation and want to feel and be treated as normal, equally others feel that their journey to pregnancy has been complex and they need to discuss at length what choices they have with regard to birth, to minimise any risk to the baby.

The clinician should be able to present choices and the rationale for why some options may be recommended. In order to be in a position to provide appropriate information, maternal and fetal surveillance should have been undertaken according to identified risk factors, to ensure that issues such as fetal growth problems, placental issues, maternal medical problems and psychological needs have been identified prior to a final planning discussion.

Where complications have developed these should be managed in line with national guidelines where available. In the UK the most pertinent guidelines are: National Institute for Health and Clinical Excellence (NICE): Hypertension in pregnancy [17], Diabetes in pregnancy [18], Management of multiple pregnancies [19] and the Royal College of Obstericians and Gynaecologists (RCOG) guideline on Placenta praevia, accreta and vasa praevia with the National Patient Safety Agency care bundle for the management of placenta praevia after previous CS [20].

The key aspects for birth planning will include:

- Timing of birth
- Method of delivery
- Fetal monitoring preferences
- Alternative options for when the unexpected happens (with particular regard to pre-term birth)
- Additional precautions that may be needed to ensure a safe birth
- Postnatal care and support

Planning and Timing of Birth in Relationship to Identified Risk Factors

Increased Maternal Age

Delayed conception has led to a worldwide increase in the age of childbearing. Additionally, ART has also offered treatment for older women to overcome infertility related to advanced age.

Induction of labour at 39 weeks in women of 35 or more with an uncomplicated first pregnancy, has been addressed in a recent trial. The primary outcome measure was delivery by caesarean section. There was no difference in this outcome between the induction at 39 weeks or usual time (41–42 weeks). The caesarean section rate was 32 and 33 % respectively. No difference in fetal outcome was seen but the trial was not sufficiently powered to look at stillbirth prevention.

This trial does not support routine induction of labour in primigravida for age alone, but does provide safety data to support women's request for induction after 39 weeks as a safe option. Interestingly the primary reason for women choosing not to be randomised was because they did not wish to be induced at 39 weeks [21].

Hypertension

The cumulative effects of advanced maternal age, primiparity, and IVF all act synergistically to increase the risk of hypertension. Advanced maternal age (>35 years) is known to be a risk factor for pregnancy induced hypertension (PIH) and gestational diabetes. These risks are much more pronounced in older women who are nulliparous and have a multiple pregnancy conceived with ART.

The aging process leads to systemic dysfunction of the endothelial cells in the vasculature and may be the pathophysiological basis for the age related increase in PIH risk. The higher incidence of pre-eclampsia hypertensive disorders in women over the age of 40 is in itself a risk factor for PET. The association between IVF and PIH is not fully understood and is discussed in more detail in Chap. 9 on maternal complications during pregnancy.

NICE guidance recommends low dose aspirin at a dose of 75 mg from 12 weeks for women with two or more of the following risk factors for PET risk reduction:

- First pregnancy
- Age 40 or more
- An interval greater than 10 years since your last pregnancy
- Significant obesity – a body mass index (BMI) of 35 kg/m^2 or more at the first visit
- Family history of PET
- Multiple pregnancy

This will cover a large number of women conceiving after ART. In addition the fertility team may have advised aspirin during pregnancy for fertility treatment reasons.

NICE guidance recommends birth within 24–48 hours for women who have pre-eclampsia with mild or moderate hypertension after 37 weeks.

Recently, investigators of the HYPITAT (Pregnancy-induced hypertension and pre-eclampsia after 36 weeks: induction of labour versus expectant monitoring: A comparison of maternal and neonatal outcome, maternal quality of life and costs) randomized trial evaluated maternal and neonatal complications in patients at 36–40 weeks' gestation who were randomized to either induction of labour or expectant monitoring. The results of this trial revealed that induction of labour at or after 37 weeks was associated with lower rate of maternal complications without increased rates of either CS or neonatal complications [22]. This data support delivery after 37 weeks in women with hypertension in pregnancy.

Consideration must be given to fetal risks, however, when the chosen route for delivery is by elective CS. Where this is the case, discussion of outcomes for the baby must be balanced when delivery is proposed earlier than 39 weeks. Corticosteroids for fetal lung maturation should be given when delivery by elective CS is planned before 39 weeks [23].

Gestational Diabetes (GDM)

GDM has been associated with pregnancies that are conceived with ART. Ashrafi et al. concluded that singleton pregnancies conceived with IVF are twice as likely to develop GDM as their spontaneous counterparts [24].

GDM is associated with adverse obstetric outcomes, including an increased risk of PIH/PET, macrosomia, shoulder dystocia, birth injuries and caesarean section. Neonatal complications include respiratory distress syndrome, hypoglycaemia and jaundice [25].

The possible reasons for this are multifactorial, but clearly the higher proportion of ART patients with advanced maternal age, obesity, multiple pregnancy and polycystic ovarian syndrome (PCOS) will contribute to this increase. However, additionally, the actual process of IVF has also been implicated. It is thought that hormones produced as a result of the ovulation induction and luteal support phases of IVF may be associated with insulin resistance. The presence of underlying metabolic and vascular factors may also be exacerbated with the hormonal stimulation used in the initial stages of ovulation induction.

In the UK, women with confirmed diabetes in pregnancy, planning for birth should be undertaken using the guidance provided by NICE [18]. The key statements are:

- Explain to pregnant women with diabetes who have an ultrasound-diagnosed macrosomic fetus about the risks and benefits of vaginal birth, induction of labour and caesarean section.
  - The RCOG guideline on "shoulder dystocia, 2012" [26] states that "infants of diabetic mothers have a two- to four-fold increased risk of shoulder dystocia compared with infants of the same birth weight born to non-diabetic mothers. Elective CS should be considered to reduce the potential morbidity for preg-

nancies complicated by pre-existing or gestational diabetes, regardless of treatment, with an estimated fetal weight of greater than 4.5 kg."

- Advise women with gestational diabetes to give birth no later than 40+6 weeks, and offer elective birth (by induction of labour, or by CS if indicated) to women who have not given birth by this time.
- Consider elective birth before 40+6 weeks for women with gestational diabetes if there are maternal or fetal complications.

Multiple Pregnancies

In the UK around 15–20 % of IVF pregnancies result in a twin birth compared to the 1–1.5 % conceived spontaneously [27]. Despite improvements in both obstetric and neonatal care, twin pregnancies have a poorer outcome compared to singleton pregnancies.

Whether twin pregnancies conceived through ART are at higher risk that those conceived naturally is not clear cut, with some studies stating a higher risk, and others citing no trend [28]. This issue is covered further in Chap. 8 on multiple pregnancy.

With regard to birth outcomes the two largest systematic reviews on the perinatal and obstetric outcomes of twin pregnancies following ART [13, 14, 29] have found conflicting conclusions. McDonald et al. [29] found that IVF conceived twins pregnancies were more likely to experience antepartum haemorrhage (APH) and disorders of placentation such as placenta praevia (PP). They were also at a slightly higher risk of being delivered by CS and babies were twice as likely to be admitted to the neonatal unit.

The controversy in the data exists mainly because most studies looking at obstetric outcomes in ART twin pregnancies have a cohort design with no matched control group and small numbers. Invariably there are few distinctions made in terms of stratifying patients according to the fertility treatment, i.e., IVF vs Intracytoplasmic sperm injection (ICSI). There is also sparse information available on the chronicity of the twins included, pre-existing maternal medical conditions, parental BMI, and smoking status.

The main birth considerations for multiple pregnancies will be:

- Vigilance for and management of suspected or actual preterm labour
- Appropriate method for birth, determined by fetal sizes, number, presentation, placental site, gestation and maternal wishes.

The twin birth study (TBS) [30] has demonstrated that in uncomplicated twin pregnancies between 32 and 39 weeks, there is no benefit in delivery by CS. In the group randomised to vaginal birth, if labour occurred 65 % of women achieved a vaginal birth. The overall vaginal birth rate for this group was 44 %, but a third of caesarean sections were performed before labour, either for maternal complications, bleeding or failed induction of labour.

Where there is a discrepancy in predicted birthweight, the rate of complications rises. Variously the rise in risk has been described as occurring with a 18, 20 and

25 % discrepancy. This does not seem to translate into delivery problems until the discrepancy is 40 %; however, given the wish to minimise any complications, it would seem reasonable to use 20–25 % as a threshold for considering CS as the better option. Interestingly, significant expected birthweight discordancy was an exclusion in the twin birth study, in the TBS, but the definition is not given in the published results.

Higher order multiple pregnancies are usually delivered by CS, at gestations of viability, simply because fetal monitoring is so much more difficult though some units will consider vaginal births for healthy triplets.

In the TBS the rate of CS after delivery of the first twin was 4.2 %. This rate is lower than that seen in many units. It is vital therefore, when counselling women regarding method of delivery, that the counselling includes the ability to provide an experienced acchoucheur if vaginal birth is planned. In particular a practitioner experienced with breech birth as even when both twins are presenting by the vertex, 20 % of second twins will change presentation after delivery of the first twin.

Units that cannot provide a safe vaginal delivery should recommend delivery by CS. It is important to recognise, however, that even when CS is planned 10 % of women may deliver vaginally and still need good quality care.

Where the first twin is breech, many units would recommend CS as the best option. In the TBS 7 % of pregnancies had a breech first twin, and no differences were seen in this group. However, given current trends CS is likely to be the choice of most women in this circumstance.

Timing of Birth in Multiple Pregnancies

Guidance as to the timing of birth for multifetal gestations varies depending on country. In the UK, NICE guidance recommends delivery at 36–37 weeks for uncomplicated monochorionic diamniotic (MCDA) twins and 37–38 for uncomplicated dichorionic diamniotic (DCDA) twins [12]. Recommended delivery for triplets is at 34 weeks.

In the USA the thresholds for twins are a week later, taking into account that although the stillbirth rate peaks at 37 for MCDA and 38 for DCDA twins, there is additional neonatal mortality in a small number born earlier. Steroid cover should be considered for MCDA twins if following NICE guidance and for DCDA if delivery is planned by CS [12].

Monitoring of Multiple Pregnancies in Labour

Electronic fetal monitoring (EFM) is usually recommended in twin pregnancies. This is not on the basis of data supporting improved outcomes, but rather because intermittent monitoring is almost impossible. Women should understand this recommendation and also that it is often easier to obtain two traces using a fetal scalp electrode for the presenting twin.

Preterm Considerations for Singleton and Twin Pregnancies

Preterm birth is commoner in ART pregnancies for a variety of reasons including:

- Iatrogenic prematurity because of maternal medical problems
- Increase incidence of growth restriction leading to both iatrogenic and spontaneous prematurity
- Higher incidence of women with uterine abnormalities
- A higher incidence for no apparent cause, but related to the underlying cause of infertility.

Preterm Multiple Pregnancies

Preterm birth is common in twins, with 40 % delivering before 37 weeks. It is now clear from the TBS that from 32 weeks' onwards, vaginal birth is as safe as CS in uncomplicated pregnancies. The literature on best method of birth at earlier gestations is much less clear. Some studies show better outcomes when delivery is by CS especially for the very low birthweight babies, but others do not support this.

When preterm birth occurs at less than 32 weeks, a full discussion taking into account fetal sizes, presentations, overall wellbeing and gestation must take place.

Whether a singleton or multiple pregnancy, multidisciplinary involvement including a neonatologist or paediatrician in the discussion is also vital, so that parents can make decisions knowing the predicted outcome at that gestation.

Discussion must include consideration of:

- Corticosteroids for fetal lung maturation
- Magnesium sulfate for fetal neuroprotection at gestations of 23–30 weeks
- In-utero transfer for neonatal care (often more of an issue for multiple pregnancies and especially higher order pregnancies)
- Fetal monitoring at the limits of viability (22–24 weeks)

Parents who have been through ART may find it especially difficult to confront issues of poor survival and deciding not to monitor a fetus in labour; however, the team need to sensitively cover whether abdominal delivery would confer advantage and the potential long term problems of a complex CS.

Other Key Issues for Birth Planning

1. Has the fertility treatment involved the use of medication that might be pertinent to birth?

(a) Steroids:

Prednisolone taken for longer than a week at a dose of 10 mg or more within three months of delivery should prompt additional steroid replacement in labour. Additional hydrocortisone 100 mg 6–8 hourly for the duration of labour is recommended or for 24 hours, if delivery is by elective CS. If steroids were taken through pregnancy up until birth the doses will need to be gradually reduced following delivery if the intention is to discontinue.

(b) Low Molecular Weight Heparin (LMWH):

Many women undergoing ART are taking LMWH throughout pregnancy at prophylactic doses. THE RCOG guidelines state [31]:

Women receiving antenatal LMWH should be advised that if they have any vaginal bleeding or once labour begins they should not inject any further LMWH. They should be reassessed on admission to hospital and further doses should be prescribed by medical staff.

Regional techniques should be avoided if possible until at least 12 h after the previous prophylactic dose of LMWH.

A postnatal risk assessment should be undertaken and LMWH prescribed for those at increased risk for thromboembolism for at least 7 days.

(c) Low dose aspirin (LDA):

Aspirin at a dose of 75 mg does not appear to increase the risk for bleeding complications during labour and so it is recommended that if this is started during pregnancy it is safe to continue until birth. There should be no contraindication to regional analgesia or anaesthesia.

2. Are there features that would need consideration for delivery by CS?

(a) This may particularly relate to women who have undergone complex uterine surgery, where pre-delivery planning is important. Also, some women may have undergone previous abdominal surgery, making access more difficult, and planning for birth in these cases is important.

(b) Confidence in placental site location and absence of vasa praevia

Placenta praevia is easily discounted by ultrasound in the third trimester. When undertaking birth planning it is worth considering screening for vasa praevia in cases where there was a previously low lying placenta that has now migrated enough for a safe vaginal birth, as ART is a significant risk factor for this life-threatening complication. This is particularly worthwhile in multiple pregnancies.

(c) Is there an increased risk for abnormal placental adherence?

When considering placental adherence some consideration must be given to women who have a scar in the upper segment. This may be particularly pertinent in women who have undergone metroplasty or myomectomy. Knowledge of the placental site in relationship to any known scar will help to inform further management.

3. Are there conditions that might lead to an increased risk of problems in labour, such as hypertension, gestational diabetes, pre-existing medical problems and ensuring specific instructions for the team are provided for labour.
4. Has there been a recent assessment of fetal wellbeing and size where additional risk factors have been identified?
   (a) Both growth restriction and macrosomia are more prevalent in ART pregnancies.
5. Is the fetus presenting by the vertex (pertinent where there are known uterine abnormalities)?

Preparation for Birth: Discussion of Choices of Place and Method of Delivery

For some women choice will be limited by safety for them and their baby, but for many women after an uncomplicated pregnancy, there will be choices of where and how to have their baby.

The clinical team should feel able to support choice where safety is not at issue. After an uncomplicated pregnancy with a well-grown baby, in a healthy mother, choices should be made available as they would be for any woman, as birth outcomes should be similar. This should include home-birth, midwifery led and consultant led care.

A discussion of views regarding what happens in labour may be needed for some women who may be keen to avoid certain interventions such as augmentation, fetal blood sampling or assisted vaginal delivery. Individualised birth plans can be compiled to cover a range of options to provide women with the confidence needed to ensure that their wishes are understood, acknowledged and agreed.

Some women will find the concept of birth too uncertain and will request elective caesarean delivery. When this occurs, as for any woman where there are no medical indications, a careful examination of the request should be undertaken. If helpful, psychological assessment with a trained person can be undertaken, but is often not necessary. In the UK, NICE [12] supports the ability of women to choose the method of birth for themselves and requires referral to an alternative clinician if the obstetrician feels unable to support this request. In many countries the literature suggests that elective CS is considered a reasonable choice for many women after ART.

Consideration of Timing of Birth

Timing for birth will be driven by identified risks and problems many of which are outlined above. Where there is no indication to consider elective induction or CS, discussion should take place regarding maternal wishes. In the UK, induction of labour between term +7 and term +14 is recommended, but there is much flexibility within this range. Some clinicians feel that because there is a higher stillbirth rate in ART pregnancies, induction should be considered at term. There is no evidence that elective induction at term increases the risk of CS, but also no evidence that where adequate surveillance has been undertaken and risk factors identified, in the uncomplicated ART population the risks of adverse outcome are any higher than the general population.

In an ideal situation, women should be provided with information to enable them to decide on birth timing for themselves within safe parameters.

Elective CS should only be planned earlier than 39 weeks with good reason, as it is clear that earlier delivery increases neonatal and post-neonatal risk.

Considerations during Labour

Fetal Monitoring

Uncomplicated term ART pregnancies with no identified risk factors should be offered a choice of monitoring as would be available to any woman, including both intermittent monitoring and continuous electronic fetal monitoring intermittent monitoring and continuous EFM. Clearly where there are risks identified that impact on the potential fetal reserve during labour, EFM should be the norm.

Women must be enabled to choose EFM in line with NICE guidance, even in the absence of any risk factors [32].

Vigilance for Complications

Unexpected complications can occur in any labour. With regard to ART pregnancies there are a few complications that clinicians should be particularly aware of. The main ones to consider are:

- Vasa praevia: Awareness if there is vaginal bleeding associated with a sudden change in fetal condition, especially if this occurs just after rupture of membranes.
- Undetected macrosomia: Macrosomia is slightly more likely in IVF pregnancies. Clinicians should document a symphysis fundal height (SFH) at the beginning of labour and be vigilant if this is more than 40 cm. If the SFH is large and progress poor, consider macrosomia. Beware if considering an assisted vaginal birth with a large SFH that shoulder dystocia may be an issue.
- Undetected growth restriction: Growth restriction is more common in ART pregnancies. In most this is detected before birth, but by no means in all. Measure the SFH on admission in labour and plot on a standard chart. If this is small recommend EFM. Be very vigilant if the EFM shows signs of potential fetal compromise.

- Hypertensive disorders: All women will have their blood pressure monitored during labour. PET can occur for the first time in labour and after and additional investigation should be instituted where there are concerns.
- Progress of labour: The risk of dysfunctional labour increases as a woman gets older. The reasons for this are unclear, but it is a consistent finding across many studies. The extent to which women having undergone ART are more at risk is unclear and it is likely that other contributors such as age, BMI, macrosomia all play a much larger part. When poor progress in labour is diagnosed all women should have the opportunity for a full discussion of the options available, including hydration, oxytocin, watchful waiting and delivery by CS. Given the paucity of evidence that oxytocin improves birth outcomes, respect for the wish of the individual woman is vital. One might expect that this discussion is always conducted before embarking on a course of action, and such would be the expectation for women after ART.

Postpartum Support

Issues of adjustment to pregnancy and beyond are discussed in greater detail in Chap. 3 on psychological issues of periconceptual period.

The adjustment to motherhood and the postnatal period in women conceiving with IVF is an emerging area of interest. Investigation of the psychological and social aspects of infertility and its treatment have consistently revealed that suboptimal reproductive health can negatively impact on the both the male and female emotional well-being and self-esteem. This thought process can continue in pregnancy and beyond delivery thereby reducing confidence in parenting ability, despite the baby being highly desired.

In their systematic review of 28 studies: Hammarberg et al [7], found mixed observations. Some studies concluded that couples conceiving with ART had a similar experience of parenting to spontaneous conception [33, 34] whereas other studies highlighted this group of women as being particularly vulnerable to difficulties [35]. The review concluded that although anxiety rates were similar between couples conceiving with ART and spontaneously, women who had undergone IVF were much more anxious about fetal health. They were also more likely to display the self defence mechanism of not believing the pregnancy and its success with fear of adverse complications occurring. This along with the idealisation of a natural birth led to a delayed adjustment to the delivery, and attachment to the baby, especially if the birth experience was divergent to the couple's expectations.

A long period of infertility and multiple unsuccessful treatment attempts have been cited as major risk factors for delay in attachment and adjustment to parenthood. The additional complication of these women delivering a pre-term or small for gestational age infant, leads to new parents having to adjust to the challenges of neonatal care. These are also influential in lowering postnatal confidence in self efficacy and parenting skills.

It is consistently noted that primiparous women who deliver a multiple pregnancy following ART have the highest rates of adjustment difficulties compared to their singleton and spontaneous conception counterparts [7]. The obstetric and psychological complications associated with CS may also be a contributory factor. There is evidence to suggest that this group of women have a higher rate of readmission to hospital with mood disturbance and infant feeding problems.

In their case control study of 200 women undergoing ART, Listijono et al. found no significant difference in postnatal depression between women conceiving with IVF and spontaneously [36]. They did, however, find pre-existing rates of depression were higher in the ART group (17 % vs 5 % p, 0.05), perhaps due to the delay in fertility.

Partner support in labour and the postnatal period has been cited as a beneficial factor in establishing a good mother-baby relationship. Women conceiving with ART have been shown to have high levels of marital satisfaction and partner support in caring for their babies. This is perhaps due to the solidarity and strong commitment that develops in ART couples who have the mutual desire to achieve parenthood.

Clinical Recommendations

The postnatal period can be emotionally and physically difficult for women who conceive with ART. There is heightened anxiety about parenting skills and adjustment post delivery. This is particularly evident in primiparous women who have a multiple pregnancy delivered by operative delivery.

Partner and family support should be encouraged so that women are not isolated in the early postnatal period. Changes in mood should be detected and explored by an adequately trained professional at the earliest opportunity so that confidence in parenting skills is maintained.

Health professionals must be ensure that they are aware of psychological subtleties in this vulnerable group of women and ensure that they are empowered and supported in their adjustment to parenthood.

Conceiving Through Art and Breastfeeding

From a maternal perspective breastfeeding can help with weight loss, postnatal depression and improve bonding with their baby [37]. Babies that are exclusively breast fed tend to have lower rates of infection, atopy and failure to thrive. The process, however, is not always automatic and can be challenging for some women.

Women conceiving with ART are highly motivated to initiate and maintain breastfeeding. The reasons for this are multifactorial and have raised issues that highlight the demographic and psycho-social differences in the way the fertility treatment seeking population view parenthood.

Demographically women who conceive with ART are on average, primiparous, older, in established relationships with their partners and more socioeconomically stable. These factors have been found to be highly psychologically protective and influential in increasing the motivation to breast feed.

For most women conceiving with IVF, a determination to succeed with breastfeeding is seen as a way of normalising or counteracting the medicalization that they may have undergone in order to conceive and indeed during labour [38].

Fisher et al. studied the trends in breastfeeding in women conceiving with ART immediately after delivery and up to 4 months post-partum [39]. In their cohort of 800 women, this study found that despite 90 % of women exclusively breastfeeding their babies in the first few day of life, only 40 % of women who conceived with IVF were maintaining this at 4 months postpartum. They also noted women who were delivered by elective CS were more likely to introduce formula milk prior to discharge from hospital and discontinue breast feeding in the subsequent 4 months. A lack of education, motivation and support by health professionals was highlighted as a contributory factor for both early and later cessation.

It is well known that women who conceive with ART are at risk of having a CS for both clinical and non-clinical reasons. They are also more likely to have a multiple gestation. A perceived disadvantage of undergoing an operative delivery is the disruption to mother and baby contact in the first hour of life. If this vital interaction is not established with early introduction of baby to the breast, then women are less likely to continue this mode of feeding [40].

The level of satisfaction with the birth experience is also highly influential in continuation of breast feeding and overall confidence in maternal caregiving. It has been found that women who have undergone ART and deliver by CS unexpectedly view their birth as an uncontrolled and negative experience. This is seen as a deviation from an idealised view of parenthood and can demotivate and affect their self-esteem [41].

Improving breast feeding rates amongst women who conceive with IVF are dependent on modifying all aspects of their antenatal and intrapartum care.

When discussing elective CS in primiparous women who conceived with IVF, discussion of feeding intention should be undertaken and measures taken to enhance skin to skin contact immediately after birth to help breast feeding initiation if the intention is to breast feed. If an emergency CS is indicated, women should be involved in the decision making where possible so that they do not feel disempowered.

Health professionals need to ensure that separation of mother and baby is minimised regardless of mode of delivery so that women feel confident with handling and breast feeding.

Hammarberg et al. highlight that there was a lack of advice and support given to women regarding breast feeding and rather than focusing on the technique, health professionals should aim to empower women [42]. The promotion of self-efficacy facilitates confidence building for all primiparous women, and particularly those conceiving with ART.

Clinical Recommendations

Women conceiving with ART are highly motivated to breast feed but can this decline if they are not adequately supported. Therefore health professionals should aim to empower women so that their confidence in establishing breast feeding is nurtured. This can involve measures such as early skin to skin contact, involvement of a breast feeding advisor and peer breast feeding support.

Women who have conceived with ART are more likely to have an operative delivery. This can have a negative impact on initiating and maintaining breast feeding. Health professionals need to be aware of this important difference and be extra vigilant in detecting delayed bonding in this vulnerable group.

Summary

The intrapartum and postnatal care of women who conceive and subsequently deliver babies following ART is complex. It is dependent on obstetric and midwifery staff being aware of the antenatal risk factors that influence delivery choices, and the psychosocial status of these patients.

The extent to which singleton pregnancies conceived after ART convey a higher risk of obstetric complications such a preterm labour, APH, abnormal placentation, dysfunctional labour necessitating CS and postpartum heamorrhage (PPH) is still not entirely clear, though in healthy pregnancies babies tend to arrive a few day earlier and are slightly smaller. Twin gestations conceived with ART have a higher incidence of perinatal mortality. The pathogenesis and mechanisms for these differences are poorly understood; however, the underlying cause of fertility and the IVF process itself may be important contributory factors.

The fertility treatment seeking population is undoubtedly getting older and there is a higher incidence of pre-existing maternal conditions such as diabetes and hypertension that will impact on the antenatal and birth events of these patients.

The postnatal course of these women should be handled sensitively as they are vulnerable to experiencing low self-esteem regarding their parenting skills and adjustment to motherhood. Therefore health professionals must provide education, support and advice to ensure the mother baby relationship is maintained.

Good communication between the fertility unit and obstetric team is key to ensuring that these women are triaged appropriately with regards to their obstetric and antenatal needs.

During labour and birth, maternity staff should know what the birth plan is, be aware of the complications that can arise and ensure clear communication with the parents. If CS is required, inclusion in decision making and good communication with the couple will reduce anxiety and improve obstetric outcomes for both the mother and her baby. The research evidence on postnatal adjustment is very variable, with many suggesting it is more difficult after ART, but equally, others showing no difference in adaptation or outcomes.

It does seem clear that postnatal depression (PND) is a common feature after ART pregnancies. The degree to which this is associated with a higher level of higher risk outcomes for PND such as being older, being delivered by CS, having a multiple or preterm birth is difficult to disentangle [41]. One of the key principles aimed at helping women in pregnancy after ART is to establish a solid framework for support during the antenatal period. Many women undergoing ART will be older, have worked most of their adult lives and may have poor social or family support networks locally. Continuity of midwifery care during the antenatal period improves mothers' confidence with the baby postnatally and is now strongly recommended in the UK. Continuation of this relationship into the postnatal period can be helpful.

Midwives on the wards and in the community need to be aware that PND is a risk, and, after birth, women and their partners should be signposted to support that is available. Breastfeeding support should also be signposted.

Prompt intervention when PND occurs can reduce the long-term effects on both mother and baby.

References

1. Human Fertilisation and Embryology Association. The HFEA guide to infertility 2007/08. London: HFEA; 2007.
2. Joels L, Wardle P. Assisted conception and the midwife. Br J Midwifery. 1994;12(9):429–35.
3. Morgan J. The assisted conception pregnancy. Pract Midwife. 2004;7(8):18.
4. Hjelmstedt A, et al. Patterns of emotional responses to pregnancy, experience of pregnancy and attitudes to parenthood among IVF couples: a longitudinal study. J Psychosom Obstet Gynaecol. 2003;24(3):153–62.
5. Younger M, Hollins-Martin C, Choucri L. Individualised care for women with assisted conception pregnancies and midwifery practice implications: an analysis of the existing research and current practice. Midwifery. 2015;31(2):265–70.
6. Windridge KC, Berryman JC. Women's experiences of giving birth after 35. Birth. 1999;26(1):16–23.
7. Hammarberg K, Fisher JR, Rowe HJ. Women's experiences of childbirth and post-natal healthcare after assisted conception. Hum Reprod. 2008;23(7):1567–73.
8. Bryan A. The psychosocial effects of infertility and the implications for midwifery practice. MIDIRS Midwifery Dig. 2000;10(1):8–12.
9. Poikkeus P, et al. Birth experience of women conceiving with assisted reproduction: a prospective multicenter study. Acta Obstet Gynecol Scand. 2014;93(9):880–7.
10. Rouhe H, et al. Fear of childbirth according to parity, gestational age, and obstetric history. BJOG. 2009;116(1):67–73.
11. Hjelmstedt A, et al. Emotional adaptation following successful in vitro fertilization. Fertil Steril. 2004;81(5):1254–64.
12. National Institute for Health and Clinical Excellence. Guidance on antenatal care for uncomplicated pregnancies (CG62). 2008.
13. Helmerhorst FM, et al. Perinatal outcome of singletons and twins after assisted conception: a systematic review of controlled studies. BMJ. 2004;328(7434):261.
14. Jackson RA, et al. Perinatal outcomes in singletons following in vitro fertilization: a meta-analysis. Obstet Gynecol. 2004;103(3):551–63.
15. Marino JL, et al. Perinatal outcomes by mode of assisted conception and sub-fertility in an Australian data linkage cohort. PLoS One. 2014;9(1):e80398.

16. Koudstaal J, et al. Obstetric outcome of singleton pregnancies after IVF: a matched control study in four Dutch university hospitals. Hum Reprod. 2000;15(8):1819–25.
17. National Institute for Health and Clinical Excellence. Guidance on Hypertension in pregnancy:diagnosis and management (CG107). 2011.
18. National Institute for Health and Clinical Excellence. Guidance on diabetes in pregnancy: management from preconception to the postnatal period (NG3). 2015.
19. National Institute for Health and Clinical Excellence. Guidance on multiple pregnancy-antenatal care of twin and triplet pregnancies (CG129). 2011.
20. Royal College of Obstetricians and Gynaecologists. RCOG guideline on placenta praevia, accreta and vasa praevia with the national patient safety agency care bundle for the management of placenta praevia after previous Caesarean section-green top guideline 27. London: RCOG; 2011.
21. Walker KF, et al. Induction of labour versus expectant management at term by subgroups of maternal age: an individual patient data meta-analysis. Eur J Obstet Gynecol Reprod Biol. 2016;197:1–5.
22. Koopmans CM, et al. Induction of labour versus expectant monitoring in women with pregnancy induced hypertension or mild preeclampsia at term: the HYPITAT trial. BMC Pregnancy Childbirth. 2007;7(1):14.
23. Royal College of Obstetricians and Gynaecologists. RCOG guideline on antenatal steroids to reduce neonatal morbidity and mortality -green top guideline 7. London: RCOG; 2010.
24. Ashrafi M, et al. Risk of gestational diabetes mellitus in patients undergoing assisted reproductive techniques. Eur J Obstet Gynecol Reprod Biol. 2014;176:149–52.
25. Cunningham FG. Williams obstetrics. 23rd ed. New York: McGraw-Hill; 2010. p. 1385.
26. Royal College of Obstetricians and Gynaecologists. RCOG guideline on shoulder dystocia -green top guideline 42. London: RCOG; 2012.
27. Human Fertilisation and Embryology Association. Fertility treatment in 2013: trend and figures. London: HFEA; 2013.
28. Caserta D, et al. Maternal and perinatal outcomes in spontaneous versus assisted conception twin pregnancies. Eur J Obstet Gynecol Reprod Biol. 2014;174:64–9.
29. McDonald S, et al. Perinatal outcomes of in vitro fertilization twins: a systematic review and meta-analyses. Am J Obstet Gynecol. 2005;193(1):141–52.
30. Barrett JF, et al. A randomized trial of planned cesarean or vaginal delivery for twin pregnancy. N Engl J Med. 2013;369(14):1295–305.
31. Royal College of Obstetricians and Gynaecologists. RCOG guideline on thrombosis and embolism during pregnancy and the puerperium, reducing the risk-green-top guideline No. 37a. London: RCOG; 2009.
32. National Institute for Health and Clinical Excellence. Guidance on intrapartum care in healthy women and babies (CG190). 2014.
33. Cox SJ, et al. Maternal self-esteem after successful treatment for infertility. Fertil Steril. 2006;85(1):84–9.
34. Greenfeld D, Caruso KS. Transition to parenthood among in vitro fertilization patients at 2 and 9 months postpartum. Fertil Steril. 2001;76(3):626–7.
35. Fisher JR, Hammarberg K, Baker HW. Assisted conception is a risk factor for postnatal mood disturbance and early parenting difficulties. Fertil Steril. 2005;84(2):426–30.
36. Listijono DR, Mooney S, Chapman M. A comparative analysis of postpartum maternal mental health in women following spontaneous or ART conception. J Psychosom Obstet Gynaecol. 2014;35(2):51–4.
37. Labbok MH. Effects of breastfeeding on the mother. Pediatr Clin North Am. 2001;48(1):143–58.
38. Barnes M, et al. Experiences of birth and breastfeeding following assisted conception. Breastfeed Rev. 2013;21(1):9–15.
39. Fisher J, et al. Assisted conception, maternal age and breastfeeding: an Australian cohort study. Acta Paediatr. 2013;102(10):970–6.

40. Difrisco E, et al. Factors associated with exclusive breastfeeding 2 to 4 weeks following discharge from a large, urban, academic medical center striving for baby-friendly designation. J Perinat Educ. 2011;20(1):28–35.
41. Fisher JR, Hammarberg K, Baker GH. Antenatal mood and fetal attachment after assisted conception. Fertil Steril. 2008;89(5):1103–12.
42. Hammarberg K, et al. Breastfeeding after assisted conception: a prospective cohort study. Acta Paediatr. 2011;100(4):529–33.

Chapter 12
Surrogate Pregnancy

Janet R. Ashworth

Introduction

A surrogacy arrangement involves one woman (the Surrogate Mother) agreeing to bear a child for another woman (the Intended Mother) or a couple (the Commissioning Parents). The majority of surrogate pregnancies will utilise assisted reproductive techniques of one sort or another, although these will not always involve health care professionals. While many of the obstetric risks are similar to those of any pregnancy achieved using assisted conception, the legal, ethical and communication intricacies involved in providing care may be outside the usual scope of practice for many obstetricians. This chapter aims to explore some of the potential issues which may be encountered by the health and social care team in the perinatal period.

The Legal Status of Surrogacy Agreements

In UK law, surrogacy is not illegal, provided that any payment is only to cover the reasonable expenses incurred by the Surrogate Mother in the course of the pregnancy (altruistic surrogacy). It is not illegal to be a surrogate, nor to ask someone to be a surrogate, but it is illegal to advertise to be a surrogate or seeking a surrogate; the editor responsible for the publication of such an advert would be the guilty party in law. The surrogacy arrangement is NOT legally enforceable. Commercial surrogacy is illegal, as is any part in its negotiation, including the offer of negotiation or compilation of information for others seeking to partake in commercial surrogacy. These points are within the Surrogacy Arrangements Act 1985 [1].

J.R. Ashworth, BM, BS, BMedSci(hons), DM, FRCOG
Department of Obstetrics and Gynaecology, Royal Derby Hospital, Derby, UK
e-mail: janet.ashworth1@nhs.net

K. Jayaprakasan, L. Kean (eds.), *Clinical Management of Pregnancies following ART*, DOI 10.1007/978-3-319-42858-1_12

All those pregnancies where a health professional is involved in the insemination in any way are governed by the Human Fertility and Embryology acts of 1990 and 2008 [2, 3].

Australian law is similar to that of the UK.

In the USA, commercial surrogacy is legal, but surrogacy itself is completely illegal in some states. In Israel, commercial surrogacy is legal but altruistic surrogacy is illegal.

It is critical therefore that the clinician is aware of how the law applies in their country, and to seek legal advice if necessary.

Prenatal Counselling

Surrogacy is a planned pregnancy which allows the opportunity for pre-conception counselling. For most prospective surrogates/commissioning parents, any advice sought prior to undertaking a surrogate pregnancy is likely to be from the legal profession, but many of the potential risks and conflicts of interest can be anticipated from a medical perspective so pre-conceptual counselling is to be strongly recommended. It affords the opportunity to fully explore the physical and emotional risks of surrogate pregnancy for the prospective surrogate, as well as to clarify the legal implications of different types of surrogacy and raise some of the possibly unanticipated dilemmas or conflicts of interest which may occur. Some aspects of the counselling will be best provided by specialist organisations, such as the British Infertility Counselling Organisation [4].

If the prospective surrogate mother is married or in a Civil Partnership, her partner should be included in the discussions and be aware with the woman of the implications (particularly emotional) for the partnership and any other children in the family. Also, provided the partner consents to the surrogacy process going ahead, he or she will have equal parental responsibility for the baby until any other legally-binding arrangements are made with the commissioning parents after the baby has been born, as in the UK he or she would be the other legal parent (along with the surrogate mother).

As for most aspects of care in a surrogate pregnancy, it is ideal that the surrogate mother and commissioning parents should have a different health professional providing care, to avoid bias in advice for either party. The ultimate responsibility of the obstetrician is unequivocally to the surrogate mother, although with her uninfluenced consent, commissioning parents may appropriately be included in some of the care or discussions.

The suitability of the prospective surrogate mother should be examined with her, and any risks from the pregnancy fully discussed. The risks are likely to be lowest in a parous woman, provided previous pregnancies have been uncomplicated, as she avoids the increased risks due to placental dysfunction (pre-eclampsia, intra-uterine growth restriction) inherent in a first pregnancy and she will have an examinable track record in pregnancy. However, certain findings in the obstetric history may be relative contra-indications to surrogacy. This would include a history of previous caesarean section with an expressed wish to consider vaginal birth (VBAC), as this would introduce a potential conflict of interest between mother and fetus, which could result in conflict between surrogate mother and commissioning parents. Any relevant medical history which may carry a risk to the fetus (known or suspected carriage of genetically transmittable disease, history of pre-term delivery or intra-uterine growth restriction, for example) should be encouraged to be disclosed to the commissioning parents and these risks factored into the care plan for the pregnancy.

As in any pre-conceptual counselling, the prospective surrogate should be encouraged to avoid smoking, alcohol and illicit drug use and should aim for a body mass index within normal range (18–25 kg/m^2), as well as to be Rubella immune, on folic acid supplementation and have relevant infectious diseases excluded (syphilis, hepatitis B and C, HIV). Any additional risk due to maternal age should be avoided by the Surrogate being ideally no older than 35 years, and she should be over the age of 18 (21 in the USA). Most licensed fertility clinics have their own guidance on acceptable age range for Surrogate Mothers [5].

The Surrogate should be encouraged to discuss all antenatal screening fully with the Commissioning Parents and reach agreement on those screening tests which will be accepted, as well as how they will proceed if screening detects a problem or an increased risk of a problem. Attitudes of both parties to risk of aneuploidy and fetal anomaly should be as clear as possible, as well as the nature of problems which would make either party wish to consider termination of pregnancy. Although such discussions will not exclude potential conflicts of interest when the time comes, they may help to avoid these being entirely unanticipated, as well as allowing either party to reconsider the surrogacy undertaking if a likelihood of being unable to find a common ground on such areas is identified.

Part of the discussion of assisted conception will need to include the differing types of surrogacy, resultant genetic relationships to the child and implication for achieving legal parenthood, as well as the medical implications for those involved and successful pregnancy rates.

Conception and Types of Surrogacy

When discussing assisted conception, the different types of surrogacy should be discussed. All surrogacy arrangements in the UK must be altruistic (although agreement of reasonable expense payments to the surrogate is permitted), as commercial surrogacy is illegal in this country. Traditional ("partial" or "gestational") surrogacy involves the sperm of the commissioning father being used for conception by intra-uterine insemination or by artificial insemination (or, more unusually by natural conception). The latter two methods may be used at home by couples agreeing a surrogate arrangement without medical involvement, and clearly carries the risk that many of the issues covered above may not have been considered. With traditional surrogacy, the Commissioning Mother has no genetic relationship to the baby.

Gestational ("full") surrogacy requires some form of in-vitro fertilization as it uses an embryo created from the egg and sperm of the Commissioning Parents. In this approach, both Commissioning Parents then achieve a genetic relationship with the baby, but at the expense of a technique with a significantly lower ongoing pregnancy rate [5], considerable cost, and invasive treatment to the Intended Mother which would not otherwise have been required. The biological relationship of the Intended Mother to the conceptus has no influence on her legal relationship to the baby, which is non-existent until a Parental or Adoption order bearing her name has been issued. This situation has recently been examined in Ireland, when an Intended Mother, who provided the egg for a gestational surrogate pregnancy wished to be recorded as the mother on the birth certificate. The High Court ruling on the application that the Surrogate Mother is the biological mother and should be recorded as the mother on the birth certificate was over-ruled by the Supreme Court judgement as contrary to statutory law [6].

It should be noted that whether the Intended Father is the donor of the sperm for the conception and whether conception is achieved via a licensed clinic may both have a bearing on legal fatherhood according to the initial birth certificate of the baby (see the section on Parental Responsibilities and Rights in this chapter).

Antenatal Care

The Surrogate Mother is the patient and has all legal responsibility for decisions about care for her or the fetus throughout the pregnancy. All providing care must respect the confidentiality of the patient and no information should be disclosed to the Commissioning Parents without the express consent of the Surrogate Mother.

As in all pregnancies, the pregnant woman has the right to accept or decline any screening, investigation or treatment during the pregnancy. It is extremely helpful if discussions about antenatal, peri-partum and postnatal care have taken place preconceptually or very early in the pregnancy, and all decisions have been documented, as this will help to minimise conflicts and misunderstandings on the part of both parties, as well as by those providing care. However, the Surrogate Mother has the right to amend any of her previously-expressed decisions regarding care, and these wishes must be respected as they would be for any other patient.

Anyone providing treatment or care during the pregnancy must satisfy themselves that consent for treatment (written or verbal) from the pregnant woman is her own, and not given as a result of coercion by others, including the Commissioning Parents.

Additional thought should be given to the potential increased risk for preeclampsia. This is likely to be highest if the surrogate is primiparous and the pregnancy is with donor gametes from both prospective parents. Although there are no data to advise aspirin at low dose (75 mg o.d.) this may be prudent in some cases. Surveillance for hypertension in the last trimester should be no less frequently than fortnightly.

Potential Areas for Conflict in the Antenatal Period

Antenatal screening and prenatal diagnosis are an area often poorly counselled for in all pregnancies. The fact that there may be at least five parties (Surrogate Mother, Partner, Commissioning Parents and fetus [one or more in multiple pregnancy!]) with differing vested interests in screening, testing and their outcomes makes early, specific counselling particularly pertinent in a surrogate pregnancy. Ideally, discussion of all options and responses to different possible outcomes would have been explored pre-conception, and the Surrogate Mother will be clear about what is wished. However, it is not uncommon in a Fetal Medicine setting to find that preconceived ideas of parents about how they will feel and react when faced with concerning or bad news turn out to be different to their response at the time. Additionally, although the Surrogate Mother is the only party with the legal right to consent to undergo any screening, diagnostic testing, or therapeutic procedures for herself or the fetus, it is the Commissioning Parents who will be anticipated to be bringing up the child, with any associated consequences of disability or limited life expectancy, so ethically the pregnant woman may wish to discuss any concerns with them, although she is not required to do so. Remember that a Surrogate Mother would have the option of terminating a pregnancy that the Commissioning Parents would have wished to continue, but also that the Surrogate carries the risk of being left responsible for a baby with long-term care requirements if the Commissioning Parents decided to end the arrangement late in the pregnancy; they have no legal obligation to take the baby should they choose not to, and termination of pregnancy, other than for life-threatening maternal or seriously disabling fetal conditions, is not permitted by UK law after 24 weeks' gestation. Again, the legal partner of the Surrogate Mother may also, with the woman's consent, wish to be party to these discussions, as he or she would carry equal parental responsibility should the Commissioning Parents decide to withdraw from the agreement and the pregnancy continue.

With good pre-conception counselling, it is reasonable for the parties involved to accept that where decisions regarding the mother's health are concerned, the Surrogate Mother should make decisions on treatment, in conjunction with the professionals providing care. Conversely, if decisions relate solely to the health of the fetus, then the Commissioning Parents would decide on management, with the understanding that the Surrogate Mother would not be compelled to accept their decision if she was not in agreement.

Intra-partum Care and Midwifery Care

In the UK, The Royal College of Midwives has guidance for the role and responsibilities of the midwife when caring for a Surrogate Mother [7] which can provide a good framework for care in other jurisdictions. These emphasise the importance of maintaining the right to confidentiality of the pregnant woman, with information only being shared with the Commissioning Parents with the express permission of the Surrogate Mother. The guidance also clarifies that in any conflict of interest, the duty of the midwife lies with the wishes of the Surrogate Mother. The guidance is also clear that the midwife must take no part in handing the baby over to the care of the Commissioning Parents; this must occur outside of the hospital after the mother and baby have gone home. However, the notifying midwife has a responsibility to notify the maternity services in the Commissioning Parents' area of the impending transfer of the baby's care, as well as giving details of the baby's birth. The Commissioning Parents' address, contact number and GP details must also be documented in the maternal and neonatal notes.

With the reported increase in incidence of surrogate pregnancies over recent years, it would be prudent for all Trusts to have access to clear guidance regarding surrogate pregnancy and the responsibilities of its employees providing care.

It is the professional responsibility of health care workers involved in care in this situation to be aware of the law as it pertains to surrogate pregnancy and to remain non-judgemental towards all participants in the surrogacy agreement.

Birth Planning

Ideally, birth planning should be done in advance, with clear documentation of the wishes of the Surrogate Mother. She may wish her choice of birth partners to include one or more of the Commissioning Parents, and will need to ensure that such plans are within the confines of what is acceptable within the setting she chooses for delivery; for example, it is common for Trusts to limit numbers of birth partners to two, with only one permitted in an operating theatre if operative delivery is required and with restricted visiting in high-dependency settings. Openness in these discussions is to be encouraged so that her wishes can be most closely adhered to with sensitivity to all parties involved.

It should be remembered that this is likely to be both an exciting and worrying time for the Commissioning Parents, and that emotions may also be different from those expected in the pregnant woman and her partner, if present. Whilst many of those directly or indirectly involved in care provision may be unfamiliar with surrogate pregnancy, breach of confidentiality by discussion of the situation with those who do not need to know the circumstances to provide appropriate care must be avoided.

Potential Conflicts of Interest Around Delivery

Birth plan formulation should involve discussion of situations where there may be conflict of interest between fetus and pregnant woman. While the responsibility of healthcare professionals is entirely to the mother until the baby is born, as in any birth, she is likely to also want to protect the interests of the baby and hence the interests of the Commissioning Parents, for whom she is performing an altruistic act. However, in some circumstances, the best interests of mother and fetus would be best served by different management. An example would include mode of delivery in very pre-term delivery with malpresentation (28 weeks breech presentation), where evidence suggests that the neonatal outcome may be better with a caesarean section, even though this may require an upper segment incision in some cases, with prejudicial effect on future pregnancies. Similarly, in the presence of severe shoulder dystocia, the consideration of damaging maternal procedures like symphysiotomy versus fetal cleidotomy or prolonged anoxia may have different implications for the mother in a surrogate pregnancy. While counselling regarding decisions for such rare events cannot be specific in advance or adequately balanced in an emergency, the possibility of being faced with such decisions is important to understand for all involved, as well as the anticipation that the choice of the Surrogate Mother may be different from that if she were planning to keep the baby.

A much more common example, and one which should be considered in advance, is if the Surrogate Mother is considering a vaginal birth after caesarean section (VBAC). While the risks of loss of life of the mother due to scar dehiscence are very small in most cases [5] and the risks of complications in this or future pregnancies from repeated caesarean sections relatively higher, the one-off risk to the fetus, for whom scar dehiscence carries a high risk of death or lifelong severe disability, is almost certainly lowest with a planned, appropriately-timed caesarean section. Added to this, the acceptance of surgery is likely to be higher in a woman anticipating having a baby to take home at the end of the process, compared to a Surrogate Mother going home with an operation to recover from and no baby to take home, whose only rewards are altruistic. Discussions about such potential conflicts of interest would ideally have been covered before a Surrogate Pregnancy was conceived in women with a previous caesarean section, but as the obstetrician may only meet the woman once the pregnancy is underway, it is important that these issues and the outcome of any prior discussions are explored in this situation.

As in all parts of the pregnancy, the wishes of the pregnant woman at the time they are expressed over-ride any previous consents, provided the staff involved in her care are as sure as they can reasonably be that they are her own informed preferences and not influenced in any way by the coercion or undue influence of others (particularly if her influencer(s) may not have her best interests as their primary motivation).

The Post-natal Period and Parental Rights and Responsibilities

After birth it is important that postnatal care of the surrogate is provided as usual and that she knows how to seek help if needed.

Following the birth of the baby and until a Parental Order or Adoption Order has been made, the Surrogate Mother is always the legal mother of the baby and has the right to make any decisions about treatment, even if these conflict with the wishes of the Commissioning Parents. If she is married or in a civil partnership, then her legal partner also has parental rights, unless he/she did not consent to the treatment resulting in the pregnancy. If the Surrogate Mother is not legally partnered, then the Intended Father may rarely be eligible to be registered as the Legal Father if all of the exacting 'fatherhood conditions' are fulfilled. Most notably, the Intended Father CANNOT be the Legal Father if he donated the sperm for the pregnancy. It may seem counter-intuitive that a genetically-related father may have less automatic legal rights than one unrelated, but it is governed by the law that a sperm donor cannot be treated as the father of a child (section 41, Human Fertility and Embryology Act 2008) [3].

Conditions for Legal Fatherhood

These are the conditions for legal fatherfood:

- The Surrogate Mother is unmarried.
- The Surrogate Mother was treated in a UK licenced clinic for the assisted conception.
- The Surrogate Mother and the Intended Father both gave written, signed consent to the Intended Father becoming the father.
- The consent was given at the time when the embryo or sperm were placed in the Surrogate Mother.
- The consent has not been withdrawn.
- The sperm used to fertilise the egg was NOT from the intended father.
- The man was alive at the time of conception.

If all of these conditions are met, then the Intended Father can be registered on the original birth certificate as the father and will share parental responsibility with the Surrogate Mother. Should there be disagreement between the Legal Father and Surrogate Mother about the baby's medical care, then legal advice should be sought.

Transferring Legal Parental Responsibility

There are two ways in which Commissioning Parents become the legal parents, these being the ONLY ways that the Intended Mother can become a legal parent following a surrogate pregnancy:

1. Parental Order
2. Adoption Order

On the issuing of either order, a new birth certificate is issued, citing the parents named in the order, and parental rights transfer completely from the Surrogate Mother to the new parents.

The Commissioning Parents must seek independent legal advice on the transfer of parental rights.

Parental Order

A Parental order is a form of expedited adoption, obtained via the family courts by parents who satisfy a number of conditions. At least one of the parents must be genetically related to the baby (sperm or egg donor) and be a couple who are over 18 years of age and married, in a civil partnership or in a demonstrable long-term, stable relationship with each other. The application for the order must be after 6 weeks (prior to which the agreement of the legal mother is not considered valid) and within 6 months of the baby's birth, and the baby must be living with the Intended Parents at that time. No payment, other than of 'reasonable expenses' must have been made, and at least one of the Intended Parents must reside in the UK and the baby must then live with them. A Parental Order cannot be obtained by Intended Parents who are both genetically unrelated to the baby, or by a single person.

Adoption Order

Adoption is the only option for Intended Parents genetically unrelated to the baby or by a single Commissioning Parent. The process of adoption is governed by the Adoption Act (1971) [8] and must be administered by a registered adoption agency.

Outcome of Surrogate Pregnancies

In the majority of cases it appears that the outcome of surrogate pregnancies is satisfactory for the different parents involved. An overview of case series found that achievement of a clinical pregnancy in gestational surrogacy ranged from 18 to 69 %, and that in a total of 158 pregnancies, only 5 had significant complications: one woman developed pregnancy-induced hypertension, one fetus had intrauterine growth restriction, two patients developed gestational diabetes, 1 patient had placenta accreta and post-partum hysterectomy (triplet pregnancy) and one had spontaneous uterine rupture in the absence of previous uterine scar (fourth parity) [5]. Clearly, embarking on a multiple pregnancy intentionally using assisted reproductive techniques will increase a number of obstetric risk factors, including prematurity and risk of placenta praevia and operative delivery.

Although a potential vulnerability of the Commissioning Parents is that the Surrogate Mother may decide not to respect the surrogacy agreement and to keep her baby, a situation in which they would have no legal redress, in practice only 4 % of Surrogate Mothers are reported to have done this.

It might be anticipated that the emotional effects of taking part in a surrogate pregnancy agreement, with the potential uncertainties for the Commissioning Parents and the eventual relinquishing of a child by the Surrogate Mother would have a detrimental effect on mental health, but there is no apparent increase in the incidence of post-natal depression in Surrogate Mothers and no recognised burden of psychiatric illness or psychological ill-effects in the Commissioning Parents [9].

Conclusion

Surrogate pregnancy is a subject that requires a clear knowledge of the physical issues presented to the surrogate as well as the legal and psychological issues that face both the surrogate and Commissioning Parents. Decisions regarding the pregnancy can only be made by the pregnant woman and careful counselling needs to be undertaken to ensure that the needs of the pregnant woman are fully understood, without coercion from the Commissioning Parents.

It is important that the teams caring for these pregnancies have a clear understanding of the roles and responsibilities of each team member, that the legal framework for the Country in which the pregnancy is pursued is followed to avoid later problems, and that confidentiality for all is maintained within the law.

Postnatally, the wellbeing of the surrogate mother must be borne in mind, though it is heartening for these women that perinatal psychiatric issues are not a larger problem than in the general population.

References

1. Surrogacy Arrangements Act 1985, Chapter 49.
2. Human Fertility and Embryology Act 1990.
3. Human Fertility and Embryology Act 2008.
4. www.bica.net.
5. Duffy DA, et al. Obstetrical complications in gestational carrier pregnancies. Fertil Steril. 2005;83:749–54.
6. Supreme Court Judgement: MR and Another v. An tArd Chlaraitheoir and others 2014 IESC60.
7. Surrogacy: defining motherhood. Position paper number 18 (HIR: 29760). Royal College of Midwives, 1997.
8. Adoption Act 1971.
9. MacCallum F, et al. Surrogacy – the experience of commissioning couples. Hum Reprod. 2003;18:1334–42.

Chapter 13
Strategies for Risk Reduction and Improving Success in Women with Medical Comorbidities

Alison Richardson and Scott M. Nelson

Introduction

Every single IVF cycle is planned and as such requires consultation with health care professionals prior to commencement. This provides a unique opportunity for preconceptual counseling, that is often not possible prior to a spontaneous conception. For most women this simply entails general advice regarding folic acid supplementation and ensuring a healthy lifestyle, balanced diet avoiding certain foodstuffs and smoking cessation. For women with medical co-morbidities, however, this preconceptual period is even more critical as it provides an opportunity to: ensure optimal control of the condition; review medication; provide adequate counselling regarding the risks of pregnancy to them and the impact of the condition on the pregnancy; and lastly modify treatment protocols to minimize risks and achieve a successful outcome.

Many of the risks associated with IVF can be avoided by reducing the risk of ovarian hyperstimulation syndrome and/or minimizing the occurrence of multiple pregnancy. For all women therefore, but especially for those with medical comorbidities, the safest way of conducting an IVF cycle is to employ an antagonist stimulation protocol with a relatively low dose of FSH, use of a GnRH agonist trigger, cryopreservation of all embryos and then elective single embryo transfer in a frozen embryo replacement cycle. Although this segmented approach may detract from the overall success rates, compromising any element of this overall strategy will incorporate an increased risk to the women with medical comorbidities.

A. Richardson, MBChB, MA, MRCOG (✉)
Division of Child Health, Obstetrics, and Gynaecology, School of Medicine,
University of Nottingham, Nottingham, UK
e-mail: Alison.richardson@nottingham.ac.uk

S.M. Nelson, BSc, PhD, MRCOG
School of Medicine, Glasgow Royal Infirmary, University of Glasgow, Glasgow, UK
e-mail: Scott.nelson@glasgow.ac.uk

K. Jayaprakasan, L. Kean (eds.), *Clinical Management of Pregnancies following ART*, DOI 10.1007/978-3-319-42858-1_13

Reducing the Risk of Ovarian Hyperstimulation Syndrome (OHSS)

Whilst all women undergoing ovarian stimulation should be considered at risk of OHSS and should be provided with verbal and written information about the condition, women at higher risk of developing OHSS include those with a high ovarian reserve, which is commonly observed in young women and those with polycystic ovaries. The stimulation strategy itself may also predispose women to OHSS for example the use of GnRH agonist control, increased exposure to gonadotrophins either through high doses or low body mass and lastly the use of a hCG trigger. In those cycles where pregnancy occurs, late OHSS is driven by the endogenous hCG and consequently OHSS risk is greater in multiple pregnancies. Whilst rare, severe manifestations of OHSS include a tendency to develop thrombosis, renal and liver dysfunction and acute respiratory distress syndrome, causing serious morbidity. It is therefore imperative that efforts are made to reduce development of this condition in women known to be at increased risk and in those with pre-existing medical comorbidities. There are multiple approaches, which may either be employed individually or in combination.

Gonadotrophin-Releasing Hormone Antagonists

Aggressive stimulation is associated with an increased rate of OHSS and should therefore be avoided in women at risk of developing the condition. Whilst assessing variability can be challenging, a woman's individual ovarian reserve can be predicted following ultrasonographic determination of her antral follicle count (AFC) and/or serum anti-Mullerian hormone (AMH) level. Although both the AFC [1] and the AMH [2] indicate a woman's ovarian reserve at any age and can be used to predict both oocyte yield [3, 4] and extremes of ovarian response [5, 6], multiple randomized controlled trials have demonstrated superiority of AMH in response prediction [7]. We can modify ovarian response by utilising either a GnRH agonist (associated with maximal follicular recruitment, side effects and significant OHSS) or GnRH antagonist approach (associated with reduced follicular recruitment and fewer oocytes and embryos but equivalent live birth rates and reduced or no OHSS) to stimulation [8, 9]. The use of a GnRH antagonist also provides the opportunity to use a GnRH agonist trigger further minimizing the risk of OHSS (see next section in this chapter). Information regarding ovarian reserve can therefore be used to effectively stratify treatment and subsequently minimise risk [10, 11].

A recent systematic review and meta-analysis attempted to evaluate the effectiveness and safety of GnRH antagonists compared with the standard long protocol of GnRH agonists for controlled ovarian stimulation in assisted conception cycles [12]. Twenty-nine randomized controlled trials incorporating 5417 women demonstrated a statistically significant reduction in the incidence of OHSS in women that were treated using GnRH antagonists compared to the long GnRH agonist protocol

(RD −0.03; 95% CI −0.05 to −0.02). This effect was maintained regardless of whether the women had polycystic ovarian syndrome (RD −0.10; 95% CI −0.14 to −0.07) or not (RD −0.02, 95% CI −0.03 to −0.01) [12]. Furthermore, since most of the studies included in this review utilised hCG to trigger final oocyte maturation, it is likely that this could be reduced even further by using a GnRH agonist trigger (see next section in this chapter).

Regarding reproductive outcomes, meta-analysis of 41 randomized controlled trials incorporating 6571 women demonstrated a statistically significant reduction in clinical pregnancy rates following GnRH antagonist compared with GnRH agonist (OR 0.84; 95% CI 0.75–0.94). Whilst meta-analysis of the nine randomized controlled trials (n = 1515 women) that reported live birth rate demonstrated a similar effect size (OR 0.86; 95% CI 0.69–1.08), confidence intervals were wider and included unity. Similar effect sizes were reported for women with polycystic ovarian syndrome, for clinical pregnancy (OR 0.87; 95% CI 0.64–1.19) and live birth (OR 0.91; 95% CI 0.67–1.22) rates.

For women with medical comorbidities there is therefore compelling evidence that the use of a GnRH antagonist protocol for ovarian stimulation is associated with a statistically significant reduction in the development of OHSS even if hCG is used for triggering. However, potentially the most important aspect of the use of GnRH antagonist for pituitary control is that it facilitates the use of a GnRH agonist to induce final oocyte maturation.

GnRH Agonist Trigger

Due to its structural and biological similarities with LH, hCG has, up until relatively recently, been the gold standard agent to induce final oocyte maturation prior to oocyte retrieval. However, because the half-life of hCG is more than 24 h [13] (compared to the half-life of LH which is approximately 1 h [14]), it exerts sustained luteotropic activity and may contribute to the development of OHSS [15]. The fact that the GnRH agonist has greater affinity for the GnRH receptor than the GnRH antagonist enables it to displace the antagonist and induce an endogenous flare in LH and FSH. This flare is adequate to induce final oocyte maturation, but is very short and therefore does not support development of corpus luteum. The initial randomised controlled trials failed to recognise the need for modified luteal support and were associated with very poor clinical outcomes and early pregnancy loss rates [16–18]. More recent studies that have modified the luteal support either by providing small levels of exogenous hVG or high levels of exogenous sex steroids or a combination of both have shown outcomes comparable to those observed with hCG triggering, but with a substantially lower but not completely negated risk of OHSS [19–23]. As a consequence, using a GnRH agonist to trigger final oocyte maturation is now the first-line approach to stimulation in many oocyte donation programmes [24, 25] and should, we recommend, be adopted routinely following stimulation with a GnRH antagonist in women with medical comorbidities.

Elective Cryopreservation of Embryos

The elective cryopreservation of all embryos and their subsequent transfer in a non-gonadotrophin stimulated cycle could be used to avoid the endogenous production of hCG observed in fresh IVF cycles [26] and therefore minimise the development of OHSS. It is well recognized that the risk of OHSS is largely avoided after an agonist trigger when embryo transfer does not occur, as observed in oocyte donors. However, despite the overwhelming evidence from observational studies, a recent systematic review on the effectiveness of elective cryopreservation of all embryos for the prevention of OHSS [27] concluded that there was insufficient evidence to support routine cryopreservation of embryos for the prevention of OHSS. The systematic review, however, only identified one randomized controlled trial of 125 women and although the difference was not found to be statistically significant, there were four cases of moderate and/or severe OHSS in the fresh embryo transfer group compared to none in the cryopreservation group (OR 0.12; 95 % CI 0.01–2.29). This highlights the issue with the focus on randomised controlled trials when larger, more powerful, observational cohort studies may provide a much stronger evidence base.

Although segmentation of IVF cycles and cryopreservation of all embryos has also been suggested as a means of improving perinatal outcomes for all women, the effect on overall success rates is unclear with several randomized controlled trials ongoing [28]. However, even if these do report a reduction in livebirth rates following elective cryopreservation of embryos, in women with medical comorbidities, the associated reduction in late OHSS would potentially outweigh any reduction.

Luteal Phase Support

Use of hCG for luteal support is no longer common practice due to its higher risk of OHSS (OR 3.62; 95 % CI 1.85–7.06) than supplementation with progesterone alone [29]. However, 1500 IU of hCG is often administered at the time of oocyte retrieval as part of the modified luteal support package after a GnRH agonist trigger. The use of even this small dose of hCG has been associated with early and late OHSS, and therefore hCG even in low doses should not be used for luteal support in women with medical comorbidities.

Other Options

Other options such as discontinuation of gonadotrophins prior to the hCG trigger [30, 31], cancellation of the treatment cycle [32], early unilateral follicular aspiration [33], the use of cabergoline [34], metformin [35] and macromolecules such as albumin [36], minimal stimulation or natural cycle IVF and in vitro maturation of oocytes [37, 38] have all been associated with reductions in the risk of OHSS but do not completely eliminate it and should not be considered first-line in women with medical comorbidities.

Reducing the Risk of Multiple Pregnancy

Pregnancy places a physiological strain on every single organ system and this is exacerbated by multiple pregnancy. The exposure of women with a higher background risk due to her pre-existing medical comorbidity to the potentially avoidable enhanced risk of multiple pregnancy is therefore inappropriate. The single most effective way to minimize multiple pregnancies following IVF is the elective transfer of a single embryo (eSET). Until relatively recently eSET was taboo because it was feared that the pregnancy rate would decrease to unacceptable levels. With the improvement of freezing technologies, the transfer of embryos one at a time is now feasible with maintenance of cumulative live-birth rates as defined by one or more infants but a vast reduction in multiple pregnancy rates [39]. It is also clear that there is no benefit in transferring more than two embryos (Fig. 13.1) [40].

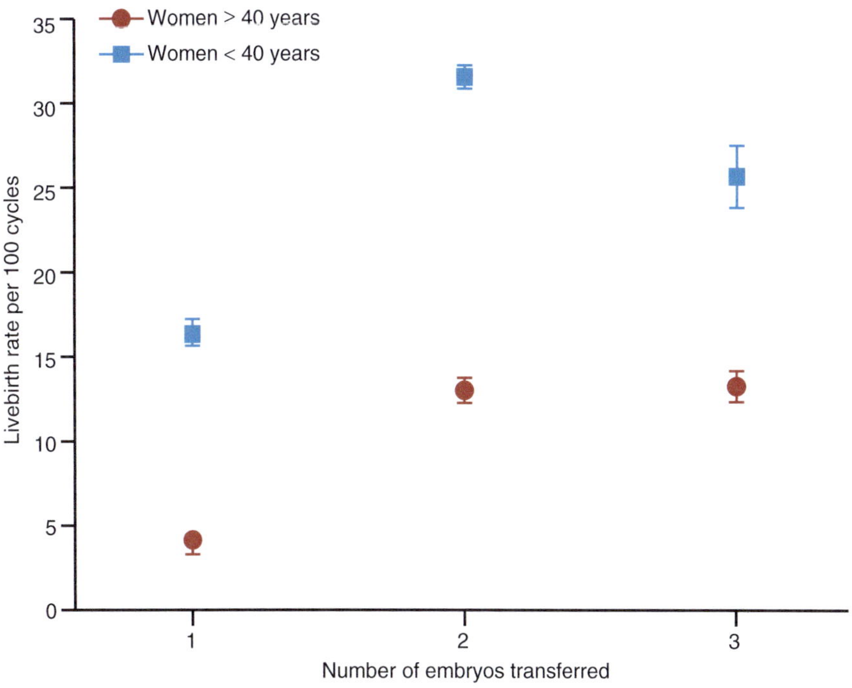

Fig. 13.1 Unadjusted live birth rate per 100 cycles by number of embryos transferred and maternal age (Reproduced with permission of Elsevier from Lawlor and Nelson [40])

Further improvements in single embryo transfer live birth rates are anticipated with the widespread adoption of blastocyst culture [41]. However, additional selection methods will be required as the association between euploid status and standard morphological grading of the embryo is limited [42]. In particular, the use of non-invasive assessment of morphokinetics, although having the potential to improve blastocyst selection above and beyond simple grading, has limited accuracy for detecting aneuploidy. Rather, invasive testing of the embryo is likely to be beneficial as analysis of blastocysts, even in women under 25 years of age is still associated with up to 30 % of blastocysts being aneuploid [43] and this increases to almost 80 % in women over 45 years of age. Accordingly, there are now several randomized controlled trials all consistently showing improved clinical pregnancy rates with comprehensive chromosome analysis of blastocysts as compared to selection based on blastocyst morphological grading alone.

Conclusion

It is now possible to manipulate and modify IVF cycles such that the risks are almost equivalent to spontaneous conception. The fact that assisted conception also provides ample opportunity to optimize medical comorbidities prior to conception should mean that affected women enter into pregnancy in the best possible health and informed state possible, with the highest chance of attaining a successful outcome.

References

1. La Marca A, et al. Age-specific nomogram for the decline in antral follicle count throughout the reproductive period. Fertil Steril. 2011;95(2):684–8.
2. Nelson SM, et al. Reference range for the antimullerian hormone Generation II assay: a population study of 10,984 women, with comparison to the established Diagnostics Systems Laboratory nomogram. Fertil Steril. 2014;101(2):523–9.
3. Chang MY, et al. Use of the antral follicle count to predict the outcome of assisted reproductive technologies. Fertil Steril. 1998;69(3):505–10.
4. Nelson SM, Yates RW, Fleming R. Serum anti-Mullerian hormone and FSH: prediction of live birth and extremes of response in stimulated cycles – implications for individualization of therapy. Hum Reprod. 2007;22(9):2414–21.
5. Broer SL, et al. AMH and AFC as predictors of excessive response in controlled ovarian hyperstimulation: a meta-analysis. Hum Reprod Update. 2011;17(1):46–54.
6. Broer SL, et al. The role of antimullerian hormone in prediction of outcome after IVF: comparison with the antral follicle count. Fertil Steril. 2009;91(3):705–14.
7. Iliodromiti S, Anderson RA, Nelson SN. Technical and performance characteristics of anti-Mullerian hormone and antral follicle count as biomarkers of ovarian response. Hum Reprod Update. 2015;21(6):698–710.
8. Macklon NS, et al. The science behind 25 years of ovarian stimulation for in vitro fertilization. Endocr Rev. 2006;27(2):170–207.
9. Fauser BC, et al. Mild ovarian stimulation for IVF: 10 years later. Hum Reprod. 2010;25(11): 2678–84.

10. Nelson SM, et al. Anti-Mullerian hormone-based approach to controlled ovarian stimulation for assisted conception. Hum Reprod. 2009;24(4):867–75.
11. Nelson SM. Biomarkers of ovarian response: current and future applications. Fertil Steril. 2013;99(4):963–9.
12. Al-Inany HG, et al. Gonadotrophin-releasing hormone antagonists for assisted reproductive technology. Cochrane Database Syst Rev. 2011;(5):CD001750.
13. Damewood MD, et al. Disappearance of exogenously administered human chorionic gonadotropin. Fertil Steril. 1989;52(3):398–400.
14. Yen SS, et al. Disappearance rates of endogenous luteinizing hormone and chorionic gonadotropin in man. J Clin Endocrinol Metab. 1968;28(12):1763–7.
15. Delvigne A, Rozenberg S. Epidemiology and prevention of ovarian hyperstimulation syndrome (OHSS): a review. Hum Reprod Update. 2002;8(6):559–77.
16. Fauser BC, et al. Endocrine profiles after triggering of final oocyte maturation with GnRH agonist after cotreatment with the GnRH antagonist ganirelix during ovarian hyperstimulation for in vitro fertilization. J Clin Endocrinol Metab. 2002;87(2):709–15.
17. Humaidan P, et al. GnRH agonist (buserelin) or hCG for ovulation induction in GnRH antagonist IVF/ICSI cycles: a prospective randomized study. Hum Reprod. 2005;20(5):1213–20.
18. Kolibianakis EM, et al. A lower ongoing pregnancy rate can be expected when GnRH agonist is used for triggering final oocyte maturation instead of HCG in patients undergoing IVF with GnRH antagonists. Hum Reprod. 2005;20(10):2887–92.
19. Humaidan P, et al. Rescue of corpus luteum function with peri-ovulatory HCG supplementation in IVF/ICSI GnRH antagonist cycles in which ovulation was triggered with a GnRH agonist: a pilot study. Reprod Biomed Online. 2006;13(2):173–8.
20. Humaidan P, et al. 1,500 IU human chorionic gonadotropin administered at oocyte retrieval rescues the luteal phase when gonadotropin-releasing hormone agonist is used for ovulation induction: a prospective, randomized, controlled study. Fertil Steril. 2010;93(3):847–54.
21. Pirard C, Donnez J, Loumaye E. GnRH agonist as luteal phase support in assisted reproduction technique cycles: results of a pilot study. Hum Reprod. 2006;21(7):1894–900.
22. Papanikolaou EG, et al. A novel method of luteal supplementation with recombinant luteinizing hormone when a gonadotropin-releasing hormone agonist is used instead of human chorionic gonadotropin for ovulation triggering: a randomized prospective proof of concept study. Fertil Steril. 2011;95(3):1174–7.
23. Engmann L, et al. The use of gonadotropin-releasing hormone (GnRH) agonist to induce oocyte maturation after cotreatment with GnRH antagonist in high-risk patients undergoing in vitro fertilization prevents the risk of ovarian hyperstimulation syndrome: a prospective randomized controlled study. Fertil Steril. 2008;89(1):84–91.
24. Hernandez ER, Gomez-Palomares JL, Ricciarelli E. No room for cancellation, coasting, or ovarian hyperstimulation syndrome in oocyte donation cycles. Fertil Steril. 2009;91(4 Suppl):1358–61.
25. Bodri D, et al. Triggering with human chorionic gonadotropin or a gonadotropin-releasing hormone agonist in gonadotropin-releasing hormone antagonist-treated oocyte donor cycles: findings of a large retrospective cohort study. Fertil Steril. 2009;91(2):365–71.
26. Amso NN, et al. The management of predicted ovarian hyperstimulation involving gonadotropin-releasing hormone analog with elective cryopreservation of all pre-embryos. Fertil Steril. 1990;53(6):1087–90.
27. D'Angelo A, Amso N. Embryo freezing for preventing ovarian hyperstimulation syndrome. Cochrane Database Syst Rev. 2012;(3):CD002806.
28. Awonuga AO, et al. Elective cryopreservation of all embryos in women at risk of developing ovarian hyperstimulation syndrome may not prevent the condition but reduces the live birth rate. J Assist Reprod Genet. 1996;13(5):401–6.
29. van der Linden M, et al. Luteal phase support for assisted reproduction cycles. Cochrane Database Syst Rev. 2011;(10):CD009154.
30. D'Angelo A, Amso N. "Coasting" (withholding gonadotrophins) for preventing ovarian hyperstimulation syndrome. Cochrane Database Syst Rev. 2002;(3):CD002811.

31. Delvigne A, Rozenberg S. A qualitative systematic review of coasting, a procedure to avoid ovarian hyperstimulation syndrome in IVF patients. Hum Reprod Update. 2002;8(3):291–6.
32. Forman RG, et al. Severe ovarian hyperstimulation syndrome using agonists of gonadotropin-releasing hormone for in vitro fertilization: a European series and a proposal for prevention. Fertil Steril. 1990;53(3):502–9.
33. Egbase PE, Sharhan MA, Grudzinskas JG. Early unilateral follicular aspiration compared with coasting for the prevention of severe ovarian hyperstimulation syndrome: a prospective randomized study. Hum Reprod. 1999;14(6):1421–5.
34. Tang H, et al. Cabergoline for preventing ovarian hyperstimulation syndrome. Cochrane Database Syst Rev. 2012;(2):CD008605.
35. Tso LO, et al. Metformin treatment before and during IVF or ICSI in women with polycystic ovary syndrome. Cochrane Database Syst Rev. 2014;(11):CD006105.
36. Aboulghar M, Evers JH, Al-Inany H. Intravenous albumin for preventing severe ovarian hyperstimulation syndrome: a Cochrane review. Hum Reprod. 2002;17(12):3027–32.
37. Edwards RG. IVF, IVM, natural cycle IVF, minimal stimulation IVF – time for a rethink. Reprod Biomed Online. 2007;15(1):106–19.
38. Edwards RG. Are minimal stimulation IVF and IVM set to replace routine IVF? Reprod Biomed Online. 2007;14(2):267–70.
39. Thurin A, et al. Elective single-embryo transfer versus double-embryo transfer in in vitro fertilization. N Engl J Med. 2004;351(23):2392–402.
40. Lawlor DA, Nelson SM. Effect of age on decisions about the numbers of embryos to transfer in assisted conception: a prospective study. Lancet. 2012;379(9815):521–7.
41. Hardarson T, Van Landuyt L, Jones G. The blastocyst. Hum Reprod. 2012;27 Suppl 1:i72–91.
42. Fishel S, et al. Live birth after polar body array comparative genomic hybridization prediction of embryo ploidy-the future of IVF? Fertil Steril. 2010;93(3):1006.e7–10.
43. Ata B, et al. Array CGH analysis shows that aneuploidy is not related to the number of embryos generated. Reprod Biomed Online. 2012;24(6):614–20.

Chapter 14
Ongoing Developments in ART and Pregnancy Outcome

Joo P. Teoh and Abha Maheshwari

Introduction

The practice of Assisted Reproductive Technology (ART) has evolved greatly since the report of the first test-tube baby more than 30 years ago. Over the years, its use has become more accessible for many in different parts of the world, especially in countries where there is a high percentage of affluent population. The number of IVF babies is estimated to be surpassing five million. In certain states in the US, it has been reported that as high as 4.5 % of infants born have been following ART conceptions [1].

Various developments and technologies have been brought into ART; some of these have been adopted widely and are becoming routine practices. Most ART laboratories are performing embryo freezing and ICSI procedures as standard; there is little doubt that these practices have transformed the performance of IVF. In recent years an increasing array of new techniques in the laboratory has been introduced, mostly with the aim of increasing the success rates of IVF. The ability to cryopreserve gametes effectively has made fertility preservation a realistic option; sperm have been regularly retrieved surgically and frozen for male factor infertility. Companies like Apple and Facebook are offering their female employees to socially freeze the eggs to widen the fertility window.

The effectiveness of some of the new developments in ART has been questioned. There are concerns that the safety data on these new technologies are lacking, and

J.P. Teoh, MBBCh, MRCOG, MRCPI, MSc, MD (✉)
Concept Fertility Centre, Subiaco, Perth, Australia
e-mail: Joo.teoh@yahoo.com

A. Maheshwari, MBBS, MD, MRCOG
Aberdeen Royal Infirmary, Department of Gynaecology,
Aberdeen Fertility Centre, Aberdeen, UK
e-mail: Abha.maheshwari@abdn.ac.uk

K. Jayaprakasan, L. Kean (eds.), *Clinical Management of Pregnancies following ART*, DOI 10.1007/978-3-319-42858-1_14

their introduction into the marketplace is mainly due to commercial interest. In this chapter we review the effect of ongoing developments in ART on the pregnancy and health of the children. The data on the safety of ART technologies are currently inadequate. Studies on pregnancy outcomes and health of the children following ART are limited due to the paucity of centralized national data registers, ethical concerns and the lack of funding [2]. On the other hand, there is an increase in the understanding of genetics and epigenetics among the public and scientists. Advances in research techniques have allowed more cutting-edge research to be carried out to assess the changes in tissues, gametes and embryos subjected to different in-vitro environment [2, 3]. As the number of children born following ART with new technologies increases, we should expect more investigations and results in this area in the near future.

ICSI

ICSI is one of the commonest techniques practiced in ART laboratories all over the world. Its application on human gametes was first reported in 1988 [4]. The main indication for performing ICSI is male factor infertility; however, there is a trend of more widespread use of this technique even for patients not presenting with male factor infertility. In 2000, 47.6 % of ART was reported using ICSI, in 2006 the proportion increased to 66 % [5]; the level of this proportion has remained the same up to now [5, 6]. For those without male factor infertility in the US, the proportion of its use has increased from 15.4 % in 1996 to 66.9 % in 2012 [6].

There is a concern that ICSI may have detrimental effect on pregnancies and children. ICSI has removed the natural selection of the fertilizing sperm, and has also allowed the transfer of gene that would not normally be passed on. The technique may also inflict physical damage to the gametes [7]. A study on constitutional DNA copy number has detected a higher rate of changes in ICSI children in comparison to naturally conceived children; however, it is difficult to ascertain whether these genetic changes have any significant phenotypic consequences to the offsprings [8]. By comparing to conventional IVF, it has been reported that ICSI does not increase the risk of major birth defects [7, 9, 10]. In comparison to naturally conceived pregnancies, ICSI pregnancies have similar mean gestational age at birth, birth weight, neonatal distress level and Neonatal Intensive Care Unit (NICU) admission [11, 12]. A few studies have looked into the longer-term development of ICSI children. The studies of cognitive abilities, socio-emotional development and motor skills scores have been reported for children up to the age of 10. It is reassuring to learn that ICSI children largely performing on par with naturally conceived children [11–14]. In one study, IVF children were detected to have better simultaneous mental processing ability compared to ICSI children [13]. Interestingly, one of the studies showed that ICSI children had better interactional ability and lower distress level than naturally conceived children [15]. A few researchers studied the health, growth, and also pubertal and endocrinological changes on ICSI children up to late puberty. Basatemur et al. studied the growth of ART children up to the age of 18 years old. They compared 143 IVF and 166 ICSI children with 173 matched naturally conceived controls and concluded that there were no significant differences in head circumference, height and weight between the groups [16]. Pubertal development by Tanner stage and age of menarche have also been studied in ICSI children by Belva et al. Development of these sexual characteristics is largely similar for singleton born ICSI boys and girls in comparison to their 14-year-old spontaneously conceived counterparts; only one difference was detected: ICSI females had less pronounced breast development by comparison [11, 17]. In the same study, the authors also reported increased central, peripheral and total adiposity in ICSI children comparing to spontaneously conceived children. In advanced pubertal stages ICSI adolescents had more peripheral adiposity. The same group has also performed other studies to assess different aspects of health effect of ICSI on children. In one paper, they compared blood pressure between ICSI boys and girls with spontaneously conceived children before and after subjecting the participants to a stress test; no detrimental blood pressure effect was detected for ICSI children in the study [18]. To complement the studies on physical characteristics, the group measured salivary cortisol in the children [19]. They related alterations in cortisol level with changes in adiposity, blood pressure and glucose tolerance. In that study of 14-year-olds, ICSI females but not males were detected to have lower salivary cortisol concentrations in comparison to spontaneously conceived children. Belva et al. have also studied salivary testosterone concentrations in pubertal ICSI boys compared with spontaneously conceived boys. As ICSI removes the process of natural selection of sperms for fertilization, some worry that this technique may increase the risk of male offsprings inheriting karyotypic anomalies or Y-chromosome microdeletions from their fathers, resulting in genital malformations or impaired testicular function. The authors used salivary testosterone level as a surrogate marker of testicular function in 14 year-old male adolescents. In this study 58 ICSI male teenagers were compared to 62 spontaneously conceived counterparts. They found that the testosterone levels for these ICSI boys conceived from men with severely compromised spermatogenesis were similar to the naturally conceived group. In other studies, no increase in male urogenital anomalies was reported for ICSI children in comparison to the background risk [20, 21]. For children who inherit Y-chromosome deletions, it is suggested that the size of the deletion is not increased in the offspring, and the extent of infertility for the children is likely to be the same as for the fathers [20, 22].

In summary, the findings of the studies regarding ICSI pregnancies and children are generally reassuring. In comparison to spontaneously conceived offspring, ICSI adolescents are at risk of developing obesity [17]. However, from this study it is difficult to ascertain whether the phenotypic pattern is due to the effect of ICSI; previous study has shown that IVF children have more peripheral adiposity in comparison to spontaneously conceived children [23]. For the application of ICSI, various sperm selection techniques have been developed, most of them still lacking evidence in proving their safety and effectiveness [24–26].

Surgically Retrieved Sperm

The application of ICSI technique has permitted the use of surgically retrieved sperm for ART treatment. It is now possible for men with obstructive azoospermia, non-obstructive azoospermia and severe oligospermia to father children using non-ejaculated sperm. Successful testicular sperm retrieval has been reported in males with Klinefelter's syndrome, and also in patients post chemotherapy [27–29]. The use of surgical retrieved sperm is not without concern. Some believe that ICSI using surgically retrieved sperm is a step further in eliminating the natural selection of suitable sperms for fertilization. In addition, sex chromosome anomalies and Y-microdeletions have been detected in more than 10 % of patients with non-obstructive azoospermia and oligospermia [30]. In testicular sperm extraction (TESE), immature testicular sperms can be extracted and used for ICSI. On the other hand, aged epididymal sperm from epididymal sperm aspiration (MESA) may contain chromosomal error [20]. It is feared that the genetic or chromosomal anomalies can be passed on to the offspring; ICSI using suboptimal sperm in theory can also have adverse effects on the pregnancies or children. Several studies reported the pregnancy outcomes of pregnancies from surgical retrieved sperm, by comparing them to ICSI pregnancies using ejaculated sperm, and also IVF and naturally conceived pregnancies. The results are largely reassuring. No significant differences have been reported in the rates of miscarriage, ectopic pregnancy, intrauterine growth restriction, maternal complications, preterm delivery, low birth weight, neonatal unit admission, perinatal mortality and infant mortality [7, 31–35]. Fedder et al. reported a lower caesarean section rate for the group of pregnancies from surgically retrieved sperm in comparison to IVF and ICSI using ejaculated sperms. [33] There is one finding of an increase in perinatal death for twins from surgically retrieved sperm when compared to ICSI using ejaculated sperm. [35] Some authors made comparison of the complications between obstructive and non-obstructive azoospermia in surgically retrieved sperms. The gestational age at birth, birth weight and neonatal outcomes are similar between these two groups [36]. There is a non-significant increase in miscarriage in the non-obstructive azoospermic group [37]. The miscarriage rate was the same regardless of whether the surgically retrieved sperm were from the testicles or epididymes [37]. In relation to fetal malformations, the results are more conflicting. The difference in results may be due to the variation in the definitions and categorizations used for different studies. Most studies reported no difference in the rate of congenital malformations [20, 34–36]. Guo et al. discovered a non-significant increase in birth defects in the TESA group (103 children) in comparison to 1008 children born after ICSI with ejaculated sperms. [32] Fedder et al. studied different groups consisting of 466 children born with surgically retrieved sperms, 8967 ICSI children with ejaculated sperms, 17,592 IVF children and 63,854 naturally conceived children [33]. By tests of variance, they reported the rate of undescended testicles and cardiac malformations in boys significantly increased from natural conception to IVF to ICSI with ejaculated sperm to ICSI with surgically retrieved sperm. In a different study, this research team also discovered an increased rate of hypospadias for children born with surgically retrieved sperm (three out of 197) [38]. However, in this study no direct comparison was made for this group of patients with children born with ICSI using ejaculated sperm.

Limited data are available on the genetic and chromosomal abnormalities for children born with surgically retrieved sperm. One study reported no difference in anomalies in pre- and post-natal karyotypes in viable ICSI pregnancies between surgically retrieved and ejaculated sperm. [35] Even for males with Klinefelter syndrome, 59 % of the embryos fertilized with testicular sperms were confirmed to have a normal karyotype [27]. Another study reported 100 % normal karyotype for 16 babies born using testicular sperms from males with Klinefelter syndrome [28]. At present there is no concern regarding the neurodevelopment of children conceived with surgically retrieved sperm. These children perform very well in the assessment of their milestones and skills [7, 34, 39]. A large number of surgically retrieved sperm samples were frozen and thawed at a later date for ICSI. It has been reported that the freezing of testicular sperm does not have any adverse effect on neonatal outcomes [28, 40].

Parents planning to undergo surgical sperm retrieval must be provided appropriate counseling. Most pregnancies resulted from this technique are uncomplicated, and the babies born are healthy. However, there are reports of an increased risk of congenital malformations; the risk can be as high as 8–10 % [20]. Males detected to have Y-chromosome deletions may also pass on the genetic malformation to the male offspring. Consideration should be made to establish a system to educate the family, and perhaps the children at a suitable age regarding the possibility of inherited infertility.

Embryo Culture Technique

Phenotypic or genotypic changes may be induced in embryos subjected to various environments in vitro. Questions have been asked about whether the culture condition, media used, or length of culture have any significant impact on pregnancies and offspring. Some authors have shown that different culture media used can affect birth weight; however, not all studies demonstrated the same effect [41, 42].

In vitro maturation (IVM) is a technique becoming more popular in ART laboratory. There is a strong argument for its use in specific populations, for example in high responders to prevent ovarian hyperstimulation syndrome. Due to the lack of RCT, the safety of this new technique introduced in the early 1990s is in doubt. Studies with small samples did not detect any increase in the risks of fetal malformations or adverse perinatal outcomes [43, 44]. In a laboratory study, Yoshida et al showed that at cleavage stage the metabolic state (oxygen consumption) of embryos resulted from IVM and controlled ovarian hyperstimulation (COH) were the same [45]. In IVM babies, no abnormality was found in the expression of imprinting genes [45]. In a different laboratorial study by Virant-Klun et al., the authors detected some changes in the gene expression profile of oocytes in IVM [46]. It is unknown whether the shifts in the gene expression profile have any effect on pregnancy outcomes and the health of offspring.

Many ART centers culture the embryos today 5/6 for blastocyst transfer, with the aim to increase the success rates. There is some evidence that blastocyst transfer results in less miscarriage [47]. However, the practice of extended culture of embryos is not without health risks. It has been shown that this technique increases the likelihood of preterm delivery with odds ratio of up to 1.32 [48, 49]. Several studies also demonstrated that the transfer of blastocysts increases the chance of monozygotic twinning [50–52].

One of the most popular new technologies in ART is the time-lapse incubator. It is claimed that chromosomal normal and abnormal embryos have different morphokinesis (kinetic behavior), and the use of time-lapse technology can differentiate these embryos and its application can improve success rates [53, 54]. A decrease in miscarriage rate has been reported with the use of this technology [55]. In theory, the use of this technology should not pose any harm as its application is not truly invasive to the embryos in culture. However, prospective studies are underway currently and the data should be studied carefully when they become available [56].

In short, to date the available data have shown that the technique and duration of embryo culture can influence pregnancy outcome. It is undeniable that there is a lack of robust studies, and the evidence to support the safety of the new techniques in ART laboratories is missing.

Embryo Manipulation

Different embryo micromanipulation techniques have been introduced in ART laboratories. One of the techniques is assisted hatching; the use of assisted hatching is increasingly common [57]. There is good evidence that assisted hatching improves clinical pregnancy rate in poor prognosis patients, including those with prior failed IVF cycles [58]. It is debatable whether this technique increases miscarriage rate [57, 59]. As this process involves the disruption of the zona pellucida, a few studies showed an increase risk of dichorionic monozygotic twinning, especially if assisted hatching is performed on day 2–3 embryos [50–52, 60]. In a study to assess the safety of assisted hatching, Zhou et al. looked at 392 infants in total. The authors concluded that it did not make any significant difference in mean gestational age, mean birth weight and mean Apgar score for either singleton or multiple gestations [61].

In preimplantation genetic screening/diagnosis (PGS/PGD), cells or polar bodies are biopsied from the embryos; logically the removal of one or more blastomeres may adversely affect the development of an embryo. However, embryonic cells are totipotential in nature and perhaps the other remaining cells in the embryo have the capacity to accomplish different developmental pathways for the embryo to grow normally [62]. The safety data of this embryo manipulative technique have been reported in a few studies. In comparison to ICSI pregnancies, the rates of intrauterine growth restriction, low birth weight, congenital malformations, neonatal hospitalization, neonatal intensive care admission and perinatal death for singletons are similar [62–66]. Fewer multiple pregnancies following PGD presented with low birth weight (<2500 g) [64]. On the other hand, there is a report of an increase in perinatal deaths in post PGS/PGD multiple pregnancies [66]. In several studies, PGS/PGD has been shown to reduce the rate of miscarriage for patients with recurrent miscarriage; this includes parents with reciprocal or Robertsonian translocation [67–70]. Research on the neurodevelopment of children following PGS/PGD has produced some interesting results. Schendelaar et al. studied 49 children born following ART with PGS, comparing them with 64 children born following ART without PGS. The authors concluded that there was no difference in the neurodevelopmental outcome of these children [71]. In a different study, a Dutch group reported that PGS is not associated with any changes in mental, psychomotor and behavioral outcomes at 2 years in children born after PGS. Scores on all tests were within normal range. However, when compared to children born after IVF without PGS, PGS children had lower neurologic optimality scores, this may be a signal of less favorable long-term neurologic outcomes in these children [72]. In a separate paper, the same group reported similar neurologic outcome before 18 months for ART children with or without PGS. At 18 months, they reported increased frequencies of dysfunction in fine motor abilities and posture, and also muscle tone dysregulation in PGS children [65].

Embryo manipulation techniques, specifically assisted hatching and PGS/PGD, may be useful in improving the ART success rates for specific groups of patients. However, one should be aware of the potential adverse effects. Reassuringly both of these techniques have not been shown to cause significant problems in pregnancy and perinatal period for the majority of patients. However, one should be cautious in applying these techniques unselectively. Assisted hatching, especially performed on cleavage stage, increases the chance of monozygotic twinning. An increase in perinatal deaths was also reported in PGS/PGD multiple pregnancies. In addition, there is also a concern regarding the long-term neurologic outcomes of children following PGS/PGD.

Fertility Preservation Techniques

The technique of oocyte cryopreservation has undergone tremendous improvements in recent years. For many years, the practice of this technique is lagging behind embryo cryopreservation due to the poor survival, fertilization and success rates [73]. Currently, the literature reports oocyte vitrification yielding comparable outcomes to IVF with fresh oocytes in some cases [74].

The practice of oocyte cryopreservation became popular in Italy between 2004 and 2009 when legal restrictions permitted no more than three oocytes to be inseminated [75]. This clinical setting encouraged significant number of experiments on oocyte cryopreservation to be carried out in order to optimally preserve the supernumerary embryos retrieved in ovarian stimulation cycles. Nowadays, the primary indications for oocyte cryopreservation are for single women at risk of losing ovarian function due to oncology treatments, systemic illnesses and genetic syndromes. It is also widely used in centers with embryo donation programs to eliminate the need to synchronize the cycles of egg donors and recipients. Many women are aware of their fertility windows; requests for social egg cryopreservation to prolong the window of fertility are becoming more common. Oocyte cryopreservation is also applicable when there is an unexpected failure to obtain sperms on the day of oocyte retrieval in a fresh ART treatment cycle [73].

The pregnancy outcomes and health of the children following oocyte cryopreservation have been reported in literatures based on over a 1000 cases. Levi Setti et al. reported a higher rate of first trimester miscarriage in pregnancies following oocye cryopreservation in comparison to fresh cycles; [75] Oktay et al. looked at pregnancies following slow oocyte freezing and reported similar finding of increasing miscarriage rate [76]. Either in comparison to spontaneous conception or fresh ART cycles, reassuringly no differences have been reported in the rates of ectopic pregnancy and congenital anomalies [75, 77–79]. Levi Setti et al. reported a higher mean birth weights in singleton and twins following oocyte cryopreservation in comparison to fresh treatment, this pattern is similar to pregnancies following embryo cryopreservation [75]. Other studies, in contrast, did not see any difference in the mean birth weight. [77, 79] The study of Levi Setti et al. also recorded 138 pregnancies from 63 patients who had pregnancies in both fresh and thawed oocyte cycles; in these pregnancies, the miscarriage rate and mean birth weight were the same [75].

The advances in in vitro maturation (IVM) have enabled the development of the technique of immature oocyte cryopreservation. Immature oocyte cryopreservation is beneficial when a high proportion of oocytes retrieved are immature following ovarian stimulation. It is also potentially useful for patients who are not suited to undergo ovarian stimulation; one example of this group of patients is girls who are prepubertal. In a recent paper, it is stated that so far only one live birth following immature oocyte cryopreservation has been recorded in the literature [80]. Another experimental technique, which is increasingly common, is ovarian tissue cryopreservation. Similar to immature oocyte cryopreservation, ovarian tissue cryopreservation can also remove the need to perform ovarian stimulation for retrieving mature oocytes. Currently over 30 cases of live births following ovarian tissue transplants have been reported [80]. Histological analyses of harvested ovarian tissues have not detected any metastatic cancers for oncology patients undergoing fertility preservation [81, 82].

Early evidence on the safety of oocyte cryopreservation is reassuring. This technique has expanded the boundary of fertility treatment. It permits a specific group of patients to do what was previously impossible; it gives them the chance to have their fertility preserved and have their own genetic children. Although immature oocyte preservation and ovarian tissue preservation are still at the experimental stage, in specific centers around the world these techniques are often being offered to patients when no other modality is available to preserve their fertility. Counseling to provide appropriate information is an important part of the process to educate the patients regarding the advantages, limitations and safety of these techniques.

Immunotherapy

Immunoregulatory drugs – namely aspirin, steroids, intravenous immunoglobulin (IVIg), low molecular weight heparin (LMWH) and anti-TNFα – are known to be administered either solely or in combinations in ART treatments. Currently the evidence to support the routine use of these agents is rather limited. It is concerning to learn that some of the side effects of immunotherapy for ART patients can be very serious. Severe systemic candidiasis following immunomodulation therapy in an ART cycle has been reported [83]. In addition, the potential teratogenicity of some of the agents has not been totally ruled out [84]. A few small studies have shown some beneficial effects of immunotherapy in ART, particularly for specific groups of patients. In a small randomized controlled trial of only 54 patients, Lambers et al. concluded that the incidence of hypertensive complications was significantly lower (3.6% vs. 26.9%) in patients who received low-dose aspirin throughout IVF treatment and first trimester of pregnancy in comparison to the placebo group [85]. However, a meta-analysis of more patients (n=268) did not show any difference in the incidence of hypertensive pregnancy complications between the two groups. The same authors also did not find any difference in the rate of preterm delivery between the groups [86]. Another study observed no benefit of aspirin in the success rates of IVF or ICSI treatments; the ectopic and miscarriage rates were similar between treatment and placebo [87]. Potdar et al. reported a lower rate of miscarriage with the use of LMWH for ART patients with recurrent implantation failure; however, the analysis includes patients with thrombophilia [88]. In a meta-analysis of randomized trials, Seshadri et al. found similar miscarriage and life birth rates between ART patients who received LMWH and placebo. In contrary, when the authors performed another meta-analysis for observational studies, an increase in live birth rate for ART patients receiving LMWH was demonstrated [89]. In relation to the use of IVIg for ART patients, this intravenous treatment has been shown to lower the miscarriage rate when compared to patients who received placebo or no treatment [90].

Conclusion

ART is entering an exciting era. New technologies and ongoing developments are opening up frontiers and changing the practice of ART. However, in the absence of robust scientific evidence, many ART practitioners are cautious in introducing any new treatments that can be potentially harmful. There is a need for adequately powered randomized controlled trials to access the safety and pregnancy outcomes for different interventions in ART. International and national bodies can help in coordinating these research areas, and also in standardizing definitions and measures to enhance the ability of the researchers and practitioners to compare and contrast the research outputs for reaching conclusions. Most practitioners are aware that they have a duty to educate and counsel the patients, and inform the patients when there is a lack of evidence for their treatments. While waiting for more clinical data to inform us of the various developments in ART, sometimes we have to stop and tell ourselves: “less is more.”

References

1. Sunderam S, Kissin DM, Crawford SB, Folger SG, Jamieson DJ, Barfield WD. Assisted reproductive technology surveillance – United States, 2011. MMWR Surveil Summ (Washington, DC : 2002). 2014;63(10):1–28.
2. Brison DR, Roberts SA, Kimber SJ. How should we assess the safety of IVF technologies? Reprod Biomed Online. 2013;27(6):710–21.
3. Kimura H, Yamagata K. Visualization of epigenetic modifications in preimplantation embryos. Meth Mol Biol (Clifton, NJ). 2015;1222:127–47.
4. Lanzendorf SE, Maloney MK, Veeck LL, Slusser J, Hodgen GD, Rosenwaks Z. A preclinical evaluation of pronuclear formation by microinjection of human spermatozoa into human oocytes. Fertil Steril. 1988;49(5):835–42.
5. Ishihara O, Adamson GD, Dyer S, et al. International committee for monitoring assisted reproductive technologies: world report on assisted reproductive technologies, 2007. Fertil Steril. 2015;103(2):402–413.e411.
6. Boulet SL, Mehta A, Kissin DM, Warner L, Kawwass JF, Jamieson DJ. Trends in use of and reproductive outcomes associated with intracytoplasmic sperm injection. JAMA. 2015;313(3):255–63.
7. Palermo GD, Neri QV, Monahan D, Kocent J, Rosenwaks Z. Development and current applications of assisted fertilization. Fertil Steril. 2012;97(2):248–59.
8. Woldringh GH, Janssen IM, Hehir-Kwa JY, et al. Constitutional DNA copy number changes in ICSI children. Hum Reprod. 2009;24(1):233–40.
9. Hansen M, Kurinczuk JJ, Bower C, Webb S. The risk of major birth defects after intracytoplasmic sperm injection and in vitro fertilization. N Engl J Med. 2002;346(10):725–30.
10. Hindryckx A, Peeraer K, Debrock S, et al. Has the prevalence of congenital abnormalities after intracytoplasmic sperm injection increased? The Leuven data 1994–2000 and a review of the literature. Gynecol Obstet Invest. 2010;70(1):11–22.
11. Palermo GD, Neri QV, Rosenwaks Z. Safety of intracytoplasmic sperm injection. Meth Mol Biol (Clifton, NJ). 2014;1154:549–62.
12. Palermo GD, Neri QV, Takeuchi T, Squires J, Moy F, Rosenwaks Z. Genetic and epigenetic characteristics of ICSI children. Reprod Biomed Online. 2008;17(6):820–33.
13. Goldbeck L, Gagsteiger F, Mindermann I, Strobele S, Izat Y. Cognitive development of singletons conceived by intracytoplasmic sperm injection or in vitro fertilization at age 5 and 10 years. J Pediatr Psychol. 2009;34(7):774–81.
14. Leunens L, Celestin-Westreich S, Bonduelle M, Liebaers I, Ponjaert-Kristoffersen I. Follow-up of cognitive and motor development of 10-year-old singleton children born after ICSI compared with spontaneously conceived children. Hum Reprod. 2008;23(1):105–11.
15. Ponjaert-Kristoffersen I, Tjus T, Nekkebroeck J, et al. Psychological follow-up study of 5-year-old ICSI children. Hum Reprod. 2004;19(12):2791–7.
16. Basatemur E, Shevlin M, Sutcliffe A. Growth of children conceived by IVF and ICSI up to 12 years of age. Reprod Biomed Online. 2010;20(1):144–9.
17. Belva F, Painter R, Bonduelle M, Roelants M, Devroey P, De Schepper J. Are ICSI adolescents at risk for increased adiposity? Hum Reprod. 2012;27(1):257–64.
18. Belva F, Roelants M, De Schepper J, et al. Blood pressure in ICSI-conceived adolescents. Hum Reprod. 2012;27(10):3100–8.
19. Belva F, Painter RC, Schiettecatte J, et al. Gender-specific alterations in salivary cortisol levels in pubertal intracytoplasmic sperm injection offspring. Horm Res Paediatr. 2013;80(5):350–5.
20. Halliday J. Outcomes for offspring of men having ICSI for male factor infertility. Asian J Androl. 2012;14(1):116–20.
21. Kallen B, Finnstrom O, Lindam A, Nilsson E, Nygren KG, Otterblad PO. Congenital malformations in infants born after in vitro fertilization in Sweden. Birth defects research. Part A. Clin Mol Teratol. 2010;88(3):137–43.

22. Silber SJ. The Y chromosome in the era of intracytoplasmic sperm injection: a personal review. Fertil Steril. 2011;95(8):2439–2448.e2431–5.
23. Ceelen M, van Weissenbruch MM, Roos JC, Vermeiden JP, van Leeuwen FE, Delemarre-van de Waal HA. Body composition in children and adolescents born after in vitro fertilization or spontaneous conception. J Clin Endocrinol Metab. 2007;92(9):3417–23.
24. Said TM, Land JA. Effects of advanced selection methods on sperm quality and ART outcome: a systematic review. Hum Reprod Update. 2011;17(6):719–33.
25. Shalom-Paz E, Anabusi S, Michaeli M, et al. Can intra cytoplasmatic morphologically selected sperm injection (IMSI) technique improve outcome in patients with repeated IVF-ICSI failure? a comparative study. Gynecol Endocrinol Off J Int Soc Gynecol Endocrinol. 2015;31(3):247–51.
26. Teixeira DM, Barbosa MA, Ferriani RA, et al. Regular (ICSI) versus ultra-high magnification (IMSI) sperm selection for assisted reproduction. Cochrane Database Syst Rev. 2013;(7):CD010167.
27. Yarali H, Polat M, Bozdag G, et al. TESE-ICSI in patients with non-mosaic Klinefelter syndrome: a comparative study. Reprod Biomed Online. 2009;18(6):756–60.
28. Greco E, Scarselli F, Minasi MG, et al. Birth of 16 healthy children after ICSI in cases of non-mosaic Klinefelter syndrome. Hum Reprod. 2013;28(5):1155–60.
29. Hsiao W, Stahl PJ, Osterberg EC, et al. Successful treatment of postchemotherapy azoospermia with microsurgical testicular sperm extraction: the Weill Cornell experience. J Clin Oncol Off J Am Soc Clin Oncol. 2011;29(12):1607–11.
30. Yuanyuan Z, Qiang D, Xiaoliang L, Wanting C, Rong H, Yanyan Z. [Screening of azoospermia factor microdeletions on Y chromosome in infertile men by QF-PCR]. Yi chuan=Hereditas/Zhongguo yi chuan xue hui bian ji. 2014;36(6):552–7.
31. Oron G, Fisch B, Sapir O, et al. Pregnancy outcome after ICSI with thawed testicular sperm from men with non-obstructive azoospermia compared to ICSI with ejaculated sperm from men with severe oligoasthenoteratozoospermia and IVF with normal ejaculated sperm. Gynecol Endocrinol Off J Int Soc Gynecol Endocrinol. 2014;30(2):103–6.
32. Guo YH, Dong RN, Su YC, Li J, Zhang YJ, Sun YP. Follow-up of children born after intracytoplasmic sperm injection with epididymal and testicular spermatozoa. Chin Med J (Engl). 2013;126(11):2129–33.
33. Fedder J, Loft A, Parner ET, Rasmussen S, Pinborg A. Neonatal outcome and congenital malformations in children born after ICSI with testicular or epididymal sperm: a controlled national cohort study. Hum Reprod. 2013;28(1):230–40.
34. Woldringh GH, Horvers M, Janssen AJ, et al. Follow-up of children born after ICSI with epididymal spermatozoa. Hum Reprod. 2011;26(7):1759–67.
35. Belva F, De Schrijver F, Tournaye H, et al. Neonatal outcome of 724 children born after ICSI using non-ejaculated sperm. Hum Reprod. 2011;26(7):1752–8.
36. Esteves SC, Agarwal A. Reproductive outcomes, including neonatal data, following sperm injection in men with obstructive and nonobstructive azoospermia: case series and systematic review. Clinics (Sao Paulo). 2013;68 Suppl 1:141–50.
37. He X, Cao Y, Zhang Z, et al. Spermatogenesis affects the outcome of ICSI for azoospermic patients rather than sperm retrieval method. Syst Biol Reprod Med. 2010;56(6):457–64.
38. Fedder J, Gabrielsen A, Humaidan P, Erb K, Ernst E, Loft A. Malformation rate and sex ratio in 412 children conceived with epididymal or testicular sperm. Hum Reprod. 2007;22(4):1080–5.
39. Wennerholm UB, Bonduelle M, Sutcliffe A, et al. Paternal sperm concentration and growth and cognitive development in children born with a gestational age more than 32 weeks after assisted reproductive therapy. Hum Reprod. 2006;21(6):1514–20.
40. Tsai YR, Lan KC, Tsai CC, et al. Pregnancy outcome and neonatal data of children born after intracytoplasmic sperm injection with a different duration of cryopreservation of spermatozoa obtained through testicular sperm extraction. Taiwan J Obstet Gynecol. 2013;52(3):329–34.

41. Eskild A, Monkerud L, Tanbo T. Birthweight and placental weight; do changes in culture media used for IVF matter? Comparisons with spontaneous pregnancies in the corresponding time periods. Hum Reprod. 2013;28(12):3207–14.
42. Carrasco B, Boada M, Rodriguez I, Coroleu B, Barri PN, Veiga A. Does culture medium influence offspring birth weight? Fertil Steril. 2013;100(5):1283–8.
43. Strowitzki T. In vitro maturation (IVM) of human oocytes. Arch Gynecol Obstet. 2013;288(5):971–5.
44. Fadini R, Mignini Renzini M, Guarnieri T, et al. Comparison of the obstetric and perinatal outcomes of children conceived from in vitro or in vivo matured oocytes in in vitro maturation treatments with births from conventional ICSI cycles. Hum Reprod. 2012;27(12):3601–8.
45. Yoshida H, Abe H, Arima T. Quality evaluation of IVM embryo and imprinting genes of IVM babies. J Assist Reprod Genet. 2013;30(2):221–5.
46. Virant-Klun I, Knez K, Tomazevic T, Skutella T. Gene expression profiling of human oocytes developed and matured in vivo or in vitro. BioMed Res Int. 2013;2013:879489.
47. Wang YA, Costello M, Chapman M, Black D, Sullivan EA. Transfers of fresh blastocysts and blastocysts cultured from thawed cleavage embryos are associated with fewer miscarriages. Reprod Biomed Online. 2011;23(6):777–88.
48. Maheshwari A, Kalampokas T, Davidson J, Bhattacharya S. Obstetric and perinatal outcomes in singleton pregnancies resulting from the transfer of blastocyst-stage versus cleavage-stage embryos generated through in vitro fertilization treatment: a systematic review and meta-analysis. Fertil Steril. 2013;100(6):1615–21.e1–10.
49. Dar S, Librach CL, Gunby J, Bissonnette F, Cowan L. Increased risk of preterm birth in singleton pregnancies after blastocyst versus Day 3 embryo transfer: Canadian ART Register (CARTR) analysis. Hum Reprod. 2013;28(4):924–8.
50. Luke B, Brown MB, Wantman E, Stern JE. Factors associated with monozygosity in assisted reproductive technology pregnancies and the risk of recurrence using linked cycles. Fertil Steril. 2014;101(3):683–9.
51. Knopman JM, Krey LC, Oh C, Lee J, McCaffrey C, Noyes N. What makes them split? Identifying risk factors that lead to monozygotic twins after in vitro fertilization. Fertil Steril. 2014;102(1):82–9.
52. Kanter JR, Boulet S, Kawwass JF, Jamieson DJ, Kissin D. Trends and correlates of monozygotic twinning after assisted reproductive technology. Obstet Gynecol. 2014;123 Suppl 1:6s.
53. Campbell A, Fishel S, Laegdsmand M. Aneuploidy is a key causal factor of delays in blastulation: author response to 'A cautionary note against aneuploidy risk assessment using time-lapse imaging'. Reprod Biomed Online. 2014;28(3):279–83.
54. Basile N, Nogales Mdel C, Bronet F, et al. Increasing the probability of selecting chromosomally normal embryos by time-lapse morphokinetics analysis. Fertil Steril. 2014;101(3): 699–704.
55. Rubio I, Galan A, Larreategui Z, et al. Clinical validation of embryo culture and selection by morphokinetic analysis: a randomized, controlled trial of the EmbryoScope. Fertil Steril. 2014;102(5):1287–94.e1285.
56. Kaser DJ, Racowsky C. Clinical outcomes following selection of human preimplantation embryos with time-lapse monitoring: a systematic review. Hum Reprod Update. 2014;20(5): 617–31.
57. Kissin DM, Kawwass JF, Monsour M, Boulet SL, Session DR, Jamieson DJ. Assisted hatching: trends and pregnancy outcomes, United States, 2000–2010. Fertil Steril. 2014;102(3): 795–801.
58. Pfeifer S, Lobo R, Sokol R, et al. Role of assisted hatching in in vitro fertilization: a guideline. Fertil Steril. 2014;102(2):348–51.
59. Carney SK, Das S, Blake D, Farquhar C, Seif MM, Nelson L. Assisted hatching on assisted conception (in vitro fertilisation (IVF) and intracytoplasmic sperm injection (ICSI). Cochrane Database Syst Rev. 2012;(12):CD001894.

60. Martins WP, Rocha IA, Ferriani RA, Nastri CO. Assisted hatching of human embryos: a systematic review and meta-analysis of randomized controlled trials. Hum Reprod Update. 2011;17(4):438–53.
61. Zhou H, Zao W, Zhang W, Shi J, Shi W. No adverse effects were identified on the perinatal outcomes after laser-assisted hatching treatment. Reprod Biomed Online. 2014;29(6):692–8.
62. Simpson JL. Preimplantation genetic diagnosis at 20 years. Prenat Diagn. 2010;30(7):682–95.
63. Eldar-Geva T, Srebnik N, Altarescu G, et al. Neonatal outcome after preimplantation genetic diagnosis. Fertil Steril. 2014;102(4):1016–21.
64. Desmyttere S, De Rycke M, Staessen C, et al. Neonatal follow-up of 995 consecutively born children after embryo biopsy for PGD. Hum Reprod. 2012;27(1):288–93.
65. Middelburg KJ, Heineman MJ, Haadsma ML, Bos AF, Kok JH, Hadders-Algra M. Neurological condition of infants born after in vitro fertilization with preimplantation genetic screening. Pediatr Res. 2010;67(4):430–4.
66. Liebaers I, Desmyttere S, Verpoest W, et al. Report on a consecutive series of 581 children born after blastomere biopsy for preimplantation genetic diagnosis. Hum Reprod. 2010;25(1):275–82.
67. Keltz MD, Vega M, Sirota I, et al. Preimplantation genetic screening (PGS) with Comparative genomic hybridization (CGH) following day 3 single cell blastomere biopsy markedly improves IVF outcomes while lowering multiple pregnancies and miscarriages. J Assist Reprod Genet. 2013;30(10):1333–9.
68. Hodes-Wertz B, Grifo J, Ghadir S, et al. Idiopathic recurrent miscarriage is caused mostly by aneuploid embryos. Fertil Steril. 2012;98(3):675–80.
69. Fischer J, Colls P, Escudero T, Munne S. Preimplantation genetic diagnosis (PGD) improves pregnancy outcome for translocation carriers with a history of recurrent losses. Fertil Steril. 2010;94(1):283–9.
70. Garrisi JG, Colls P, Ferry KM, Zheng X, Garrisi MG, Munne S. Effect of infertility, maternal age, and number of previous miscarriages on the outcome of preimplantation genetic diagnosis for idiopathic recurrent pregnancy loss. Fertil Steril. 2009;92(1):288–95.
71. Schendelaar P, Middelburg KJ, Bos AF, et al. The effect of preimplantation genetic screening on neurological, cognitive and behavioural development in 4-year-old children: follow-up of a RCT. Hum Reprod. 2013;28(6):1508–18.
72. Middelburg KJ, van der Heide M, Houtzager B, et al. Mental, psychomotor, neurologic, and behavioral outcomes of 2-year-old children born after preimplantation genetic screening: follow-up of a randomized controlled trial. Fertil Steril. 2011;96(1):165–9.
73. Cutting R, Barlow S, Anderson R. Human oocyte cryopreservation: evidence for practice. Hum Fertil (Camb). 2009;12(3):125–36.
74. Paramanantham J, Talmor AJ, Osianlis T, Weston GC. Cryopreserved oocytes: update on clinical applications and success rates. Obstet Gynecol Surv. 2015;70(2):97–114.
75. Levi Setti PE, Albani E, Morenghi E, et al. Comparative analysis of fetal and neonatal outcomes of pregnancies from fresh and cryopreserved/thawed oocytes in the same group of patients. Fertil Steril. 2013;100(2):396–401.
76. Oktay K, Cil AP, Bang H. Efficiency of oocyte cryopreservation: a meta-analysis. Fertil Steril. 2006;86(1):70–80.
77. Chian RC, Huang JY, Tan SL, et al. Obstetric and perinatal outcome in 200 infants conceived from vitrified oocytes. Reprod Biomed Online. 2008;16(5):608–10.
78. Noyes N, Porcu E, Borini A. Over 900 oocyte cryopreservation babies born with no apparent increase in congenital anomalies. Reprod Biomed Online. 2009;18(6):769–76.
79. Wennerholm UB, Soderstrom-Anttila V, Bergh C, et al. Children born after cryopreservation of embryos or oocytes: a systematic review of outcome data. Hum Reprod. 2009;24(9):2158–72.

80. Levine JM, Kelvin JF, Quinn GP, Gracia CR. Infertility in reproductive-age female cancer survivors. Cancer. 2015;121(10):1532–9.
81. Oktay K, Oktem O. Ovarian cryopreservation and transplantation for fertility preservation for medical indications: report of an ongoing experience. Fertil Steril. 2010;93(3):762–8.
82. Fabbri R, Vicenti R, Magnani V, et al. Cryopreservation of ovarian tissue in breast cancer patients: 10 years of experience. Fut Oncol (London, Engl). 2012;8(12):1613–9.
83. Akhanoba F, MacDougall J, Mathur R, Hassan W. Severe systemic candidiasis following immunomodulation therapy in in vitro fertilisation-embryo transfer (IVF-ET). BMJ Case Rep. 2014;2014. pii: bcr2013203202.
84. Clark DA. Anti-TNFalpha therapy in immune-mediated subfertility: state of the art. J Reprod Immunol. 2010;85(1):15–24.
85. Lambers MJ, Groeneveld E, Hoozemans DA, et al. Lower incidence of hypertensive complications during pregnancy in patients treated with low-dose aspirin during in vitro fertilization and early pregnancy. Hum Reprod. 2009;24(10):2447–50.
86. Groeneveld E, Lambers MJ, Lambalk CB, et al. Preconceptional low-dose aspirin for the prevention of hypertensive pregnancy complications and preterm delivery after IVF: a meta-analysis with individual patient data. Hum Reprod. 2013;28(6):1480–8.
87. Siristatidis CS, Dodd SR, Drakeley AJ. Aspirin is not recommended for women undergoing IVF. Hum Reprod Update. 2012;18(3):233.
88. Potdar N, Gelbaya TA, Konje JC, Nardo LG. Adjunct low-molecular-weight heparin to improve live birth rate after recurrent implantation failure: a systematic review and meta-analysis. Hum Reprod Update. 2013;19(6):674–84.
89. Seshadri S, Sunkara SK, Khalaf Y, El-Toukhy T, Hamoda H. Effect of heparin on the outcome of IVF treatment: a systematic review and meta-analysis. Reprod Biomed Online. 2012;25(6):572–84.
90. Li J, Chen Y, Liu C, Hu Y, Li L. Intravenous immunoglobulin treatment for repeated IVF/ICSI failure and unexplained infertility: a systematic review and a meta-analysis. Am J Reprod Immunol. 2013;70(6):434–47.

Index

K. Jayaprakasan, L. Kean (eds.), *Clinical Management of Pregnancies following ART*, DOI 10.1007/978-3-319-42858-1

MIX
Papier aus verantwortungsvollen Quellen
Paper from responsible sources
FSC® C105338

If you have any concerns about our products,
you can contact us on
ProductSafety@springernature.com

In case Publisher is established outside the EU,
the EU authorized representative is:
Springer Nature Customer Service Center GmbH
Europaplatz 3, 69115 Heidelberg, Germany

Printed by Libri Plureos GmbH
in Hamburg, Germany